Clinical Skills
The Essence of Caring

*Edited by Helen Iggulden, Caroline MacDonald
and Karen Staniland*

Open University Press

London Boston Burr Ridge, IL Dubuque, IA Madison, WI New York San Francisco St. Louis
Bangkok Bogotá Caracas Kuala Lumpur Lisbon Madrid Mexico City Milan Montreal New Delhi
Santiago Seoul Singapore Sydney Taipei Toronto

Clinical Skills

The Essence of Caring

Includes €DVD. T019755

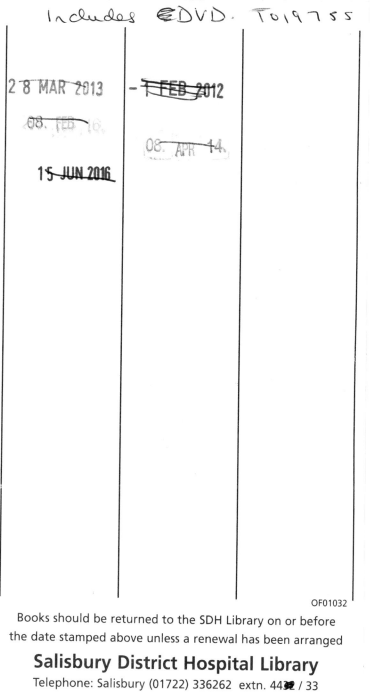

Books should be returned to the SDH Library on or before
the date stamped above unless a renewal has been arranged

Salisbury District Hospital Library

Telephone: Salisbury (01722) 336262 extn. 4432 / 33
Out of hours answer machine in operation

Clinical Skills: The Essence of Caring
Helen Iggulden, Caroline MacDonald and Karen Staniland

ISBN-13 978-0-33-522355-8 (pb)   978-0-33-522356-5 (hb)
ISBN-10 0-33-522355-9 (pb)   0-33-522356-7 (hb)

  Open University Press

Published by McGraw-Hill Education
Shoppenhangers Road
Maidenhead
Berkshire
SL6 2QL
Telephone: 44 (0) 1628 502 500
Fax: 44 (0) 1628 770 224
Website: www.mcgraw-hill.co.uk

British Library Cataloguing in Publication Data
A catalogue record for this book is available from the British Library

Library of Congress Cataloguing in Publication Data
The Library of Congress data for this book has been applied for from the Library of Congress

Commissioning Editor: Rachel Crookes
Development Editor: Karen Harlow
Product Manager: Bryony Skelton
Senior Production Editor: James Bishop

Typeset by YHT Ltd, London

Printed and bound in Great Britain by Bell and Bain Ltd

The **McGraw-Hill** Companies

Dedication

We would like to dedicate this book to our families,
friends and colleagues as, without their help, support and
encouragement it would not have been possible.

Helen Iggulden
Caroline MacDonald
Karen Staniland

Brief table of contents

Detailed table of contents

Guide to the interactive Media Tool DVD

Included with this book is a free Media Tool DVD containing a wealth of invaluable resources to help you get the most out of your clinical skills education. It offers interactive material, including video clips, images, animations and self-test material to cover every aspect of clinical skills in an exciting and accessible way.

When you access the DVD on your computer, you will find the following sections:

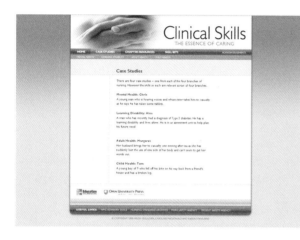

Case studies

In this section you will find **four** patient case studies, one on each of the four nursing branches: adult health, child health, learning disability and mental health. Each includes a number of video clips, self-test questions and extra resources such as animation clips and slideshows. **There is a full guide to the case studies in this section, to help you navigate the DVD and get the most out of the resources!**

Chapter resources

In this section you will find a link relating to each of the chapters in the textbook. Each link also relates to one of the benchmarks of the *Essence of Care* document which sets the standard to which all fundamental care should be given. Each chapter topic breaks down into the series of factors and statements which comprise it and contains questions, links or other resources to help you understand the background and context in which it is based. It also contains the external websites referred to in the boxes in that chapter.

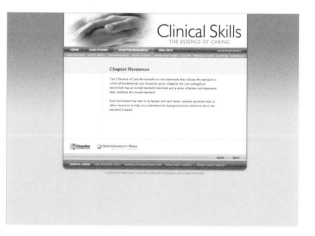

Skill sets

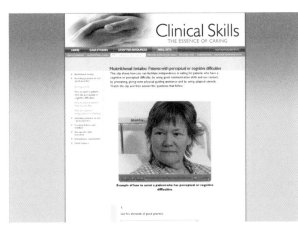

In this section you will find seven skill sets covering most of the skills taught in the first and second year nursing programmes. These are:

- **Risk and comfort**
- **Nutritional intake**
- **Infection control and hygiene**
- **Meeting elimination needs**
- **Wound care**
- **Observations**
- **Administration of medicines**

Each skill set breaks down into a list of the skills contained in that set. These are then presented as video demonstrations and narrations, followed by questions and links to background and follow-up material.

Using the book and the DVD together

You will find references to all of these sections throughout the textbook, but the case studies in particular are heavily integrated into the book so that their relevance to all of the different topics and skills can be fully explored.

While all the material on the Media Tool DVD and in the textbook makes sense stand-alone, you will get the most value from each when you use them together. The simplest way to do this is to read through the book and refer to the appropriate section of the Media Tool DVD when instructed. You could then go back and work through the DVD again; this will make sure you have examined everything and will also test how much you have remembered.

Case studies

The Media Tool DVD includes four patient case studies which are also featured throughout the textbook. As you work through chapters you will come across Activity boxes, where you will be prompted to watch clips on the DVD and answer questions/complete activities based on them.

For example, in Chapter 3 on page 42, Activity 3.9 asks you to watch a clip from the Margaret case study and then answer a question.

Activity 3.9

Go to the Media Tool DVD, select **Case Studies** and then **Adult Health (Margaret)**, then **Margaret in pain.** Watch the video clip **Margaret has an injection for pain** and then identify all the measures the nurse takes to determine that she is about to give the medication to the correct patient. Compare your answers to those at the end of the chapter.

To view updates to the Media Tool DVD, please visit **www.openup.co.uk/clinicalskills**

Please turn over for a case study guide, introducing the patients, and summarizing the resources you will find on the DVD for each case study.

Case Study Guide

Child branch case study: Tom

Introduction to Tom

Tom is 9 years old. Yesterday he was riding his bike home from his friend's house; it was dark and he had no lights on his bike. He was late and he knew his mum would be angry with him for staying out so late. As he cycled at speed round the corner, he was hit by a car and thrown off his bike. The police and ambulance were called by the driver of the car. Although Tom was conscious, he doesn't remember very much except that he had really bad pain in his leg and arm.

Tom was transferred to the local A&E by ambulance. In the ambulance he was given some gas to breathe to take away his pain. It made him feel like he was floating. In A&E the nurse had to get a pair of scissors and cut off Tom's jeans. He started to cry because he knew that his mum would be really mad with him now.

Tom's leg was really hurting him, he kept crying out, so the doctor came and gave him an injection in his leg. The injection hurt but then he began to feel very sleepy and the pain was better.

Case study learning opportunities

This case study focuses on the needs of a child confined to bed for a period of time. In a series of clips of everyday practical care we show the context of clinical skills and interventions and how the nurse and child interact to negotiate care. The nurse demonstrates skill in forming a relationship with the child and uses her professional knowledge together with clinical tools, interaction and visual observation to promote Tom's well-being. The main areas covered are:

- **Taking and recording his vital signs**
- **Assessing and managing his pain**
- **Ensuring he is not bored**
- **Recognizing and taking opportunities to promote his health and healing**

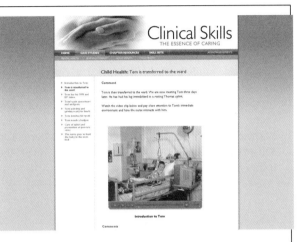

On the Media Tool DVD (found at the back of the book) you will find the full case study. It includes the following resources for Tom's case study.

Case study video clips

Tom's story is told through a sequence of video clips, which you can work through in your own time. There are nine video clips which cover the following:

- **Taking TPR and BP**
- **Communicating with Tom**
- **Pain assessment and management**
- **Administering drugs to children**
- **Meal time**
- **Self-care**
- **Elimination needs**
- **Privacy and dignity**
- **Care of a splint**

Keypoints lectures

The **Keypoints lecture** and **Extra resources** will give you the background you need in relation to Tom's case study and help deepen and expand your knowledge. The resources for Tom's case study cover child development, the management of a child in pain and also the clinical presentation and assessment of fractures. On the DVD you will find resources on:

- Child development
- Fractures
- The cardiovascular system
- Seeking consent
- Pain assessment
- Why take TPR and BP?
- Nutrition

- Creating a child-friendly environment
- Safety issues
- Communicating with children
- Respecting individuality
- Assessment and record keeping
- Drug administration
- Drug calculation
- Infection control
- Health promotion
- Privacy and dignity

Self-tests

Tom's case study includes a number of opportunities to test your knowledge, with multiple-choice and text answer questions on different aspects of care. Using the DVD you can test yourself on your knowledge and get feedback on your answers. The self-tests available for Tom's case study cover the following topics:

Mental health case study: Chris

Introduction to Chris

Chris is a psychology student at university. His friends have noticed that he has not been attending lectures or doing any of his coursework, which is out of character. They come home one day to find he has barricaded himself in his room. When they talk with him, he makes no sense to them, saying things like they're all against him; they've been putting stuff in his food. After a few days of not being able to get him out, they call his sister. They break down the door and find Chris cowering in a corner crying, and looking very dishevelled. He tells his sister that he thinks he has taken an overdose of paracetamol. His sister takes him to the local A&E department.

Case study learning opportunities

This case study focuses on the needs of a young man who is hallucinating and who thinks he might have taken an overdose of paracetamol. In a series of clips, Chris moves through three care settings and meets with varying approaches from healthcare staff in responding to his needs. In A&E the nurse interacts with him skilfully to elicit vital and relevant information about when he thinks he might have taken the tablets. She also responds efficiently to his sister's fear of blood and Chris's apprehension about having blood taken. While he is in the medical emergency unit Chris doesn't want to take his coat

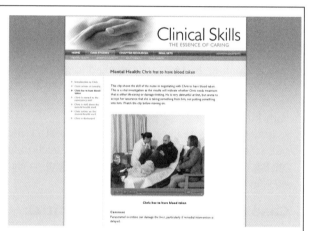

off, and he is generally suspicious. The practical procedures involved and covered in the case include:

- Taking TPR and BP
- Taking blood
- Administering an intravenous infusion
- Transferring a patient through to the mental health ward

In this case study all of the above skills are placed in the context of a reluctant and suspicious patient. Interpersonal communication skills are key elements in negotiating life-saving care with Chris.

On the Media Tool DVD you will find the full case study. It includes the following resources:

Case study video clips

Chris's story is told through a sequence of video clips, which you can work through in your own time. There are seven video clips covering the following:

- **Chris arriving in the A&E department**
- **Taking a blood sample**
- **Admission to the medical ward**
- **Assessing Chris**
- **Good practice: transferring Chris to the mental health unit**
- **Bad practice: transferring Chris to the mental health unit**
- **Discharge**

Keypoints lectures

The **Keypoints lecture** and **Extra resources** will give you the background you need in relation to Chris's case study and help deepen and expand your knowledge. The resources for Chris's case study cover psychosis and the Mental Capacity Act, management of a potential overdose, effective communication with mental health patients and risk assessment. On the DVD you will find resources on:

- **Psychosis**
- **Understanding psychotic experience**
- **Mental Capacity Act**
- **Functions of the liver**
- **Managing a potential overdose**
- **Risk of harm to others**
- **Personal space**
- **Observing a patient**
- **Risk assessment**

Self-tests

Chris's case study includes a number of opportunities to test your knowledge, with multiple-choice and text answer questions on different aspects of care. Using the DVD you can test yourself on your knowledge and get feedback on your answers. The self-tests cover the following topics:

- **Taking and recording vital signs**
- **Prioritizing care**
- **Attitudes and mental health**
- **Providing reassurance**
- **Negotiating with patients**
- **Routines and decision-making**
- **Prevalence of overdose**
- **Communication and personal space**

Learning disability case study: Alex

Introduction to Alex

Alex is a man who has a learning disability. He lives with his mother who has become ill and she is no longer able to assist him. Recently Alex has also become ill and has been diagnosed with diabetes. He is temporarily in an assessment unit while his needs are assessed.

Case study learning opportunities

This case study focuses on interpersonal skills and empowering people with a learning disability. The **Keypoints lectures** and **Extra resources** links to background information on diabetes will help you. The main areas covered are:

- **Personal space**
- **Appropriate and inappropriate communication with someone with a learning disability**

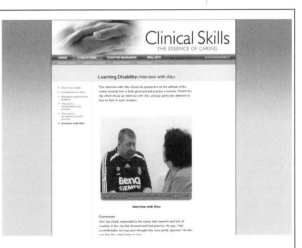

- **Self-care: explaining how a patient can manage their own condition**

On the Media Tool DVD you will find the full case study. It includes the following resources.

Case study video clips

Alex's story is told through a sequence of video clips, which you can work through in your own time. There are five clips covering the following areas:

- **The nurses arriving to visit Alex**
- **The nurses communicating with Alex: good practice**
- **The nurses communicating with Alex: bad practice**
- **The nurses manage inappropriate hugging**
- **Interview with Alex**

Keypoints lectures

The **Keypoints lecture** and **Extra resources** will give you the background you need in relation to Alex's case study and help deepen and expand your knowledge. The resources for Alex's case study provide a background on learning disability and diabetes. On the DVD you will find resources on:

- **Learning disabilities**
- **Diabetes**
- **Communication**
- **Health promotion and learning disability**
- **Empowerment**

Self-tests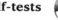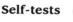

Alex's case study includes a number of opportunities to test your knowledge, with multiple-choice and text answer questions on different aspects of care. Using the DVD you can test yourself on your knowledge and get feedback on your answers. The self-tests cover the following topics:

- **Personal space**
- **Attitudes**
- **Behaviour in social situations**

Adult health case study: Margaret

Introduction to Margaret

Margaret is brought to A&E by ambulance at 7.30 p.m. one July evening, accompanied by her husband. He tells the receiving nurse and registrar that he dialled 999 when Margaret mentioned that she couldn't feel her left leg, dropped a cup of tea for no apparent reason and was unable to pick it up. She had said she felt a bit light-headed. When she arrives at the department she is extremely agitated and has a very bad headache. At this stage, Margaret's medical diagnosis is not the important part of this case study. As a student nurse, you must concentrate on the nursing assessment and care. The video clips link together and follow Margaret through the various stages of her hospital journey.

Case study learning opportunities

This case study focuses on the needs of an adult confined to bed in the acute stage of her illness. She has an episode of incontinence of urine which upsets her, her verbal communication is impaired, and she seems to be in pain. In this series of clips of everyday practical care we show the context of

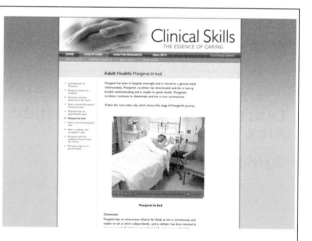

clinical skills and interventions to meet her needs in the acute stage and how the nurse, Margaret and her husband interact to negotiate care. The nurse demonstrates skill in communicating with Margaret and uses her professional knowledge together with clinical tools, interaction and visual observation to promote Margaret's well-being and involve her husband. The main areas covered are:

- **Taking and recording her vital signs**
- **Assessing and managing pain**
- **Meeting elimination needs**
- **Assisting with personal and oral hygiene**

- Preventing the development of pressure ulcers
- Communicating with a patient when their conscious level is reduced

On the Media Tool DVD you will find the full case study. It includes the following resources.

Case study video clips

Margaret's story is told through a sequence of video clips, which you can work through in your own time. There are nine video clips in total:

- Margaret and her husband in A+E
- Margaret and her husband on the ward
- The nurse checks Margaret's blood pressure
- Margaret has an injection for pain
- Margaret in bed
- The nurse checks Margaret's skin
- The nurse explains the nasogastric tube to Margaret
- Margaret and her husband choose from the menu
- Margaret's food arrives

Keypoints lectures

The **Keypoints lecture** and **Extra resources** will give you the background you need in relation to Margaret's case study and help deepen and expand your knowledge. The resources provide the necessary background in relation to meeting the needs of a patient with a reduced level of consciousness. On the DVD you will find resources on:

- Acutely ill patients in hospital
- Rationale for taking and recording vital signs
- Causes and symptoms of a stroke
- NICE guidelines on falls prevention
- Tutorial on the cardiovascular system
- Tutorial on taking blood pressure
- Fluid balance charts
- Assessment of pain
- Pressure ulcer prevention and assessment
- Malnutrition screening tool

Self-tests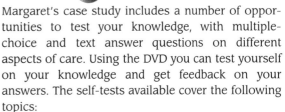

Margaret's case study includes a number of opportunities to test your knowledge, with multiple-choice and text answer questions on different aspects of care. Using the DVD you can test yourself on your knowledge and get feedback on your answers. The self-tests available cover the following topics:

- Health and safety: falling out of bed
- Settling a patient in a ward
- Administering pain relief
- Reassuring patients
- Pressure ulcer prevention
- Infection control
- Privacy and dignity
- Community care

Guide to using the book

Learning objectives

The aim of this chapter is to help you to explore the role of the nurse in relation to record keeping. Throughout the chapter we will also be referring to the case studies on the accompanying Media Tool DVD. Please watch the video clips as directed as these will reinforce your learning and expand upon the information provided in this book.

Learning objectives

These summarize the knowledge, skills or understanding you should have acquired after working through a chapter and related sections of the Media Tool DVD.

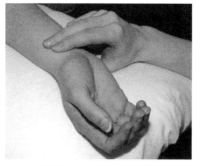

Figure 3.7 Location of the radial pulse

Figures and tables

A number of figures, photographs and tables are provided to help you to visualize the concepts and procedures explained.

Box 2.5 Grice's conversational maxims

The maxim of 'quantity'
- Be as informative as necessary
- Do not be overly informative

The maxim of 'quality'
- Do not say something you believe to be false
- Do not say something for which you lack evidence.

Boxes

Boxes break up the text and contain extra information relevant to the topics discussed. They come in a variety of different formats, some explaining procedures, some containing transcripts and some presenting weblinks to useful resources.

Activities

These boxes ask you to undertake a brief exercise, often related to the Media Tool DVD, or other information offered in the text, to help consolidate your learning. Some of the answers are found at the end of the chapter.

Scenarios

Scenario boxes are included in each chapter to examine more varied real-life examples and to set the scene for further analysis.

Summary and key points

This section summarizes the knowledge you should have gained from each chapter, particularly useful for revision and for tracking your learning.

Custom Publishing Solutions: Let us help make our content your solution

At McGraw-Hill Education our aim is to help lecturers to find the most suitable content for their needs delivered to their students in the most appropriate way. Our **custom publishing solutions** offer the ideal combination of content delivered in the way which best suits lecturer and students.

Our custom publishing programme offers lecturers the opportunity select just the chapters or sections of material they wish to deliver to their students from a database called Primis at www.primisonline.com

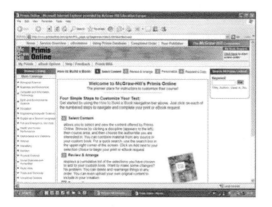

Primis contains over two million pages of content from:

- textbooks
- professional books
- case books – Harvard Articles, Insead, Ivey, Darden, Thunderbird and BusinessWeek
- Taking Sides – debate materials

Across the following imprints:

- McGraw-Hill Education
- Open University Press
- Harvard Business School Press
- US and European material

There is also the option to include additional material authored by lecturers in the custom product – this does not necessarily have to be in English.

We will take care of everything from start to finish in the process of developing and delivering a custom product to ensure that lecturers and students receive exactly the material needed in the most suitable way.

With a Custom Publishing Solution, students enjoy the best selection of material deemed to be the most suitable for learning everything they need for their courses – something of real value to support their learning. Teachers are able to use exactly the material they want, in the way they want, to support their teaching on the course.

Please contact your local McGraw-Hill representative with any questions or alternatively contact Warren Eels **e:** warren_eels@mcgraw-hill.com.

Make the grade!

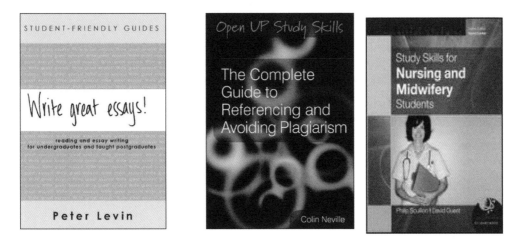

30% off any Study Skills book!

Our Study Skills books are packed with practical advice and tips that are easy to put into practice and will really improve the way you study. Topics include:

- Techniques to help you pass exams
- Advice to improve your essay writing
- Help in putting together the perfect seminar presentation
- Tips on how to balance studying and your personal life

www.openup.co.uk/studyskills

Visit our website to read helpful hints about essays, exams, dissertations and much more.

Special offer! As a valued customer, buy online and receive 30% off any of our Study Skills books by entering the promo code **getahead**

Acknowledgements

Publisher's acknowledgements

Our thanks go to the following reviewers for their comments at various stages in the development of both the text and the Media Tool DVD:

Pat Berridge, Birmingham City University
Jacqui Carr, University of Nottingham
Sue Faulds, University of Southampton
Anne Gallagher, Queen's University, Belfast
Jackie Hunt, Oxford Brookes University
Chris Jordan, Nursing Student, University of York
Rosalyn Joy, Bournemouth University
Bridget Malkin, Birmingham City University
Lorna Martin, Queen's University, Belfast
Ian McGrath, RMIT, Australia
Anne McQueen, University of Edinburgh
Lesley Nickless, Bournemouth University
Karen Ousey, University of Huddersfield
Jacqueline Rattray and team, Cardiff University
Robin Richardson, University of Central Lancashire
Andrea Shinnick, Birmingham City University
Heather Short, University of the West of England.

We would like to extend our thanks to various organisations for reproduction of material, including:
NHS Grampian
Huntleigh Healthcare
www.bradenscale.com
WileyBlackwell
Elsevier (Content in Skills boxes in Chapter 10, Box 10.7, Box 10.8, Activity 10.15 and Box 10.9 reproduced with permission from Walker S. (2007) Chapter 21, 'Elimination – faeces' in Brooker C, Waugh A (2007) 'Foundations of Nursing Practice', Elsevier, London).

Finally, we would like to thank John Matta for all his hard work and support.

If you have any questions about the Media Tool DVD or need any help using it please contact enquiries@openup.co.uk.

Editors' Acknowledgements

We would also like to thank and acknowledge the help of the Sid Merrakech and his team in the Educational Media Services Department at The Robert Gordon University, Simon Hardaker and Andy Stevenson in the Learning Technology Centre, University of Salford and Ben Mollo and Denis McGrath, the Learning Technologists in the Faculty of Health and Social Care at the University of Salford. Also, thanks to the cameraman Chris Tivey, all those who took part in the filming, Rachel Crookes and Karen Harlow for keeping us on track and to all those who gave permission to reproduce copyright material.

Every effort has been made to to trace and acknowledge ownership of copyright and to clear permission for material reproduced in this book. The publishers will be pleased to make suitable arrangements to clear permission with any copyright holders whom it has not been possible to contact.

Foreword

Ensuring the highest quality of patient care is a key government priority, and one they share with patients, the public and staff alike. The special contribution nurses make to quality has been recognised by Professor Lord Darzi of Denham, in his next stage review report 'A High Quality Care for All'. He highlighted the importance of improving the standard of patient care in three prime areas: effectiveness, safety and patient experience. Nurses using this package will be schooled into incorporating each of these aspects into their learning from their earliest days. It makes a unique contribution to nursing practice in drawing together the fundamentals of caring, as described in the Essence of Care benchmarking system, with their practical application in real situations that will be familiar to all.

Nurses are in a commanding position to influence the quality of care, the clinical outcomes achieved, and the experience patients have while they are receiving services. There in all settings, at all times of the day and night, it is the nurse who sets the tone, standards and norms of the care setting. Equally, it is likely to be the nurse who is first to notice all is not well with a patient. It is the nurse who observes, listens, and initiates the action required. Nurses must be confident, technically competent practitioners – but more than that, they must be able to create a healing environment in which care and compassion are exemplified by kindness, gentleness, empathy and understanding.

They must have regard for all in their care, while treating each patient as an individual with a unique perspective on their own situation. For this demanding role, nurses need careful pre-registration preparation, and opportunities for continuous learning. This package will help them navigate both the art and science of nursing. It shows nurses how they can be clinically effective while, crucially, helping them to consider the patient's perspective and what it may be like to be a recipient of care.

In utilising the Essence of Care as a framework for acquiring competence in clinical skills, the authors have ensured that nurses using this book will be familiarised with its ethos of defining the quality of interventions and experience from the patient, public and user point of view. Teaching nurses from their earliest days not only to care for, but also care about, the people who use their services, will enable the profession to continue to enjoy the confidence of the public and to attain the highest aspirations it sets for itself. The mix of materials used will suit all learning styles and will help more seasoned nurses as well as those at the start of their career, and will help make learning a satisfying and motivating experience, surely an ultimate goal of all educators.

Maureen Morgan
Professional Officer for Policy & Practice,
Department of Health.

Preface

Clinical Skills: The Essence of Caring is an exciting, innovative and evidence-based nursing skills textbook. The book provides the essential information that students require to help develop their competence in clinical skills using the best available evidence. It is primarily aimed at the first-year student nurse, but can be used as a reference source by all pre-registration students and may be particularly useful for 'return to practice' post-registration students.

The book and accompanying Media Tool DVD will also help students with the achievement of the Essential Skills Clusters introduced by the NMC in September 2008.

The book takes the student nurse on an interactive journey through fundamental clinical skills in preparation for the delivery of nursing care to patients in different care settings and with different care needs. The Essence of Care initiative, which arose from a commitment to help improve the quality of what are described as fundamental and essential aspects of patient care, provides the framework for the book. Each chapter considers one of the identified benchmarks, apart from health promotion, as this is a theme that relates to all aspects of care and is mentioned throughout.

The book is accompanied by a Media Tool DVD comprising video clips of skills, case studies, scenarios and activities to support the student in their clinical skills development. The unique element in this package is the integration of the book with the Media Tool DVD. This approach means that the Media Tool DVD can be used to capitalize on a variety of learning styles and strategies. We recognize that practices can vary, so it is intended that the video elements are used as a basis for classroom or placement discussion. Unlike most other skills resources, it fully supports students working on their own, before class, or before placement. Students often find it difficult to relate theory to practice, particularly prior to the first clinical placement, and this book offers a unique way to help them do this.

New health policies have important implications for power structures and the relationships between nurses and patients. These changes can cause intense pressures on time to care. The emphasis throughout the book therefore is on 'caring'. It is evident that most skills books concentrate on procedures and it is often this kind of isolation from real practice that can cause students to focus too much on the skill and forget about the person they are caring for. The accompanying Media Tool DVD demonstrates the caring and compassionate behaviour expected of nurses as they perform clinical skills today.

A great advantage is that this resource is flexible. It can be used in class, as an adjunct to, or in preparation for, classroom activity and is available as a resource or revision tool to the student when they might wish to refer to it while on their clinical placements. Lecturers and those who teach clinical skills can use the accompanying DVD independently to the book to support clinical skills teaching. There are video clips of the fundamental nursing skills taught to a first-year student and more! There are also four case studies that can be used to link theory to practice in the classroom. These alone are a fantastic resource for teaching. A unique feature of the book is that as well as good practice, the DVD also demonstrates what is considered to be *bad* practice, for discussion and group work purposes in clinical skills teaching.

This book adds a further unique dimension to current nursing texts and is the first to bring together evidence-based practice and the essence of caring.

Helen Iggulden, Caroline Macdonald and Karen Staniland

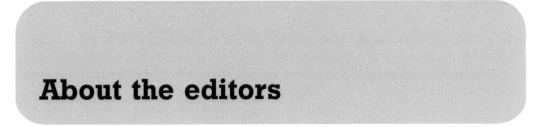

About the editors

Helen Iggulden MSc, BA (Hons), PGCE, RGN. Lecturer, School of Nursing, Learning Technology Fellow, Faculty of Health and Social Care, University of Salford.

Helen has a background in general nursing with a special interest in neurology and neuro-rehabilitation. She has worked in nurse education for 17 years and has a keen interest in developing flexible learning resources.

Caroline MacDonald MSc, PGCTLT, BSc, RGN. Senior Lecturer for Clinical Skills Development, School of Nursing and Midwifery at the Robert Gordon University, Aberdeen.

Caroline is responsible for clinical skills development and has strategic responsibility for the Clinical Skills Centre within the Faculty of Health and Social Care. Caroline's main interests are clinical skills, simulation and interprofessional education.

Karen Staniland PhD, MSc, BSc (Hons), Cert Ed, RCNT, Dip N (Lond), RN, RM. Senior Lecturer/Open Learning Lead, School of Nursing, Faculty of Health and Social Care, University of Salford.

Karen is involved with the promotion of flexible, work-based and e-learning in nursing. Her main research interests lie in healthcare quality improvement at the bedside in relation to clinical governance and *The Essence of Care*.

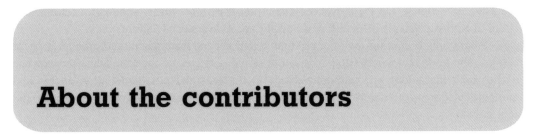

About the contributors

Alison Brown MSc, BSc (Hons), RGN, RNT. Lecturer/Programme Leader, School of Nursing and Midwifery, Faculty of Health and Social Care, Robert Gordon University, Aberdeen.

Alison Brown is Programme Leader of the post-registration Specialist Practice nursing courses. She also teaches moving and handling and cancer nursing on the pre-registration nursing courses and is the lead for moving and handling teaching across the Faculty of Health and Social Care, liaising with our partners in practice. Her particular areas of interest are rehabilitation, self-care and cancer nursing.

Ruth Chadwick MSc, BA, RGN, RSCN, RNT, FETC. Associate Dean Teaching, in the Faculty of Health and Social Care at the University of Salford.

Ruth Chadwick's work focuses upon enhancement of the student learning experience for a wide range of pre- and post-registration health and social care practitioners and individuals pursuing related disciplines. Her particular areas of interest are the healthcare needs of homeless individuals and dementia care.

Elizabeth Collier MSc, BSc, RMNPGCE. Lecturer in Mental Health School of Nursing, Faculty of Health and Social Care, University of Salford.

Elizabeth Collier is currently registered as a PhD student at the University of Salford studying the effect of long-term mental ill health on the achievements and goals of older adults. She works with both pre- and post-registration nursing students on diploma and degree programmes as well as contributing to interprofessional teaching in mental health. Her particular areas of work and interest are evidence-based practice, promoting mental health, mental health and ill health of older adults and dementia education in specialist and non-specialist settings.

Calbert H. Douglas PhD, MSc, BSc (Hons). Senior Lecturer in Planning Sustainable Environments and Environmental Management at the University of Salford.

Dr Douglas's healthcare-related research covers patient-centred built healthcare environments and health impact assessment. His other research areas cover environmental management and environmental investment, corporate social responsibility and sustainable development.

Mary R. Douglas MSc Health Services Research, BSc (Hons), RGN. Head of Learning and Development at Salford Royal NHS Foundation Trust, Salford.

Mary R. Douglas leads on supporting the breadth of the student experience and ensuring the provision of high quality multiprofessional clinical learning environments. Her research includes patient-centred built healthcare environments and professional and practice development.

Jane Ewen MSc, Pg Cert THE, RGN. Education Facilitator within the Professional and Practice Development Unit in NHS Grampian, Honorary Lecturer at Robert Gordon University, Aberdeen.

Jane Ewen has a background in cardiac and general medical adult nursing and has worked in practice development for the past ten years. Her interests include pre- and post-registration nurse education, role development and adult nursing.

Frances Gascoigne MSc, BSc (Hons), MA PG (Advanced Diploma), RGN (PhD thesis pending). Lecturer/Programme Leader, School of Nursing, Faculty of Health and Social Care, University of Salford.

Frances Gascoigne is Programme Leader for the MA in Human Relations and leads the dissertation module for the masters programmes. She leads and teaches the application of life sciences for the MSc Advanced Practice programme and teaches both physiology and pathophysiology to the pre- and post-registration degree and diploma students. Her particular areas of interest include inter- and intra-communication along with experiential learning and personal growth.

Margaret Hutson MPA, BSc (Hons), PG Dip (Nursing), RGN, SCM, RCNT, RNT. Lecturer, School of Nursing and Midwifery, Faculty of Health and Social Care, Robert Gordon University, Aberdeen.

Margaret Hutson works within the practice team focusing on the support of student learning in practice settings across Grampian in both the NHS and private sectors. The clinical assessment of pre-registration student nurses is a particular area of interest and research activity for Margaret.

Pamela Kirkpatrick MSc, PgcHELT, MA (Hons), BA, RM, RGN. Lecturer in Nursing and Joint Course Leader for the BA Public Health Nursing (District Nursing) course at the School of Nursing & Midwifery, Robert Gordon University, Aberdeen.

Pamela Kirkpatrick's interests include public health, community nursing, wound care, health psychology and sexual and reproductive health.

Elizabeth Millar BN, RGN. Sister, Cardiology Department, Aberdeen Royal Infirmary.

Elizabeth Millar is a Ward Sister in the Cardiology Department. Prior to this, her background was in general medicine, endocrinology and trauma orthopaedics. Her main interests are improving direct patient care, mentoring and supporting pre- and post-registration nursing students and engaging in new initiatives for the benefit of patients, their relatives and staff within NHS Grampian.

Naomi Sharples RNLD, RMN, BA (Hons) Linguistics and Deaf Studies, MBA, PGCE. Directorate Manager for the Mental Health and Learning Disability Nursing Team, School of Nursing, Faculty of Health and Social Care, University of Salford.

Naomi Sharples is currently studying for a professional doctorate in health and social care. Naomi has worked in mental health services for deaf people, focusing her career on organizational management, leadership and interpersonal communication. She attained her Practitioner in Neurolinguistic Programming in 2002 and her Master Practitioner in 2004. In 2000, she led the first Deaf People's Access to Nurse Education Programme. The University of Salford remains one of the leaders in providing access to nurse education for deaf people.

Melanie Stephens MA, BSc (Hons), DipN, RGN. Lecturer, and Strategic Lead for Collaborative Learning across staff/student communities, School of Nursing, Faculty of Health and Social Care, University of Salford.

Melanie Stephens co-leads the cross-faculty collaboration learning agenda. She is module leader for a pre-registration diploma programme and a post-qualifying module in tissue viability. Melanie's particular interests are in tissue viability, collaboration for better patient learning outcomes, medical ethics and law.

Susan H. Walker MA, BSc (Hons), PGCE, RGN. Lecturer in Nursing/Clinical Skills, School of Nursing, Faculty of Health and Social Care, University of Salford.

Susan H. Walker leads the development and delivery of clinical skills, teaching both pre- and post-registration students across a number of modules. Her background is in A&E care, with particular interest in acute illness management, holistic assessment and nursing management and leadership, as well as clinical skills.

Seán Welsh RGN, RN (Mental Health), DipN, BSc (Hons), PGCHERP, RNT. Lecturer in Mental Health in the School of Nursing, Faculty of Health and Social Care at the University of Salford.

Seán Welsh has a background in forensic child and adolescent mental health. His most recent publication is a chapter in the forthcoming book *Foundation Degree Development and Research: Case Studies* (University of Salford Publications, 2008).

Clinical skills: the essence of caring

1

Caroline MacDonald and Karen Staniland

Chapter Contents

Welcome to *Clinical Skills: The Essence of Caring*. This is a new, exciting and innovative evidence-based nursing skills textbook that will provide you with the essential information you need to develop your clinical skills. Not only that, but the Media Tool DVD provides extra resources such as videos and self-test material designed to enhance your learning and skills development. The book and DVD together will take you on an interactive journey which will help you provide nursing care for patients in different care settings and with different care needs.

In this chapter we will explain what's at the heart of clinical skills and how this book is designed to help you become proficient as you develop those skills. However, before we do that, we thought it would be useful to examine the idea of 'caring', which is a theme that runs throughout the book. We will also give some history and context to *The Essence of Care* and show how this relates to the book and Media Tool DVD.

Introduction to caring

'Caring' is a term that should be synonymous with nursing. Most students choose to go into nursing because they have a desire to 'care' for other people. However, while some nurses might be skilled, there is not always much evidence to show that they 'care'. On the Media Tool DVD you will find video clips which demonstrate both good and bad practice, as well as patient case studies that show positive patient outcomes. The resources on the Media Tool DVD are designed to show you the type of behaviour that is expected when you carry out your evidence-based practice in relation to clinical skills and working with

patients. These are the 'benchmarks' for good practice, modelled on *The Essence of Care* document which we will discuss later in this chapter. Before doing this however, it is important to understand what we mean by 'evidence' in this context, and how this relates to your practice and care.

Introduction to evidence

According to Traynor (1999), any professional group seeks to establish a unique body of knowledge. Traynor emphasizes the importance of nurses being able to identify evidence to justify their practice, in order for that practice to be credible. Early surveys of nursing concerning whether research was used in clinical practice indicated that it was not utilized to any great extent (Bircumshaw 1990). This may have been due to the requirements of nursing as a profession (Mackay *et al.* 1987; Witz 1992), or the result of a more altruistic notion of providing the most appropriate and humane care. It is also evident that nurses encounter barriers in practice in terms of locating, appraising and implementing research findings (Retsas 2000).

Although there are many definitions of evidence-based practice, evidence-based care and evidence-based medicine, Sackett *et al.* (1997: 2) have defined the term 'evidence-based practice' as 'the conscientious explicit and judicious use of current best evidence about the care of individual patients'. It is noticeable that the emphasis here is on 'current best evidence', not 'research evidence', and this has implications for nursing.

A study by Appleby *et al.* (1995) recognized a clear lack of nursing evidence to inform practice. This study

1

acknowledged that in respect of information for nurses working in the community, of the evidence base for 79 per cent of activities relating to the medical profession, only 15 per cent related to an evidence base within nursing. The conclusion was that the evidence base for nurses in the community was very limited. Work by French (2002) suggests that there is little evidence to support the existence of evidence-based nursing as a distinct construct or process. French concludes that evidence-based practice is commonly a euphemism for information management, clinical judgement, professional practice development or managed care, and that the term adds little more to the existing long-standing tradition of quality assessment and research-based practice. He further argues that nurses must avoid the inefficiency brought about by the intense enthusiasm, followed by sad disenchantment associated with attempts to introduce innovation into healthcare.

Nevertheless, the development of evidence-based healthcare and the availability of information and advances in technology, have clearly widened the portals for providing an evidence base for practice, together with learning opportunities for both the organization concerned and its staff. To this end, many national service frameworks and guidelines have been developed which set standards for all healthcare professionals. *The Essence of Care* was one of these initiatives.

The Essence of Care

The Essence of Care initiative (DoH 2003) related to the commitment made in *Making a Difference*, the national nursing, midwifery and health visiting strategy (DoH 1999). The document proposed a process known as 'benchmarking', through which healthcare professionals could identify best practice and improve existing practice via a structured comparison and sharing of information about patient care within a set framework. The result of such comparisons produced the final set of benchmarks for good nursing practice that are identified and utilized in this book.

The Essence of Care is a long document (175 pages), and takes what is described as a 'qualitative' approach. Various types of evidence were used to establish the benchmark standards, including national guidelines, policies, systematic reviews and large-scale studies. It is stated that 'Patients, carers and professionals

worked together to agree and describe good quality care and best practice' (DoH 2003: 7). While *The Essence of Care* document is essentially a toolkit for practitioners, it is the final agreed benchmarks that are at the heart of this book and the Media Tool DVD. The benchmarks are relevant to all healthcare professionals involved in providing direct care, but *The Essence of Care* is primarily nursing-led. The toolkit considers an evidence base for practice, in the attempt to measure the quality of care, using a hierarchy of evidence. The anticipation was that by explicitly stating each benchmark, practice quality in those designated areas would improve. The final benchmarks were derived from consideration of what patients wanted from care: 'The elements were identified by patients and professionals as crucial to the quality of a patient's care experience' (Ellis 2001: 1202).

In the context of nursing, benchmarking is a method of identifying the best nursing provision within a ward or department, measured along a qualitative continuum. *The Essence of Care* arose from a commitment to help improve the quality of what are described as fundamental and essential aspects of patient care. Eight aspects of care were originally identified:

- continence, bladder and bowel care;
- personal and oral hygiene;
- food and nutrition;
- pressure ulcers;
- privacy and dignity;
- record keeping;
- safety of clients with mental health needs in acute mental health and general hospital settings
- principles of self-care.

Since its inception, there have been additions to the original eight aspects of care: communication in 2003, promoting health in 2006 and environment in 2007. You will find a chapter on each of these topics within the book, apart from health promotion, as this is a theme that relates to all aspects of care and is referred to throughout the chapters.

The Essence of Care was about supporting practitioners to achieve the standards that patients want in fundamental aspects of care, recognizing that clinical governance is concerned with the quality of the whole healthcare experience for the patient (Ellis 2001), and advancing the clinical governance agenda (Castledine

2001). There is still a requirement to develop an 'evidence-based culture' in selecting a strategic direction for evidence-based practice, and then to apply and evaluate the appropriate use of the subsequently developed skills.

Clinical skills and evidence-based practice

Currently, evidence-based practice and evidence-based nursing have a very strong emphasis in the clinical governance agenda of quality improvement (Elcoat 2000). The Nursing and Midwifery Council (NMC) code of conduct (2008: 7) states that 'You must deliver care based on the best available evidence or best practice'. *The Essence of Care* benchmarks provide a suitable basis for clinical skills using observable standards of good practice on the wards.

Everything that you do as a nurse revolves around clinical skills, whether it is communicating with a patient, changing a wound dressing or administering medication. Carrying out these clinical skills proficiently, and using the best available evidence to inform your practice, is vital to ensure a high quality experience for the patient. In this book, you may see a clinical skill described in a different way to that which you were taught at university or on clinical placement. This doesn't mean that what you learned was wrong. There are times when there is more than one way to carry out a clinical skill correctly and safely using the best available evidence. It is vital as students that you question practice and keep your knowledge and clinical skills up to date using the best available evidence (NMC 2008).

All clinical skills are interlinked. This is evident in something as simple as the skill of oral hygiene. For example, when undertaking any oral hygiene activity with a patient you need to wash your hands prior to and following the procedure, communicate with your patient throughout and then record the care given to the patient. This one skill incorporates communication, hand washing, oral hygiene and record keeping.

Gaining competence in clinical skills is complex, and this book will help you to focus on individual skills and then link them together to provide holistic nursing care to your patients in any care setting. The Media Tool DVD is designed to help you make those links and put them into practice throughout your nurse educa-

tion, on placement and later when you are a qualified nurse.

The idea behind this book and the accompanying Media Tool DVD is that it links *The Essence of Care* theory to real nursing practice. By using the DVD you will have access to patient case studies, video clips of clinical skills, online and text-based activities, and a whole lot more. The book and the DVD can be used independently, but the real value of this resource package comes when both elements are used together. See page xiv for a guide to the Media Tool DVD, the textbook features and how to get the most out of them. By the time you have worked through this book, completed all the activities and used the Media Tool DVD, you will indeed be equipped with the clinical skills you need to enable you to deliver high quality patient care.

Skills clusters

It is important to note that the NMC, which has a duty under the Nursing and Midwifery Order 2001 to set standards for education programmes, has recently produced what are known as 'skills clusters'. These are identified as the *Standards of Proficiency for Pre-registration Training* (NMC 2004) (otherwise known as 'Nursing Standards'). The NMC introduced 'essential skills clusters' into pre-registration training in September 2008 to complement the achievement of the existing NMC outcomes and to produce a safe and effective practitioner. This book and Media Tool DVD will help you to both identify the basic skills under the existing *Essence of Care* benchmarks and put them into the context of the local essential skills cluster requirements of your programme. These requirements will vary depending on your education provider.

This is a UK-wide textbook, and you will encounter different transcultural caring practices relating to clinical skills depending on where you work, who you nurse and in relation to different sources of evidence. For example, in Scotland, the Scottish Intercollegiate Guidelines Network (SIGN) develops Scottish national clinical guidelines, whereas in England the National Institute for Health and Clinical Excellence (NICE) has this responsibility. The important thing to remember is to use the best evidence available to you and to ensure that it is from a reliable source.

Clinical skills and the student nurse

There are currently a number of major changes taking place within the National Health Service (NHS). For example, the shift away from acute hospital-based services and towards care based in the community (Scottish Executive 2007). Such changes have necessitated a shift in the role of nurses. Role development is welcomed, but it must be emphasized that skills previously in the domain of other professionals, for example, doctors, are complementary and do not replace the traditional skills of caring that are the cornerstone of nursing (Scottish Executive 2007). This book is an important one as it allows you to develop your clinical skills with an emphasis on caring, while at the same time meeting the needs of a changing NHS.

According to Benner's 'Stages of Clinical Competence', as a first-year student nurse you will be considered a 'novice', developing your repertoire of clinical skills under direct supervision (Benner 1984). As you progress through your course you will move to 'advanced beginner', aiming for 'competence' by the end of your undergraduate programme. As you move towards competence in clinical skills, the supervision from your mentor will become increasingly indirect (NMC 2007). It is, however, very important that you always work within the limits of your competence and do not undertake any aspect of care that you are not qualified to carry out.

Developing your clinical skills is an exciting part of your nursing education, and this book and the accompanying Media Tool DVD are an essential resource to help you. We hope you enjoy it!

References

Appleby, J. Walshe, K. and Ham, C. (1995) *Acting on the Evidence: A Review of Clinical Effectiveness. Sources of Information, Dissemination and Implementation*. Birmingham: NAHA.

Benner, P. (1984) *From Novice to Expert: Excellence and Power in Clinical Nursing Practice*. Menlo Park, CA: Addison-Wesley.

Bircumshaw, D. (1990) The utilization of research findings in clinical nursing practice, *Journal of Advanced Nursing*, 15: 1272–80.

Castledine, G. (2001) New benchmarking toolkit reveals nursing's essence, *British Journal of Nursing*, 10(6): 410.

DoH (Department of Health) (1999) *Making A Difference: Strengthening the Nursing, Midwifery and Health Visiting Contribution to Health and Social Care*. London: HMSO.

DoH (Department of Health) (2003) *The Essence of Care: Patient-focused Benchmarking for Health Care Practitioners*. London: The Stationery Office.

Elcoat, D. (2000) Clinical governance in action: key issues in clinical effectiveness, *Professional Nurse*, 18(10): 822–3.

Ellis, J. (2001) Introducing a method of benchmarking nursing practice, *Professional Nurse*, 16(7): 1202–3.

French, P. (2002) What is the evidence on evidence-based nursing? An epistemological concern, *Journal of Advanced Nursing*, 37(3): 250–7.

Mackay, L., Soothill K. and Melia, K. (eds) (1998) *Classic Texts in Health Care*. Oxford: Butterworth Heinemann.

NMC (Nursing and Midwifery Council) (2004) *Standards of Proficiency for Pre-registration Training*. London: NMC.

NMC (Nursing and Midwifery Council) (2007) *Standards for Medicines Management*. London: NMC.

NMC (Nursing and Midwifery Council) (2008) *The Code, Standards of Conduct, Performance and Ethics for Nurses and Midwives*. London: NMC.

Retsas, A. (2000) Barriers to using research evidence in nursing practice, *Journal of Advanced Nursing*, 31(3): 599–606.

Sackett, D.L., Richardson, W.S., Rosenberg, W. and Haynes, R.B. (1997) *Evidence-based Medicine: How to Practise and Teach EBM*. Edinburgh: Churchill Livingstone.

Scottish Executive (2007) *Better Health, Better Care: A Discussion Document*. Edinburgh, Scottish Executive.

Traynor, M. (1999) *Managerialism and Nursing*. London: Routledge.

Witz, A. (1992) *Professions and Patriarchy*. London: Routledge.

2

Communication

Helen Iggulden and Naomi Sharples

Chapter Contents

Learning objectives

The aim of this chapter is to draw attention to the importance of effective communication and interpersonal skills in developing a *therapeutic relationship* with patients. The chapter will also help you to engage in the appropriate nursing interventions when communicating with a patient. Throughout the chapter we will also be referring to the chapter resources, skill sets and case studies in the accompanying Media Tool DVD. Please watch the video clips as directed as these will reinforce your learning and expand on the information given here. After reading this chapter and interacting with the Media Tool DVD you will be able to:

- Identify the background anatomy and physiology for verbal and non-verbal aspects of communication.
- Choose appropriate aspects of non-verbal communication such as eye contact, voice modulation, interpersonal space and body posture to help develop a rapport and a therapeutic relationship with patients.
- Modify word choice to interact with patients in jargon-free communication.
- Recognize and respond to opportunities for communicating with patients, respecting their privacy and dignity and taking into account their communication needs.
- Value the importance of information sharing between the patient, carer and interprofessional team in coordinated care.
- Identify the resources available to aid communication between patients and healthcare professionals and ensure patients are empowered to communicate.

Introduction

Good communication skills are identified as a key element in *The Essence of Care* benchmarks (DoH 2003). Good communication skills will enable you, as a student, to interact empathically and therapeutically both verbally and non-verbally with people in various physical or mental states. As a student, you will need to develop a range of communication skills while under the supervision of your mentor on clinical placement, some of which are illustrated by examples on the Media Tool DVD and in the case studies.

This chapter addresses both verbal and non-verbal communication, including body language and personal space. The relationship between communication and culture is also emphasized. There is a strong focus on the importance of *interpersonal skills* in communication throughout the chapter. The role of communication when sharing information and in coordinating care will also be highlighted.

Background physiology and communication

Despite the fact that we generally think of communication as verbal, non-verbal communication accounts for a large percentage of human interaction. Body language such as facial expression, eye contact, vocal tone, pace and pitch, gesture and body posture can convey both attitude and emotion which we process much more speedily than language.

Communicating non-verbally

Small almond-shaped groups of neurons sited at the base of the brain are known as the the *amygdala* and are the 'engine room' for the expression of emotion in body language. The amygdala release neurochemicals that fix our emotional experiences onto our memories and initiate bodily changes and movements. This process is faster than the process that produces language and affects the sound of our voices, the way our hands and face move, our breathing rate and even the colours in our skin. All these changes give the listener clues to our emotional state, but until we become self-aware we are often unconscious of our own body language and the effect it has on others.

Communicating verbally

Learned language, on the other hand, is usually stored in the left hemisphere of the higher brain. A simple model (see Figure 2.1) shows that words begin in *Broca's area* of the brain; signals are sent to the sensory cortex which in turn travel to the basal ganglia and onwards to the lungs, the larynx and the mouth, or the arms, face and hands if you are, for instance, using signing (sign language). Then the word or utterance is produced. It is perceived by the listener using the visual cortex and the auditory centres of the brain; meaning is decoded in *Wernicke's area* and then understood by the listener.

Scenario 2.1

A 17-year-old boy who has fallen from a tree has sustained an eye injury and a fractured right arm. He is displaying signs of hypovolaemic shock, with low blood pressure and a rapid pulse. How might his communication skills be affected in each of the following areas?

- Upper limbs and hands
- Body language
- Sensory input
- Language skills
- Motor skills
- Speech production
- Social skills

You can find some suggested answers to this scenario at the end of the chapter.

How are communication and culture linked?

Good cross-cultural communication enhances your nursing practice by:

- building the patient's confidence in the nurse–patient relationship;
- improving patient safety and clinical outcomes;
- making more effective use of time spent with your patient;
- increasing patient satisfaction and decreasing stress for both you and your patient (Pullen 2007).

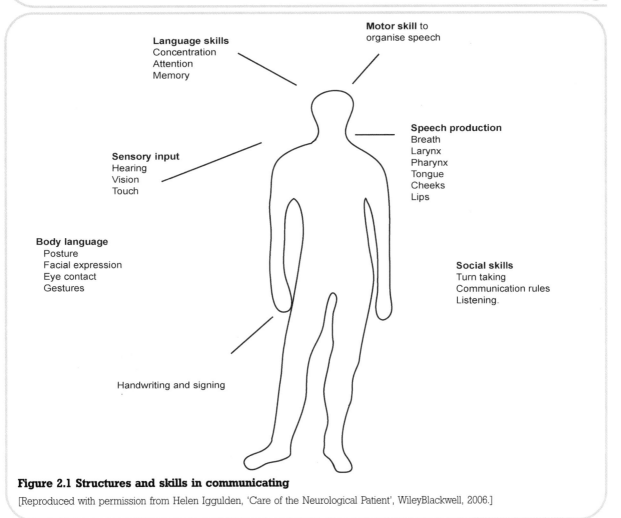

Language skills
Concentration
Attention
Memory

Motor skill to
organise speech

Speech production
Breath
Larynx
Pharynx
Tongue
Cheeks
Lips

Sensory input
Hearing
Vision
Touch

Body language
Posture
Facial expression
Eye contact
Gestures

Social skills
Turn taking
Communication rules
Listening.

Handwriting and signing

Figure 2.1 Structures and skills in communicating
[Reproduced with permission from Helen Iggulden, 'Care of the Neurological Patient', WileyBlackwell, 2006.]

How we express ourselves is fundamentally linked to our culture, beliefs and values, our status and our language skills. *Culture* is the learned and shared patterns of behaviour and information that a group uses to generate meaning among its members. However, these can be highly individual and we need to be careful not to stereotype people or make assumptions based on a person's gender, race, nationality, religion, sexual orientation or age. *Beliefs* are the assumptions that we hold about ourselves, about others in the world and about how we expect things to be. *Values* are about how we have learned to think things ought to be and how people ought to behave. *Status* is in the context of social interaction is the relative rank that an individual holds in a given society and in relation to others. *Language skills* are our listening, speaking, signing, reading and writing skills in the mother language or in a second, third or foreign language. Lis-

tening, visual perception and reading are *receptive* skills, and speaking, signing, gesturing and writing are *productive* skills. *Language abilities* are needed for good interpersonal communication, but are not the same as interpersonal skills, although the two are closely connected. Box 2.3 on page 9 lists some typical interpersonal skills.

Communication models

The principles of interpersonal and social communication can be represented in models of communication. 'Models' are simplifications that help us understand the components and processes of experiences such as communication. For example, think about the London Underground map. This 'model' is nothing like the actual Underground network, but displays a simplistic interpretation of the system in a model so that routes can be understood easily. Communication models can also represent how we send messages to, and understand messages from, others. Some models identify a sender, a message and a receiver, using arrows to indicate the direction of communication. Depending on the complexity of the model they also represent other factors that might affect the meaning of the message. Figure 2.2 shows a very simplified model for one-way communication. A sender sends a message and the receiver receives it. The receiver then becomes the sender.

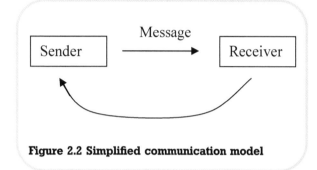

Figure 2.2 Simplified communication model

However, life is not that simple, and Berlo's (1960) model of communication (see Table 2.1) draws attention to the dynamic relationship between the sender and the receiver. This model recognizes the importance of the relationship between the people who are communicating and their awareness of each other, culturally and socially. The receiver is seen as equally important as the sender in making the meaning of the communication clear.

In this more complex model, the 'elements of a message' are the code, content and treatment. How these elements are packaged together forms the 'structure' of the message. The code is the system of symbols we choose to use to present the message. The content of the message is the material chosen to put into the message and the treatment is how we choose to produce it. For example, think of a person in difficulties in a boat, waving frantically at a passing ship. The elements are packaged together using the visual gestural code of arms outstretched, moving left and right arm at the same time out to the side and up above the head repeatedly. The content is the force and speed of the arm movements and the timing of those movements. Strong and rapid arm movements that go on for some time say something very different from a gentle arm movement that stops after a couple of repetitions – such a movement is more likely to say 'hello' rather than 'please help me'. Finally, the treatment in this case represents an almost universal request for assistance. If any of the elements of the message were changed slightly, it could easily mean something else. A different arm movement, for example, might signify 'keep away'.

Berlo's model takes into consideration the communication skills, attitudes, beliefs, knowledge base, social system and culture of the person sending the message and that of the person receiving it. It clearly demonstrates how complicated communication really is.

The feedback loop

What is missing from Berlo's model, however, is the feedback mechanism crucial to communication. Both the sender and receiver look and listen for feedback throughout the communication process. Feedback

Table 2.1 Berlo's model of communication (Berlo 1960)			
Sender	*Message*	*Channel*	*Receiver*
Communication Skills	Elements	Hearing	Communication Skills
Attitudes	Structure	Seeing	Attitude
Knowledge	Code	Touching	Knowledge
Social System	Treatment	Smelling	Social System
Culture	Content	Tasting	Culture
Message $\longrightarrow$			

helps us to know if our message is correctly or incorrectly formed. When people give us an expected response to our message, we can generally presume that the message is understood. When the response is not as expected, the sender must consider a number of reasons for this and adapt their communication appropriately. Box 2.1 shows some examples of unexpected responses.

Box 2.1 Examples of unexpected responses

- Blank stare from the listener
- Listener not behaving as requested
- Laughing where humour was not intended
- Taking offence where humour *was* intended
- Message distorted and changed when relayed to others
- Listener focusing on one area of the message and missing the area felt to be most important
- Message inadvertently triggers a memory in the listener that is unrelated to the message

---

Interpersonal skills

It is very easy to assume that information about language and communication is 'obvious' because we communicate constantly and, most of the time, effectively. Reading about communication is often comfortable because we are so used to the process. However, conscious communication happens less often. It is this 'mindful' communication that is the most challenging and most important aspect of communication for nurses. Lack of 'mindfulness' when communicating can create tension and anxiety in others.

Box 2.2 presents a transcript from a video clip on the accompanying Media Tool DVD; only the scenario and words are given here; there is no indication of any non-verbal communication.

It is clear from the previous example that language is much more than just speech – it also involves interpersonal skills. Box 2.3 lists, in a nursing context, the kinds of interpersonal skills that we mean.

Body language

Body language is an important aspect of communication. It has been suggested that body language

---

Box 2.2 Transcript from the video clip

Sound of clattering wheels. The patient is asleep in bed. Nurse enters the room pushing a Dinamap machine. She walks to the patient and shakes her.

Nurse: Mrs Bennet? Mrs Bennet? Oh hello, I've just come to do your observations, OK? I am just going to do your blood pressure if that's OK? Thanks very much. Oh that's a nasty cough you've got there isn't it? This'll just feel a bit tight on your arm . . . if I can just have your wrist . . . that's fine. Thanks very much, I am just doing your pulse. Oh it's all right. Right, I am just going to do your temperature now. Just turn your head that way a bit now, my love, thanks very much . . . just keep still if you can.

Mrs Bennet: Oh, it's tight, this.

Nurse: Oh, it'll be alright love.

Mrs Bennet: Oh, it is tight.

Nurse: Yes, yes, yes, just leave it alone for a minute.

Box 2.3 What are interpersonal skills?

- Self-awareness
- Active listening
- Empathy
- Having a range of communication styles and knowing when each style is most appropriate
- Sensitivity to others, their individuality and their contributions
- Ability to observe, assess the styles, preferences, knowledge, skills, abilities and shortcomings of others and develop rapport
- Ability to build strong and effective relationships with others based on trust, honesty and integrity
- Ability to delegate, give direction, appraise/ evaluate, give feedback
- Ability to help resolve conflict diplomatically
- Ability to offer support and encouragement

Activity 2.1

Go to the Media Tool DVD, select **Skill Sets**, then **Observations**, then **Temperature Taking**, then watch **Temperature Taking, poor practice**. It will be clear that from a visual point of view body language, manner and attitude are a significant part of an interaction, and you may see more to the interaction now than can be identified just from the transcript.

You can see that the nurse does not introduce herself, she does not ask for consent, she tells the patient what she is going to do, she restrains her, she is rough, she does not make eye contact and she does not respond to Mrs Bennet's discomfort. Her tone of voice and manner are impatient. This is why the practice is unacceptable.

Activity 2.2

Using the list of interpersonal skills in Box 2.3, read the following transcript from **Temperature Taking, poor practice**. What does the nurse do in this case that conveys respect? What interpersonal skills do you think the nurse is demonstrating? Make a note of your answers.

Nurse: Good morning.

Mrs Bennet: Good morning, nurse.

Nurse: My name's Dawn. I'm going to be looking after you today.

Mrs Bennet: All right.

Nurse: I need to do your observations if that's ok?

Mrs Bennet: Yes, that's fine.

Nurse: Do you remember having them done in accident and emergency?

Mrs Bennet: Not really, no.

Nurse: OK, then. Well, what we need to do is measure your temperature, your pulse, the amount and the rate that you're breathing and your blood pressure.

Mrs Bennet: Right. OK.

Nurse: You don't remember them in A&E? OK. What I'm going to do first is your blood pressure. It involves putting a cuff around your upper arm and then it gets a bit tight; we set a machine doing it automatically. When it's pumping up you'll feel a bit uncomfortable, you might get some pins and needles in your fingers but that's quite normal. It will release after about a minute and the feeling should come back, OK? So what I need to do is just lift your gown up a little bit, I'm not going to expose too much of you [*nurse applies the cuff*]. All it does, is it slides round until it fastens automatically. I don't need you to do anything, just to lie there, but be comfortable. Are you all right there?

Mrs Bennet: Yes.

Nurse: OK. Is your hand going to be all right there? Do you want to rest it? Maybe on you?

Mrs Bennet: OK [*machine begins to bleep*].

Nurse: You'll hear the machine bleep as it pumps up.

Mrs Bennet: Oh, it's noisy, isn't it?

Nurse: It is a little bit, that's all, and there's lots of figures on, don't be worried by those.

Mrs Bennet: But what do they do?

Nurse: What they do, they measure when your heart's contracting and when it's relaxing, that's how we measure your blood pressure. So every time your heart takes a beat, that's what it does. And then it gives us some numbers and that's what we write down.

Mrs Bennet: Right.

Nurse: You might have had it done in the past, maybe in the old-fashioned way, little machine at the side of your bed. Yeah.
Are you OK? Quite comfortable there?

Mrs Bennet: Yes.

Nurse: So you'll hear it clicking and you'll hear it pumping up.

Mrs Bennet: It goes down slowly?

Nurse: It does, yes, yes, eventually. OK, are you getting that funny feeling in your fingertips? OK, that's it. Do your fingers feel all right?

Mrs Bennet: Is it OK?

Nurse: It is yes. Your pulse is a little bit high but that's probably due to the chest infection that the doctors think you've got, and that's why you've been admitted. So what we'll need to do is check that again in about four hours' time.

In this instance you can see that the nurse greets Mrs Bennet, introduces herself and asks for consent for the procedure, which Mrs Bennet gives. She explains what she is going to do and any discomfort that Mrs Bennet might feel. She checks that Mrs Bennet is comfortable and answers her questions in terms that she can understand, and gives her feedback on her pulse rate. The nurse demonstrates active listening skills and empathy, and is able to explain things in a way that Mrs Bennet can understand. She is sensitive to Mrs Bennet, able to offer her support and encouragement, and inspires her trust. This is clear from the ease with which Mrs Bennet asks questions.

provides the listener with about half of the overall message along with additional information about trustworthiness, mood, and of course health status (Jennings and Haughton 2002).

Body language is the non-verbal whole-body aspect of communication. People express themselves through their bodily movements and these add to the utterances they make to communicate. While we can work on body language to promote better understanding by other people, a more useful skill is a proper understanding of how speech and body language interact to produce meaning.

A simple example of body language in action is the concept of a 'closed' or 'open' posture. Although this is a generalization, people who 'close themselves off' by, for example, crossing their legs or folding their arms, while curving inwards at the waist, give an impression of self-protection – their body language is telling the observer not to come too close. In the still photograph from the Chris case study (Figure 2.3), you can see very

pronounced protective body language. In addition, the nurse who is standing in the foreground has her hands on her hips, which may indicate either readiness, impatience, or even aggression.

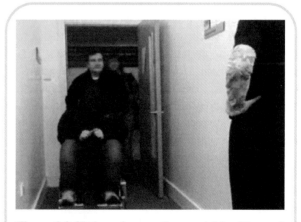

Figure 2.3 Chris arrives on the mental health ward – bad practice

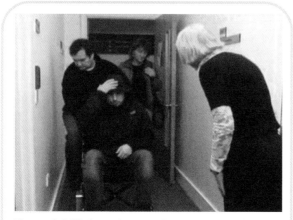

Figure 2.4 Chris arrives on the mental health ward – good practice

On the other hand, a person with open arms and relaxed legs, who is leaning forward towards their interlocutor, is giving the opposite impression: they are relaxed, open to dialogue and give no sense of needing to protect themselves. The body language suggests that they are approachable and open to contact.

If you now look at Figure 2.4, you will see that here the nurse greeting Chris is adopting a very different posture: she is leaning forward and her arms are placed unthreateningly at her sides. It is clear that she is open to communication. Her head is inclined, which demonstrates interest, but she is keeping her distance, showing respect for Chris's personal space. This also enables Chris to see her clearly from his seated position, and she him. Were she to stand too close she would either have to kneel to look under Chris's hood, which would be intrusive, or Chris would have to look up at her, suggesting subordination.

When you watch the video clip on the Media Tool DVD you will appreciate how much the nurse's tone of voice and manner of speaking add to this picture of visual openness. You may also notice several other aspects of her body language. She extends her hand to Chris to show respect, but seeing he is not going to take it she quickly withdraws it and continues introducing him to the ward, regardless of the fact that Chris is ignoring her. This is because, unlike a personal situation in which the nurse might feel snubbed, in this clinical situation it is a way of assessing Chris's emotional state.

There are a number of aspects of body language that are worth considering in your practice, and these are examined below.

Genuiness and sincerity

While it is a useful tool, we must exercise caution and avoid generalizing about a person purely on the basis of their body language. From our own perspective, the important thing is to be *congruent* – i.e. does our body language match our message? Incongruence, where our body language doesn't appear to match what we say, can lead lead to mistrust in the listener.

Smiling

False smiles

For instance, we can often recognize a 'false smile' when we receive one. We know that it is false because when one does not actually feel happy it is difficult to engineer a full smile that incorporates the muscles around the eyes. When we see unsmiling eyes and smiling mouths we feel unsure about the person's emotions, thoughts and intentions.

Polite smiles

The professional or polite smile has been called a 'pan-American' smile (Seligman 2002). This type of smile is used by people attending to others in a customer care sense rather than to convey true happiness.

Genuine smiles

Genuine, full-face smiles that reach the eyes are referred to as 'Duchenne smiles' after Guillaume Duchenne, who first discovered how to stimulate facial nerves utilizing electricity. He identified the nerves used to smile and, significantly, how nerves around the eyes were engaged when expressing true happiness. Such smiles are a genuine response to a pleasurable emotion or feeling.

Eye contact

Box 2.4 How we use eye contact

- To regulate conversation
- To regulate intimacy levels
- To communicate interest or disinterest
- To gain feedback
- To express emotions
- To influence others

Activity 2.3

Look at Figures 2.5 and 2.6 from the Alex case study on the Media Tool DVD. Think about the difference between the two images.

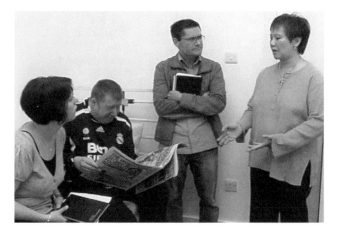

Figure 2.5 The nurses visiting Alex demonstrate bad practice

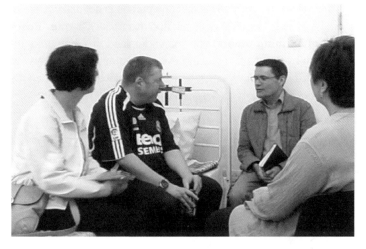

Figure 2.6 The nurses visiting Alex demonstrate good practice

You will notice that in the first image the patient, Alex, is being talked over and no one can make eye contact with him because he is reading a newspaper! In Figure 2.6 the seating is arranged to include all members of the group so that they can make good eye contact. Everyone is on the same level; this is an important communication feature that promotes equity in relationships.

Eye contact is an important aspect of face-to-face communication. Box 2.4 indicates how we use eye contact. We tend to drop eye contact when we have finished speaking. We also drop eye contact when we are distracted, lose interest in what the *other* person is saying or when we do not respect them.

Gazing and staring

There is a difference between gazing and staring. Gazing means looking in the general direction of a person's face, while staring can be seen as threatening. We may stare when we are concentrating on what someone is saying, but we (and they) know this looks

Activity 2.4

Look at Figure 2.7. What can you tell from the eye contact between these two people?

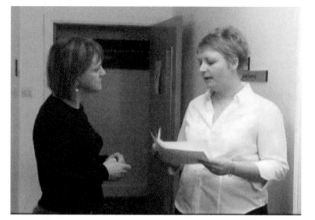

Figure 2.7 Shirley asks for her blood results – poor nursing response

As we pointed out in the section on communication models, communication is dynamic and it is also a process. From a still image such as this, all we can truly say is that one person is not making eye contact with the other. If you watch the video clip on the Media Tool DVD (you can find this under **Chapter Resources-Mental Health Needs-Assessment of risk of harming others**) you will understand that the nurse (in the white shirt) is attempting to end the interaction by frequently breaking eye contact and looking away while she is speaking. Shirley is just as intent on continuing the conversation in order to achieve her goal and tries very hard to get eye contact from the nurse, to the point of almost ducking under the nurse's face in her fervent attempts at engagement.

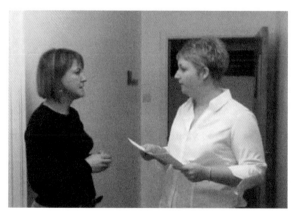

Figure 2.8 Shirley and the nurse make eye contact – good nursing response

Figure 2.8 shows a still shot from a second video clip, demonstrating much better eye contact. It shows that the nurse has positive eye contact which helps Shirley to feel heard and she remains relaxed, trusting and confident in the belief that the nurse is listening and attending to her.

and feels very different from an angry stare. Patients often gaze at nurses as they go about their work, sometimes as a way of trying to attract their attention.

Eye contact and cultural differences

Eye contact behaviour is different in different cultures. It is important to know whether avoiding eye contact is considered rude for the other person or a sign of respect. Direct eye contact can show that you are listening or that you are challenging the authority of the speaker, depending on the situation. Most English people make eye contact at the beginning of a conversation and then let their gaze drift to one side periodically to avoid staring at someone continually, which might make them feel uncomfortable – colloquially referred to as 'staring the person out'. In South Asia and many other cultures, direct eye contact is regarded as aggressive and rude, while eye contact between men and women can be regarded as flirtatious. Some cultures, such as British culture, are 'low look' societies, because watching people overtly is seen as intrusive and rude. In 'high look' cultures such as Italy or Spain, being watched is not a problem. You need to be aware of your style in communicating with your patients and be ready to pick up any feedback. A mismatch with eye contact rules can severely affect the relationship between listener and speaker.

Speaking and body language

It is not just what we say but the way we say it that imparts emotion. Clearly, the tone of our voice has a considerable impact on the emotional message we are communicating. Again, however, we have to be wary of sweeping generalizations. Nevertheless, we do hear and see people's emotional states in their voice and in their hand shapes. Angry people will increase the loudness of their voice, their lips may tighten and their larynx will be tense, resulting in strong, clear tones. Often their skin changes colour – angry people may go very red in the face or even 'white' with rage. People who are sad will speak more quietly, with a more relaxed larynx, tongue and lips which changes the 'shape' of the sound; it becomes subdued, less defined and slightly more muffled. Very sad people may exhibit pallor to their skin. Happiness creates much more of a sing-song quality in the voice which relates directly to the physiology of our emotions.

Body language and hearing impairment

A hearing impairment or deafness can occur at any time in our lives for various reasons. The gravity of the hearing loss and the medical and educational support services available will determine how a person goes about addressing such a loss. Some people choose to learn sign language and therefore access the world through visual communication. Others choose to address their hearing loss through amplification technology such as hearing aids, cochlear implants or brain implants, which are linked to a body-worn receiver.

People who experience hearing impairment or deafness rely heavily on facial expression, lip patterns and body language in order to access as much of the conversation as possible. It is important to remember that people without a hearing impairment or deafness also rely heavily on these components of language and communication, but for them, sound waves are also used. Therefore, if you take away some, or all, of the sound waves, people will naturally rely more on visual cues. As a result, people who communicate using very few gestures, only a small level of lip movement and limited facial expression will create more of a communication problem for those suffering from a hearing impairment. Conversely, people who use *pantomime* in an effort to help a deaf or hard of hearing person understand them, may also complicate matters due to the over-extension of facial expression, abnormal lip patterns and gestures that belong to a game of 'charades' rather than universal gestures that are fully accessible to all.

Sign languages are a fully developed forms of communication with a set of specific hand shapes which take on specific orientations to the body, located in a specific place in space. Sign languages utilize timelines to show the audience when something may have happened or be about to happen, over how long, and how far in the future or past. They also have non-manual features which show movements of the face, head and trunk, all of which have specific meanings, and all of which work together to create a signed utterance. *British Sign Language* (BSL) is the first or preferred language for about 50,000 hearing-impaired people in Britain and you will most likely come across at least one patient who uses BSL during your nursing career. In such cases it is vital to work with qualified BSL interpreters within the healthcare setting to

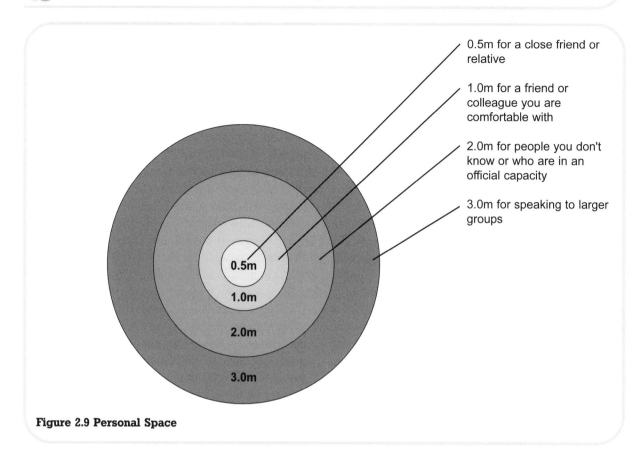

0.5m for a close friend or relative

1.0m for a friend or colleague you are comfortable with

2.0m for people you don't know or who are in an official capacity

3.0m for speaking to larger groups

Figure 2.9 Personal Space

ensure the deaf person has full access to, and understanding of, their care.

Personal and social space

Where we physically position ourselves in relation to the listener or listeners (known as *proxemics*) adds another dimension to our communication skills. Clearly, turning our back to the speaker gives the very strong impression that we are disengaging from the process unless we have to turn our back due to environmental constraints. In such a situation it should still be possible to turn the head and/or shoulders to show that we are still listening.

Standing too close to the other person can make them feel very uncomfortable; again we need to be aware of cultural norms. The more comfortable we are with the other person, the closer we tend to accept them standing (or sitting). However, standing too far away from a person will send a strong message that you may not trust, like or respect them. If as a clinician it is necessary to give someone space, that physical

space can be balanced by your use of the appropriate register of language (which we will discuss in the next section) and demonstration of empathy.

A general guide for acceptable proximity shown in Figure 2.9 is:

- 0.5m for a close friend or relative;
- 1.0m for a friend or colleague you are comfortable with;
- 2.0m for people you don't know or who are in an official capacity;
- 3.0m for speaking to larger groups.

Distance is dictated by personal comfort, your relationship with the other person and the number of people being spoken to. We also need to consider proxemics in regard to people who use wheelchairs, or who are constrained by their health situation. However, health professionals often have to break commonly held principles of distance because of the clinical situation. For example, in Figure 2.10 you can see that the nurse is very close indeed to Chris, well within the interpersonal range of 1m. The nurse is

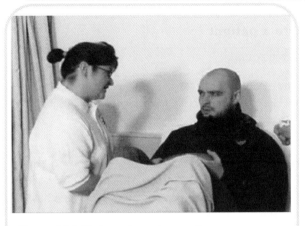

Figure 2.10 Chris arrives at casualty

speaking continually, giving information and checking understanding. Her aim is to gain compliance as quickly as possible because time is not on Chris's side if he has taken an overdose. The nurse has to utilize her communication skills to speed up the development of trust and rapport in order to get a blood sample from Chris in a very challenging situation. You will also note when you watch this video clip on the Media Tool DVD that the nurse:

● utilizes closeness to encourage a sense of trust – because this proximity is usually reserved only for people we trust;
● makes sure that her voice is gentle and kind, maintaining a consistent speed and intonation that expresses care;
● makes sure that her movements and gestures reflect the care in her voice (she is congruent);
● keeps up the pressure for Chris to comply with the blood test because of the serious nature of the clinical situation.

Words and word choice

Now that we have considered the physiological aspects of communication, aspects of body language, eye contact and proximity, we will look at the language we use when communicating and what impact this has.

Sociolinguistics provides us with a great deal of evidence regarding the sociological basis of language. It offers information regarding the 'registers' or 'styles' people use. These are called 'language registers'. Language registers are ways of speaking and com-

municating according to a given culture, occupation or profession, social setting, social class or group norm. For example, the way we communicate with our peers in a relaxing environment is very different from the language we choose to use in a formal clinical setting. Some examples of this are identified in Table 2.2.

Table 2.2 Examples of alternative language registers	
Formal	*Informal*
Sutures	Stitches
Myocardial infarction	Heart attack
Hypertensive	High blood pressure
Tachycardia	Rapid heart beat

Healthcare practitioners need to be able to switch from one register to another – formal to informal. When you are communicating with professional healthcare colleagues it is usual to use 'professional language', but you may need to seek clarification from interprofessional colleagues as each discipline has its own jargon, register and acronyms. You will need to be able to express clinical information using a client's or patient's 'register' to ensure informed consent and that the expected outcome is clear. See Activity 2.5 for an example of a patient's register.

Activity 2.5

Go the media tool and select **Case Studies**, then **Mental Health (Chris)**, then **Chris arrives at casualty**. Then scroll down to watch the second video clip on this page, **Chris has to have blood taken**. The nurse in A&E is taking blood from Chris for a full blood analysis. Despite the fact that Chris is concerned and a little nervous, the nurse maintains an open posture with eye contact and provides a jargon-free explanation of the procedure. As you will see, Chris feels free to ask questions and his eye contact remains active, because he is engaged with the process.

Activity 2.6 A nurse explains IV cannulation to a patient

Read the transcript and note the comments that follow. Do you agree?

Nurse: Right. I'm just going to take a moment to prepare my equipment and then I'll put a cannula in and take you through the procedure. So, is there anything you would like to ask me about the procedure while I just prepare the equipment?

Patient: Does it hurt?

Nurse: You will have some discomfort, but only for a moment, just while we get the needle in position. So, what I'm going to do now is just put this tourniquet on. It will feel quite tight initially and I'm going to place it below your elbow in the first place because I want to look at the veins in the back of your hand and along this area here [*motions to patient's forearm*]. OK. So tell me again, have you had a cannula sited before?

You can see that the nurse explains that there will be some discomfort and, again, the conversation has good quality, quantity, manner and relation.

Openness, honesty and transparency

All health professionals need to develop and maintain the skills that support openness, honesty and transparency. Trustworthy communication with patients, families, colleagues and carers is fundamental to efficient and effective care delivery and management (Burke 2003). *Openness* refers to the amount of information that is provided, and *honesty* refers to the trustworthiness of that information. *Transparency* refers to the clarity of the information provided. When openness, honesty and transparency are lost, anxiety and anger may soon follow. While we consider our skills in terms of being open, honest and transparent, we should always think about the needs of the listener. A model that illustrates this extremely well is known as 'Grice's conversational maxims', and is outlined in Box 2.5 (Chapman 2005).

Activity 2.6 shows how these elements are at work in explaining the procedure of intravenous (IV) cannulation to a patient.

Box 2.5 Grice's conversational maxims

The maxim of 'quantity'
- Be as informative as necessary
- Do not be overly informative

The maxim of 'quality'
- Do not say something you believe to be false
- Do not say something for which you lack evidence

The maxim of 'relation'
- Make sure what you are saying is relevant to the conversation

The maxim of 'manner'
- Avoid being obscure or difficult to understand
- Do not say something that is ambiguous – i.e. that could be taken in more than one way
- Be to the point
- Be organized in what you are saying

Establishing rapport: active and empathic listening

As we have already seen, there are numerous ways of establishing a connection with another person that facilitate therapeutic engagement. From the negative examples, we can also clearly see how quickly and easily this engagement, or its potential, can be damaged.

Rapport

Rapport is the connection that we have with another person. When we are in rapport with someone, we have a sense of relationship with them. This connection helps the interpersonal process to develop, which in turn enables people to care for others, to educate, to inform and to involve those people necessary to the

Box 2.6 Techniques to help develop rapport

Questioning

Ask two or three initial questions to which you know the answer is yes; this helps to build a positive start. For example, 'So you came in today?', 'Yes', 'And you live at 23 Stables Lane?' 'Yes.' This is better than asking, for example, 'When did you come in?' and 'Where do you live?'

Pacing and matching

Pace your patient by matching them in subtle ways. You can mirror their body posture, their facial expression, their head tilts, their hand gestures, the pitch of their voice pitch, and its rhythm, tone, volume and speed. One of the most subtle forms of rapport-building is to match a person's breathing. This helps you to tune in to your patient's emotional state and makes them aware (non-verbally) that you have done this.

These techniques can be adapted to the circumstances according to the age of the patient and their level of understanding. Sometimes a person is either physically or emotionally unable to answer the generating questions. In these circumstances, it is vital that you use all possible means to develop a connection. It may be that you have to be far more attentive to the person's non-verbal cues – for example, eye contact, gaze direction, pointing – anything in fact that indicates contact/communication. Sharing day-to-day activities always helps to promote a good relationship and establish rapport.

---

healthcare of patients, clients or carers. In our home lives, rapport enables our friendships and relationships; it also helps us to negotiate a good deal with sales people, or them to clinch a deal with us. Rapport relies on shared language and understanding. When people are in rapport, they find connection through common interests, humour, situations, likes and dislikes. There are degrees of rapport, so it is useful to think of it as a scale where 0 is no rapport and 10 denotes excellent rapport:

0	**2**	**4**	**6**	**8**	**10**

No rapport   *Excellent rapport*

Building rapport with patients

Rapport is created by gently mirroring and matching body movements and postures, facial expression, tone

of voice, speed and volume of speech. The more of these behaviours match between two people, the more likely it is that they will like each other, feel rapport and be interested in what each other is saying (Griffin and Tyrrell 2003). Several techniques can help develop rapport quickly, such as questioning, pace and matching, all shown in Box 2.6.

Empathy

Empathy is the emotional connection between people. While rapport deals with language, interests, commonality and personal space, empathy goes deeper and involves one person feeling some of the emotions of another. This emotional connection can rarely be total, but by utilizing our skills of perception and assessing the physiological status of the other person, we should be able to consider their circumstances and then utilize our own memories and experiences to align ourselves to some extent with their emotions.

Empathy can be seen in many everyday clinical situations – for example, when you are feeding a patient or client: you may find that you open your own mouth at the moment you want your patient to take in food. 'Infectious' laughter, colloquially known as 'the giggles', is another good example. Laughter can spread throughout a group, even if the joke is not shared by everyone in that group. However, emotion is

Activity 2.7

Go to the Media Tool DVD and select **Skill Sets**, then **Nutritional Intake**, then **Venepuncture**. Watch the clip **Angela has blood taken**. What does the nurse do to establish rapport? Make a note of your answers and compare them to those at the end of the chapter.

communicable rather than infectious. So, if we put empathy on the same type of scale as rapport, we can identify a useful level of empathy where the healthcare practitioner can be a resource for the individual without over-empathizing.

0	2	4	6	8	10
No empathy					*Complete empathy*

Where there is no empathy, the nurse will have no appreciation of how the patient perceives their situation. There will be a lack of warmth between the two people and no sense of connection. We often identify this as 'coldness' in an attempt to describe the emotional distance encountered. This distance leads to a lack of trust, openness and honesty because to be trusting, open and honest in this situation could leave a person very vulnerable.

At the opposite end of the scale we have complete empathy. While it is generally accepted that this is virtually impossible, we are encouraged to 'walk in the shoes' of the other person in order to fully understand how they feel. However, over-empathizing is not resourceful for healthcare practitioners as it can create an unhealthy reliance on the part of the practitioner on the patient or client. The practitioner develops a need for the other person which disables their ability to be an effective resource, and this can result in a loss of professional perspective.

To function at a level of 5 or 6 is the optimum. This level of empathy enables us to perceive the world through the other person's eyes, to see and feel their happiness, confusion, fear, anxiety or love. This knowledge is useful for practitioners as it allows them to present information in a way that is more likely to be understood by the patient, client or carer. It supports a trust that is necessary for healthcare to be effective and efficiently managed. It gives the care-giver an insight into their ability to form a therapeutic alliance and how effective that alliance is.

Self-awareness

Nurses have varying amounts of time to develop therapeutic relationships with their patients, depending on how much and for how long they come into contact with them. An encounter may be very rapid, such as an appointment in a GP's surgery, or in an outpatients' department for one brief episode of care, or it may be in a hospital over the course of a shift, for a day or two, a week, several months or even, in arenas of long-term care, years. Whatever the situation, developing a successful therapeutic relationship always requires self-awareness (Rowe 1999).

To be aware of 'you' is a complex concept. Self-awareness is a positive skill, because there is a correlation between our ability to be self-aware and our ability to be resourceful for others and develop a therapeutic relationship (Sundeen *et al.* 1998). Self-knowledge and understanding help us to appreciate all our facets and the deeply-held values and beliefs that form us as individuals. They help to develop the understanding we need to engender rapport and empathy with other people (Jack and Smith 2007). We can develop self-awareness, but only if we understand that we are becoming self-aware. At times this can be uncomfortable. Self-awareness requires a number of self-acknowledgements that are interrelated, as indicated in Table 2.3.

How does self-awareness work?

If I feel I have a very good relationship with my friend, but my friend is very critical of my sense of dress, I would need to use my senses, my values and beliefs about my dress sense, and think about the image I want to portray. I would then need to compare this to the views my good friend expressed. As a result I might make a conscious decision to ignore my friend's opinion and to rely on my own understanding of myself. Alternatively, I might decide to take on board the criticism and adjust my dress accordingly. I may take this information further and ask myself if the benefit of the friendship is worth the critical comments about my dress sense. The further I consider the information and the more positions I utilize for this consideration, the more awareness I develop of myself and my position in relation to image, friends and criticism.

Self-awareness in clinical situations

In clinical situations a self-aware nurse is able to manage his or her feelings and emotions, rather than being overwhelmed by them. For example, nurses in a palliative care setting need to be aware of the equal input that patients have in the communication process. Patients will quickly pick up any signals that the nurse

Table 2.3 Self-awareness and self-acknowledgement

Mode	Examples	Function in self-awareness
Physiological senses	Happiness Sadness Curiosity Fear Anxiety Confidence Assertiveness	What it feels like in your body What it feels like when it is absent Where it is when it is at its most intense Where it is when it is just emerging
Sensory experiences	Sight Sound Taste Touch Smell Balance	When we are conscious of environmental and internal inputs that provide information
Internal dialogue and thoughts	These express our inner ideas, understandings and responses to external and internal stimuli	Accepting these thoughts as information. Consciously finding meaning in our ideas and their sources, which assists our awareness of self
Our values and belief systems	If I am aware of my spiritual beliefs I may be able to empathize with someone who shares similar beliefs or understand that if someone does not share my beliefs I should find other ways of building rapport and empathy. Where people hold different values and beliefs, understanding each other's position is crucial to the relationship. *Understanding* is not the same as *believing*, it is showing respect for different positions	Give meaning to our self-concept and develop our self-awareness. In this respect our thoughts, internal dialogue, values and beliefs can be influenced by external sources
External information and feedback	The opinions of other people Your employment status Your financial position Your relationships with family and friends Your hobbies and interests Your spiritual associations	We use external feedback to consider and contrast our internal feedback and vice versa

is uncomfortable in communicating with dying patients and their families (Dunne 2005).

Recognizing opportunities and sharing information

Many of the factors that contribute to the opportunity for communication involve aspects that as a student you have no control over. Part of your skill in communicating lies in how well you can identify opportunities for communication. Opportunities often happen informally while you are carrying out direct and indirect patient care. They can occur when patients arrive, while you are helping someone to have a wash, helping them go the lavatory, making their bed, giving out medicines or walking down the ward. These opportunities need to be recognized, but also need to take into account the environment that you are in and the patient's privacy and dignity, along with the previously agreed role and ground rules that you have established with your mentor.

Cross-cultural communication

In cross-cultural communication, the first step is your awareness of your own cultural beliefs (Pullen 2007). Knowing what these are will help you to identify any prejudices or tendencies you may have to stereotype people. You also need to be aware of the patient's cultural norms in relation to body language, eye contact and personal space. Pullen (2007) suggests the following when communicating with a person from a different culture who does not speak, or speaks only a little, of your language:

- Approach slowly and wait for him or her to acknowledge you (rushing in may exacerbate the patient's fear of the unknown).
- Greet the patient using his or her title and last or complete name.
- Smile, point to yourself and say your name.
- Sit down in a chair next to the patient.
- Don't fidget or look at the clock.
- Use simple words, such as 'pain' or 'hurt' rather than, for example, 'discomfort'.
- Short, simple phrases, such as 'Do you hurt?' or 'Do you have pain?' are the most effective.
- Avoid using medical jargon and slang terms.
- Use gestures and simple actions to pantomime words while verbalizing them. For example, instead of saying, 'Are you cold and in pain?', mime or gesture while saying, 'Are you cold?' and then say, 'Do you hurt anywhere?'
- If you know any words in the patient's language, use them to show that you're aware of and respect his or her culture.
- Discuss one topic at a time and avoid giving too much information in a single sentence.
- To assess the patient's understanding, have them repeat instructions, demonstrate the procedure or act out the meaning.
- To reinforce your message, provide easy-to-read material with basic illustrations appropriate to the patient's, educational level, experiences and back-

ground. Make sure you provide concrete, specific and relevant information.
- Document the communication strategies you have used and the patient's response in the appropriate record.

Communicating with young people and children

When communicating with children and young people, you need to be very aware of yourself and how you may be presenting yourself and your attitudes. Box 2.7 lists key communication skills for communicating with young people and children as identified by Westwood (2007).

> **Box 2.7 Communicating with young people and children**
>
> - Listen carefully.
> - Ask questions to verify the child's story and listen for what is left unsaid.
> - Use lots of eye contact and be ready to share information about yourself.
> - Explain possible treatment options and ask for the child's preferences.
> - Use your intuition so as to play sensitively with the child.
> - Be confident in yourself when confronted with parents' distress.
> - Be empathetic about the situation.

> **Activity 2.8**
>
> Go to the Media Tool DVD and select **Case Studies**, then **Child Health (Tom)**, then watch the clip **Tom painting and getting ready for lunch**. Notice how the nurse listens to Tom and negotiates with him. Also, notice how she again negotiates with him about how he can improve his calcium intake, even though he doesn't like plain milk!

Communicating with unconscious patients

When a patient is unconscious or has low awareness, it is vitally important to be courteous and kind, to use

Activity 2.9

Go to the Media Tool DVD, select **Case Studies**, **Adult Health (Margaret)**, and then watch the clip **Nurse checks Margaret's skin.** What do you notice about the way the nurse communicates with Margaret? Compare your observations with the answers at the end of the chapter.

touch and the correct pitch and tone of voice to convey empathy and give information. Hearing is the last sense to go when a patient has a reduced level of consciousness.

Assessing communication needs

An assessment of a patient's or client's communication needs is usually carried out by a qualified nurse or a speech and language therapist. This should include the identification of any resources or further assessment as required. Information should be recorded in the patient's notes and any treatment/interventions included in the care plan. Refer to Chapter 3 for more information on this.

Information sharing

In the spirit of openness, honesty and transparency, information should be shared with patients, both verbally and in writing. It needs to be in different formats – for example, leaflets, audio cassettes, books, intranet, signed and subtitled videos, large print text and BSL interpretations, or translated into an appropriate language to meet the needs of the local community. Other resources such as leaflets, posters, library facilities, information technology, adaptations and accessible information media should be available for patients and/or carers to use.

Resources to aid communication and understanding

There should be a range of resources such as interpreters, hearing loops, text phones, pictures, books, toys, Braille and multi-lingual literature available, and staff should be able to support patients and carers in using them. It may be useful to check with your clinical area for the local policies in respect of this.

Assessment to identify principal carer

A suitably trained professional should assess, with the patient's consent, who is the principal carer, what the care involves and whether extra resources are needed. Patients and carers also need to know who they should contact first if they have any questions regarding care. Good relationships with carers require exactly the same interpersonal skills as working with patients, clients or children.

Empowering patients and carers

This includes supporting patients and carers both practically and psychologically and making them aware of their rights to benefits, services and other help from support groups and charities. A risk assessment should indicate what kind of support plan will help, with clear arrangements for crisis intervention. See also the section on risk assessment in Chapter 6.

Coordination of care

A named professional should take the lead in order to ensure well-coordinated care. Patients and carers should be able to identify who is coordinating the care and the other key agencies providing care should also know who that person is. Nurses should explain all the care options and listen to and act on any wishes the patient expresses, if these are feasible. You may find, as a student giving everyday care, that patients will communicate openly with you. You need to communicate such information to the care team as part of your handover report. The patient's record should be available to them within appropriate safeguards to ensure confidentiality is maintained. Patients should participate in multidisciplinary case reviews, person-centred planning, the single assessment process and discharge planning. Care plans should be understandable by all care providers, be free of jargon and demonstrate interprofessional working and collaboration.

All healthcare professionals should be able to anticipate a patient's needs, provide them with advocacy and gain explicit consent. They should give patients sufficient time to communicate their needs and preferences and use technology when necessary in order to meet those needs – for example, electronic prescriptions, electronic environmental controls and adapted telephones or videophones. Patients' and or carers' views should be listened to, valued, respected and acted upon (NMC 2008).

It is the responsibility of healthcare professionals to be flexible and to modify and change their behaviour based on new understandings of a patient's wishes. Patients should collaborate as far as possible in their care planning and the care philosophy should reflect a positive approach to the patient's and carer's involvement.

Summary and key points

This chapter has covered many important aspects of communication, which is a fundamental clinical skill that applies to every other area discussed in this book. Now that you have read the chapter and completed the activities in relation to communication and interpersonal skills, it is important to remember the following key points:

- Your body language indicates your attitude and emotional state more forcefully that your words.
- Use self-awareness and various techniques such as eye contact, voice modulation and pacing to establish good rapport with patients.
- Use your awareness of body language and eye contact to pick up on opportunities to communicate with patients.
- Choose your words to give patients information and explanations that are jargon-free and in the correct register of language.
- Recognize and value the contributions that patients make to their care.
- Make yourself familiar with the services and resources that empower patients and aid understanding in your healthcare setting.

References

Berlo, D. (1960) *The Process of Communication: An Introduction to Theory and Practice* New York: Holt, Reinhart & Winston.

Burke, L. (2003) Promoting prevention skill sets and attributes of health care providers who deliver behavioral interventions, *Journal of Cardiovascular Nursing*, 23(June): 17–47.

Chapman, S. (2005) *Paul Grice: Philosopher and Linguist.* Basingstoke: Palgrove.

DoH (Department of Health) (2003) *The Essence of Care: Patient-focused Benchmarking for Health Care Practitioners.* London: The Stationery Office.

Dunne, K. (2005) Effective communication in palliative care, *Nursing Standard*, 20(13): 57–64.

Griffin, J. and Tyrrell, I. (2003) *Human Givens.* Chalvington: Human Givens Publishing.

Jack, K. and Smith, A. (2007) Promoting self-awareness in nurses to improve nursing practice, *Nursing Standard*, 21(32): 47–52.

Jennings, J. and Haughton, L. (2002) *It's Not the Big that Eat the Small, it's the Fast that Eat the Slow.* New York: Collins.

NMC (Nursing and Midwifery Council) (2008) *The Code, Standards of Conduct, Performance and Ethics for Nurses and Midwives.* London: Nursing and Midwifery Council.

Pullen, J. (2007) Tips for communicating with a patient from another culture, *Nursing*, (October): 48–9.

Rowe, J. (1999) Self-awareness: improving nurse-client interactions, *Nursing Standard*, 14(8): 37–40.

Seligman, M.E.P. (2002) *Authentic Happiness.* New York: Free Press.

Sundeen, S., Stuart, G., Rankin, E.A.D. and Cohen, S. (1998) *Nurse-client Interaction: Implementing the Nursing Process.* St Louis, MO: Mosby.

Westwood, C. (2007) Connecting with children: nursing sick children can be stressful but hugely rewarding, *Nursing Standard*, 21(31): 62–4.

Answers

Activity 2.7

You can see that the nurse gets onto the floor so that she is at the same height as Angela; she asks questions to which she knows the answer is yes. However, Amber seems to turn this into a guessing game, which the nurse plays for a little while before getting on with the procedure.

Activity 2.9

You will probably have noted that the nurse uses a very gentle tone of voice and a light touch. She speaks slowly and clearly and explains exactly what she would like to do and what sensations Margaret will feel. Notice that Margaret is interacting with her eyes and facial expression to indicate her consent.

Scenario 2.1

Upper limbs and hands. If he is right-handed his gesturing may be impaired and he may have difficulty signing the consent to any treatments.

Body language. He may be in pain and his body language could indicate this.

Sensory input. His vision may be impaired because of his eye injury and this may affect his ability to write.

Language skills. Hypovolaemic shock may affect his attention span, concentration and memory.

Motor skills. If he is in hypovolaemic shock, he may be slower at responding or may be restless.

Speech production. If he is in hypovolaemic shock his voice may be weak because he is short of oxygen. His speech may be difficult to understand.

Social skills. His normal social skills may be affected by his fear and his pain. He may be discourteous , short-tempered or aggressive. However, traumatic experience affects people differently and he may be quiet, withdrawn and very reluctant to interact.

3

Record keeping
Margaret Hutson and Elizabeth Millar

Chapter Contents

Learning objectives

The aim of this chapter is to help you to explore the role of the nurse in relation to record keeping. Throughout the chapter we will also be referring to the case studies on the accompanying Media Tool DVD. Please watch the video clips as directed as these will reinforce your learning and expand upon the information provided in this book. After reading this chapter and interacting with the Media Tool DVD you will be able to:

- Identify key features of all nursing records.
- Accurately record vital signs observations.
- Check and record relevant information to ensure the safe administration of medicines.
- Complete nursing records with the information required to reduce the risk of pressure ulcer development.
- Identify the issues surrounding confidentiality, security and access to patient/client records.
- Recognize the potential of the integration of incidental records and lifelong records.

Introduction

Record keeping is an integral part of nursing care. The two go hand in hand, one unable to exist without the other. Just think about how many times during a span of duty nurses have to record information about the patients in their care and how many times they use a computer keyboard for the same purpose. As well as recording information about patient care, the nurse also retrieves previously recorded information in order to carry out nursing care safely, effectively and efficiently.

This chapter begins by discussing features of all records including the general principles associated with record keeping, communication, use of abbreviations, style and content. The chapter then moves on to place these features within a nursing context and illustrate best practice in record keeping, by focusing on three key areas of nursing practice: vital signs, administration of medicines and the prevention/management of pressure ulcers.

A chapter on record keeping would be incomplete without the inclusion of information relating to confidentiality, security and access to healthcare records. This section may appear complex on first reading, particularly given the range of related legislation and the legal differences between the four countries of the UK. It is, however, all very relevant to the roles and responsibilities of the registered nurse. The chapter concludes by covering information relating to integration. In terms of record keeping, integration applies to the recording of evidence that the patient or their carer has been involved in the decision-making processes relating to their care and management. Integration also applies to record keeping across professional and organizational boundaries and issues concerning the holding of lifelong records.

The importance of record keeping

It is extremely important that you understand the basic principles of all record keeping. This section is not intended to be prescriptive in terms of how to complete every form, chart or piece of paper you will come across during your nursing career; however, it will facilitate your understanding and development of the basic principles used when undertaking any record keeping. The term 'nursing paperwork' is intended to cover general nursing notes, the multidisciplinary pathway (integrated professional pathway), patient-held records and medical notes that specialist nurses may use during consultations.

The NMC (2008b) provides guidance on the basic principles within the code of conduct for nurses and midwives. In addition to this, the NMC published an advice sheet for records and record keeping in 2007 (NMC 2007), which is currently being updated. In these documents the importance of competent record keeping is very clear for all nurses to see.

Activity 3.1

Visit www.nmc-uk.org.uk and download the advice sheet for record keeping by clicking on 'Advice by topic' and 'R' for 'record keeping'. Read this document before proceeding any further with this chapter.

Record keeping is an integral part of nursing, midwifery and specialist community public health nursing practice. It is a tool of professional practice and one that should help the care process. It is not separate from this process and it is not an optional extra to be fitted in if circumstances allow.

(NMC 2007: 1)

Regardless of where the nurse works as a student, or as a qualified member of staff, it is likely that they will come across colleagues for whom 'doing the paperwork' is perceived as an unnecessary part of their shift. However, the statement above makes it clear that

Box 3.1 Key facts about record keeping

- Ten per cent of cases referred to the NMC Professional Conduct Committee in 2007–8 related to issues concerning failure to maintain accurate records (NMC 2008).
- If it has not been recorded, it did not happen.
- Competent record keeping reflects competent nursing practice.
- Competent record keeping is indicative of a skilled nurse.

administering medications, undertaking therapeutic activities, or spending time listening to your patients is not deemed to be any more important than completing all the relevant paperwork. The completion of the paperwork should be given the same priority in terms of workload time management as the other activities nurses undertake. If a nurse does not document a drug they have administered or a dressing they have changed, then another nurse on the following shift may assume that these procedures have not been carried out and do them again. The potential harm to the patient is obvious.

Principles of record keeping

The basic principle in record keeping is that *if it has not been recorded, it has not been done*. This can initially sound like a rather harsh stance against nurses and the care they provide, however, it is not a principle agreed on by the NMC alone, but also by precedents set in law (NMC 2007). Furthermore, the NMC believes that the quality of record keeping is a reflection of the standard of nursing practice. We therefore cannot emphasize enough that record keeping should *not* be viewed as something that is done if time allows.

Good record keeping is an indicator of a skilled nurse. The antithesis is a nurse who is inaccurate, careless or inconsistent in their record keeping; this being the case, they may display those same traits in their general performance (NMC 2007). It is vital to work as a team: if every nurse completes the appropriate paperwork at the appropriate time, this will not leave some nurses having to renew all the assessments, forms and care plans every time they return to a shift on duty. If a nursing colleague is failing to complete the appropriate paperwork, then they are failing in their professional capacity by ignoring the NMC code of professional conduct (NMC 2008b).

The NMC states that 10.37 per cent of cases referred to the Professional Conduct Committee for the year 2007–8 related to issues concerning failure to maintain accurate records, an increase of 3 per cent on the previous year (NMC 2008a).

Communication

Nurses employ a variety of methods when delivering a handover from shift to shift – for example, verbal, face-to-face, recorded and pre-printed forms. Regardless of the mode of delivery it is very important that the information handed over at these times is also detailed in the nursing notes.

When challenged, or asked to check details relating to the care of a patient, the first place a nurse will look are the nursing notes. It is also common practice to see other healthcare professionals – for example, medical staff, pharmacists, physiotherapists, occupational therapists, dieticians and social workers – reading the nursing notes to gain more information about the patients with whom they are involved. Every entry in the nursing notes is of equal importance regardless of profession or grade.

Unfortunately, when communicating through the nursing notes, not all staff consider carefully enough the exact words used and the order of those words. This can lead to some embarrassing statements that may have made sense at the time, but subsequently could be judged inappropriate. Here are some examples, taken from Lederer (2000): 'the skin was moist and dry'; 'on the second day the knee was feeling better and by the third it had completely disappeared'; 'the patient had had no rigors or shaking chills, but her husband states that she was hot in bed last night'. It should be noted that it is impossible to verify these statements as actual transcriptions.

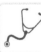

Activity 3.2

For some light relief, you can access further examples on the following website: www.snopes.com/humor/lists/doctors.asp.

Abbreviations

Within the nursing profession you will come across many abbreviations. There may be a time and place for them but they are no use whatsoever if you do not understand what they mean or, more dangerously, if you mistake their meaning. Individual hospitals or community health authorities may have their own local policy on whether and what abbreviations are acceptable. Some specialized areas have their own recognized list of abbreviations that can be used within that department. Good practice determines that the abbreviation be written in full the first time it is used and the abbreviated form thereafter.

Caution must be taken when a nurse moves between specialities or different geographical sites. Dimond (2005a) highlights the need for care with abbreviations because some can have double meanings. For example:

- PID: pelvic inflammatory disease or prolapsed intervertebral disc?
- DOA: dead on arrival or date of admission?
- Pt: patient, physiotherapist or part-time?
- NFR: not for resuscitation or neurophysiological facilitation of respiration?
- NAD: nothing abnormal discovered or not a drop?

Nurses must also be careful that they do not transfer their own abbreviations, developed to aid report taking, into the nursing notes where no one else may understand them.

Box 3.2 Writing nursing notes

- Where possible, involve the patient when writing the nursing notes.
- Your notes should be concise, avoiding irrelevant information or a rambling style.
- Entries should be written in indelible ink at all times. Local policy will state whether this should be black ink only. Black ink does not fade as rapidly as blue and photocopies better than any other colour, and is therefore usually the colour of choice.
- If an error is made it should be scored out with a single line, with 'ERROR' written over it, signed and dated by the person changing the entry. Never use correction fluid to hide what has been written; regardless of how silly the mistake was, you could still be accused of hiding or changing information.
- Do not leave blank spaces between entries even if a colleague forgets to write in something or to give an indication of a new shift or a new day. Blank spaces can be abused by someone desiring to falsify the record by entering details at a later date following an adverse incident or complaint.

Style and content

Entries into healthcare records have progressed a great deal over the last 20 years or so, owing largely to the right of patients to access their records. As this access developed and became more widely known, it was recognized that it was unacceptable to write insulting, rude and inappropriate subjective comments about patients, for obvious reasons (Dimond 2005b). By and large this rarely happens in the modern clinical setting, however, nurses have to be mindful that, depending on local policy or speciality, patients can usually access and read their nursing notes. Avoiding inappropriate comments protects the nurse from challenges of unprofessional behaviour.

When writing a report covering a shift or an event, Wood (2003) advocates communicating by referring to your senses – for example, stating what 'I felt', 'I saw' and 'I heard'. This helps prevent the use of meaningless words or phrases such as 'appears to ... ' or 'had a good day ... '. Why did they have a good day? It is important to state why you felt this was the case. Dimond (2005b: 192) points out that the patient may have had a 'good day' because they slept for most of the shift – perhaps not bothering the staff. A more accurate record would state something along the lines of 'Patient slept for most of the time between 22.00 and 06.00 hours and was clearly in no discomfort'. Always be precise and don't make assumptions about events you did not witness. For example, instead of 'appeared to have fallen out of bed', use a factual statement such as 'I found the patient lying on the floor in a position consistent with having fallen out of bed'.

In addition, entries must be:

- *Accurate.* If, for example, you are referring to an event that happened earlier in the shift, ensure that the times and details are consistent with those recorded elsewhere. If a patient has a dizzy episode and falls, with the result that you take their blood pressure and pulse, ensure that the same time is recorded on the accident/incident reporting form as in the nursing notes and that it can be evidenced by the time of the blood pressure and pulse check on the observation chart.
- *Written as soon as possible after the event.* If you are writing about a significant incident that happened earlier in the shift you should make reference to

that time in the entry. Much of the finer detail can be lost after the first 24 hours following an event. Ensure that every entry has an accurate time using the 24-hour clock, even if writing about an earlier event.

- *Dated with the day, month and year.* The date should be written for the first entry after 12 midnight and thereafter on every new page used, unless local policy states differently.
- *Legible.* Remember that colleagues have to be able to read every entry. If you know your handwriting is difficult to read, try to ensure that your records are not written in a hurry, resulting in further deterioration in legibility.
- *Signed.* At the end of every entry you must ensure that you sign, not initial, your name. Local policy will determine if the name should be printed above the signature on every entry at the start of each new shift or for the first entry only. Some departments have signature sheets to allow easy identification of all the staff involved with that patient. Ease of identification is very important if someone is attempting to trace a member of staff to help with the investigation of a complaint. In many areas, entries are made by permanent and temporary staff, students, those working for nursing agencies and those from other professions.

Record keeping and vital signs

In order to maintain their registration, every nurse must be competent in undertaking a range of different clinical skills. It is of equal importance that the nurse produces a competent record of the findings after undertaking any given skill. Gathering data about a patient's *vital signs* is an important part of nursing care and one that is often delegated to the student nurse (Davidson and Barber 2004). It is fundamental that you know how to obtain, interpret, record correctly and report the findings of any normal or abnormal vital sign.

Vital signs provide important information about a patient that can determine both nursing interventions and medical treatment. Recording a patient's vital signs on admission provides a baseline for future measurement. It can assist with disease diagnosis, monitoring of treatment, and pre- and post-operative assessment. Zeitz and McCutcheon (2006) identify the

patient observations that are traditionally considered under the umbrella term of 'vital signs' and these are listed in Box 3.3.

Box 3.3 Vital signs

- Blood pressure
- Pulse rate
- Temperature
- Respiration rate
- Oxygen saturation level

The charts used to document vitals signs will vary between wards, specialities, hospitals and other care settings, however, regardless of such variations, the principles underpinning how and what is documented remain the same.

When a nurse is required to take the vital signs, sometimes referred to as 'the *observations*' or 'the *obs*', they must be aware of the particular vital signs that are routinely checked in that specific care setting. In addition to this, the nurse must also understand *why* these particular signs have to be checked at that point in time. Is it the 'routine' time for vital signs to be checked or does the patient require further assessment for another reason – for example, because they have returned from theatre, had some other intervention or been administered a new medication? The nurse must know the correct procedure to measure vital signs, be aware of the normal values for their patient and what may cause a deviation from that norm. These areas will be covered for each vital sign later in the chapter.

The recording chart

The chart on which the results of the vital signs check are recorded must include the relevant patient identity details. These comprise name (first name and surname), date of birth, and unit number (see Figure 3.1. for a sample recording chart). These details must be visible and legible before any information is recorded on the sheet. If these details are not recorded and the sheet is misplaced the potential for harm to that patient or another could be significant. Think, for example, about the implications if a patient's medicine

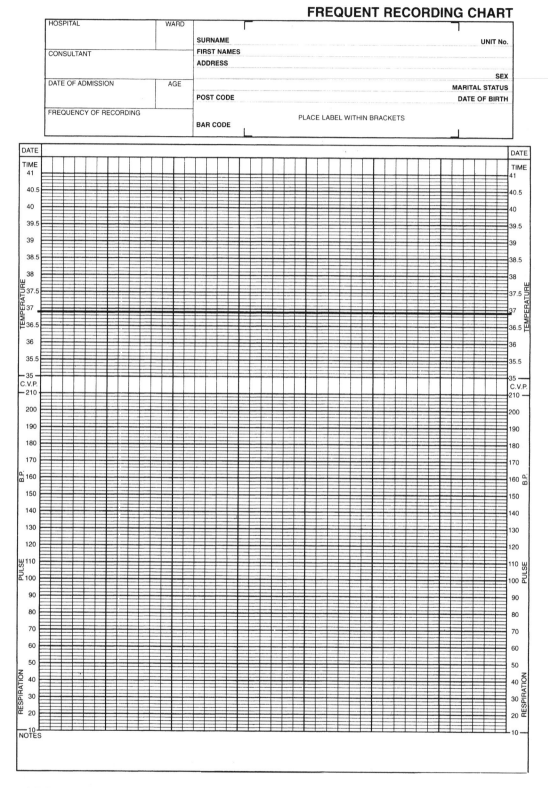

Figure 3.1 A sample recording chart

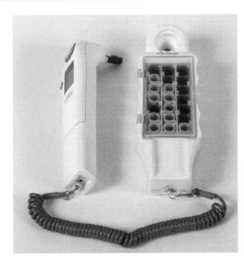

Tympanic thermometer

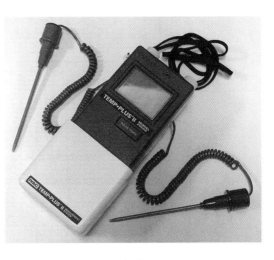

Electronic thermometer

Figure 3.2 Commonly used thermometers

therapy was altered, based on a high blood pressure reading that was in fact recorded from another patient.

The date should be clearly written, recording when the vital sign was taken. This record should comprise the day, month and year – for example, 29.11.2008. The time of the vital sign check should also be noted, using the 24-hour clock.

Recording the actual time

If the nurse is undertaking a routine check of vital signs, they should record the *actual* time and not the *routine* time. For example, if children on a medical ward are meant to have their vital signs checked at 10.00 hours, a nurse looking after four of them would clearly be unable to check all four at exactly 10.00 hours. In this instance, the nurse should record the actual times, for example, 09.55, 10.00, 10.10, 10.15 hours. The recording of set times in advance is poor practice and should be avoided at all times. Consider how you would explain the following situation: you take a patient's blood pressure at 21.45 hours and record it as being carried out at 22.00 hours (the routine time). The patient's condition then deteriorates rapidly and they have a cardiac arrest at 21.55 hours – five minutes *before* the 'official' reading was taken.

Recording temperature

The principle of always recording the actual time also extends to regular temperature checks on a post-operative patient. If the patient requires a temperature check every 15 minutes, avoid writing in the preset times – there is no need to slavishly adhere to these. For example, if the preset times would have been 13.00, 13.15, 13.30 and 13.45 hours and the nurse first attends the patient at 12.50, then it follows that next check will be at 13.05. However, if that nurse was delayed and attended that patient at 13.10, that would be the time they would document, and the next time to reassess the patient would be 13.25, and so on.

Accurate temperature measurement is important as it can indicate various disease processes including infection (Hooper and Andrews 2006). A patient's temperature can be measured in several locations but most commonly it is taken in the tympanic membrane in the ear or orally using an electronic thermometer. Figure 3.2 shows two commonly used thermometers.

The normal temperature for an adult is approximately 37ºC. In healthy children, body temperature tends to be slightly higher (Childs 2006).

When recording a patient's temperature, a dot should be placed on the chart. This single dot should then be connected to the previous temperature recording with a single line. Following this practice

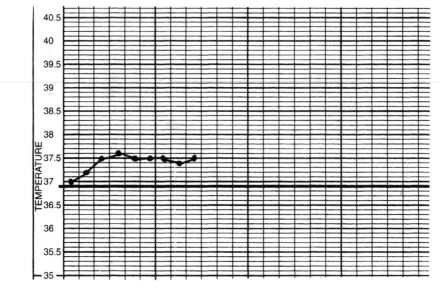

Figure 3.3 Example of temperature recording

allows a graph to develop and therefore any trend can easily be identified, as shown in Figure 3.3. The record may also include the location on the body where the temperature was taken, for example, axilla, for consistency.

Activity 3.3

To help you put the theory into context, go to the Media Tool DVD, click on **Skill Sets**, then **Observations**, to bring you to the **Taking temperature** page. Work through the temperature recording section before reading any further.

Recording blood pressure

Before you take on any skill it is vital that you have the underpinning theory to support your practice. In preparation for this section please revise the anatomy and physiology of the heart and then undertake Activity 3.4.

Measurement

Blood pressure can be measured manually or electronically, but it is best as a student to become proficient at taking a manual blood pressure reading using a

Activity 3.4

Go to the Media Tool DVD, select **Skill Sets**, then **Observations**, then **Pulse rate recordings**, and then click on the link at the bottom of the page for a tutorial on the cardiovascular system.

manual *sphygmomanometer*. Often machines do not give accurate readings and indeed if a patient's blood pressure is very high or very low, the electronic machines may not read it accurately (British Hypertension Society 2006). It is also important to select the correct cuff size to fit around the patient's arm, otherwise this may affect the reading. To take the blood pressure manually you will need the equipment shown in Figure 3.4.

The actual 'how' to record a blood pressure varies in practice with little guidance found in nursing textbooks, and you are bound to experience variations in practice. Some nurses record a blood pressure with a dot, marking the systolic and diastolic measurements. Others use an upward arrow head (^) to mark the systolic and a downward head (ˇ) to mark the diastolic, while others use the (ˇ) to mark the systolic and (^) to mark the diastolic. The tip of the arrow head points to the actual measurement figure. Some

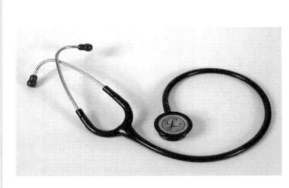

Stethoscope (alcohol-wiped clean)

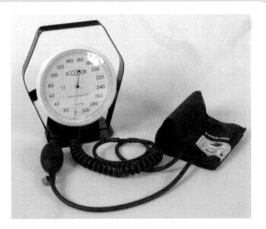

Sphygmomanometer with appropriately-sized cuff

Figure 3.4 Equipment required for manual blood pressure reading

nurses use a dotted line (---) to join the dots or arrow heads while others use a solid line (—). In practice, all are acceptable as long as the method is consistent and the actual measurement can be quickly and easily identified. See Figure 3.5 for a sample recording chart with a blood pressure example.

In some areas of practice, depending on a patient's condition, further information about the blood pressure is required on the recording chart – for example, whether the blood pressure was taken from the right or left arm, whether the patient was lying, sitting or standing, when a blood transfusion was commenced, or when the patient returned from theatre or was given a test dose of medication. Regardless of what words are written on the recording chart, they should be legible and not obstruct the easy reading of the blood pressure measurement.

Recording the pulse

The pulse can be located at several points on the body, as shown in Figure 3.6. The most common point to measure the pulse rate is the radial pulse. An easy way to remember the location of the radial pulse is to follow down the line of the thumb. Figure 3.7 shows more clearly where to locate this pulse.

When taking a patient's pulse you need to ensure that the patient is sitting or lying in a comfortable position and is relaxed. Although you would have explained the procedure, in order to gain informed consent, it is very important that you explain what you are doing as you proceed.

To obtain an accurate pulse rate, you must count the number of beats that you can feel for *one full minute*. In an emergency situation, if you have to obtain a pulse reading speedily, you can check for 30 seconds and multiply your answer by two to get a reading for one minute. Box 3.4 shows what the normal pulse values are for adults and children.

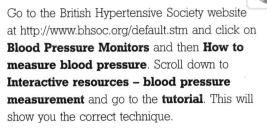

Activity 3.5

Go to the British Hypertensive Society website at http://www.bhsoc.org/default.stm and click on **Blood Pressure Monitors** and then **How to measure blood pressure**. Scroll down to **Interactive resources – blood pressure measurement** and go to the **tutorial**. This will show you the correct technique.

Once you have watched the tutorial, access and read the British Hypertension fact file 01/2006 via the following link: http://www.bhsoc.org/bhf_factfiles/bhf_factfile_jan_2006.doc.

Then go to the Media Tool DVD, select **Skill Sets**, then **Observations**, and then click on **Blood pressure recording**. Watch the narrated video clip of a nurse measuring the blood pressure using an electronic device.

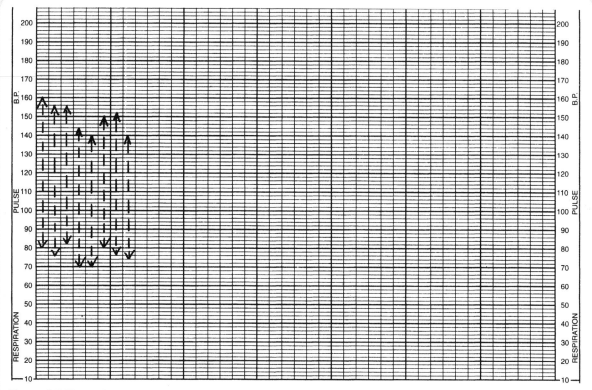

Figure 3.5 Example of blood pressure recording

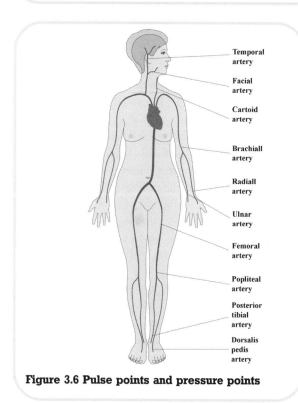

Figure 3.6 Pulse points and pressure points

Temporal artery
Facial artery
Cartoid artery
Brachiall artery
Radiall artery
Ulnar artery
Femoral artery
Popliteal artery
Posterior tibial artery
Dorsalis pedis artery

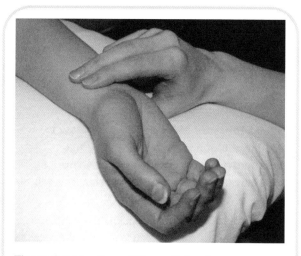

Figure 3.7 Location of the radial pulse

When a nurse undertakes a manual pulse check they are not only counting how many times the pulse beats per minute but are feeling to see if the pulse is regular or irregular and whether it is strong or weak. This provides information about the patient's condition and

Box 3.4 Normal pulse rates

- Adult: 60–100 beats per minute
- Child: 100 beats per minute
- Infant: 120–160 beats per minute (Boyle 2003)

Activity 3.6

Go to the Media Tool DVD, select **Skill Sets**, then **Observations**, and watch the narrated video clip of taking a pulse on the **pulse rate recording** page.

it may be appropriate to record the results. Good practice would advocate that the dot that marks the pulse rate is joined, by a single line, to the previous pulse recording as shown in Figure 3.8. It is important

to remember that a patient's pulse may not fall within normal limits but may still be 'normal' for that particular patient, as in Scenario 3.1.

Scenario 3.1

John is 24, and normally extremely fit and healthy. He is an elective admission for an inguinal hernia repair. His vital signs are obtained on admission to the ward and his pulse rate is 55. For John, a pulse rate of 55 is acceptable because he is young, fit and very healthy. If John were 75 and was a new admission to a general medical ward with unexplained fatigue, a pulse rate of 55 would be of concern due to the patient's age and condition, so would need to be reported to the nurse in charge.

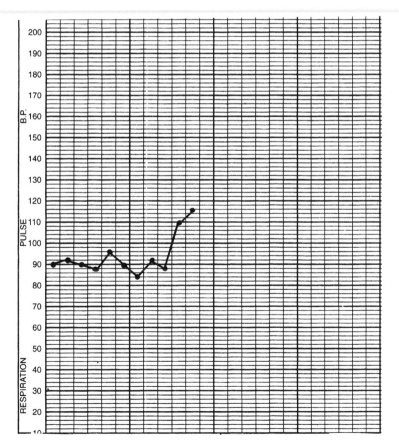

Figure 3.8 Example of pulse recording

Recording respiration and oxygen saturation

The introduction of *oxygen saturation monitors* has not diminished the importance of checking respiration rates. The measurement of a patient's respiration rate is vital as often, if a patient is unwell, there will be a change in the respiratory rate before there is a change in the other vital signs. Despite this, respiration is often not measured with sufficient frequency (Butler-Williams *et al.* 2005), and that frequency may depend on the nature of the care setting. A baseline recording of respiration rate on admission to the clinical area is always recommended. When measuring the respirations, you must count for one full minute. When you become more experienced in this skill, you can combine the respiration with the pulse measurement. In this case you would feel for the pulse for 30 seconds and then count the respirations for the other 30 seconds. If there are any abnormalities noted with either measurement you would re-check that measurement for one full minute.

The nurse should also be observing and, in some instances, recording the rhythm, depth, breath sounds and use of accessory muscles of respiration, as well as the rate of respirations. If the nurse is recording the *oxygen saturation levels*, this should be done concisely, clearly and with the appropriate information. Recording that a patient has 100 per cent oxygen saturation is meaningless without knowing whether or not the patient is receiving oxygen therapy and, if so, the prescribed percentage and oxygen delivery system in use. Figure 3.9 shows respirations accurately recorded.

Local policy for record charts

There is currently no standardized recording chart used within the UK. This is further complicated by the fact that different ward areas record additional infor-mation about the patient in other areas of the chart – for example, if they are experiencing any type of pain and, if so, where that pain is located and what score they would give that pain; information on wound sites; and peripheral pulse checks following local procedures. In the light of this it is recommended that individual wards devise a local policy for the completion of record charts with a full explanation as to the information required and where it is to be recorded.

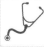

Activity 3.7

When you are on clinical placement, access and read the local policy for the completion of record charts. It is your responsibility as a student nurse to familiarize yourself with any such policy.

Further documenting of vital signs

The information given in this section is good practice for the completion of the recording chart. It must not be forgotten that if the reading of the vital sign is out of normal limits for that area, this, and any action taken, must also be recorded in the nursing notes.

Many areas have now introduced *early warning scoring systems* (see Figure 3.10). The aim of this type of system is the early identification of deterioration in a patient's condition so that appropriate and timely action can be taken.

Record keeping and the administration of medicines

Accurate and detailed record keeping in relation to the administration of medicines is crucial if patient safety is to be preserved. The nurse must take into account legal requirements, professional guidelines, national

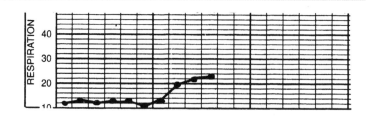

Figure 3.9 Example of respiration recording

SEWS CHART -
Acute Care Areas

SEWS KEY	0	1	2	3

Name

Age

Gender Male/Female

Unit No.

Date of Birth

Ward

Chi No.

Date

RESPIRATORY RATE	35 30 25 20 15 8	
OXYGEN SATURATION PATIENTS PREMORBID O2 STATS _____ %	96 90 85 Inspired 02%	
TEMPERATURE	39° 38° 37° 36° 35° 34°	
BLOOD PRESSURE **SEWS SCORE uses Systolic BP** PATIENTS PREMORBID BP ____ / ____	210 200 190 180 170 160 150 140 130 120 110 100 90 80 70 60 50	
CVP	170 160 150 140 130 120	
HEART RATE	110 100 90 80 70 60 50 40 30	
NEURO RESPONSE	A V P U	

Urine output <30 mls/hr for 2 hours	>30mls/hr
	<30mls/hr
SEWS Score (Score with all obs):	
Doctor/H@N Team called (tick)	
Pain Score (0-4) (Not part of SEWS)	
Nausea Score (0-3) (Not part of SEWS)	

Form - ZEE 502
CGO Ref 080076

Figure 3.10 Example of an early warning scoring system

Scenario 3.2

Read the following patient case studies and undertake the instructions in relation to **one** of them.

The adult

Desmond Brown is a 55-year-old man who has been admitted to an orthopaedic ward on 10 September 2008 at 23.00 hours. He has a fractured tibia and fibula. On admission his vital signs were as follows: temperature 36.8°C; pulse 92; blood pressure 144/96; respirations 24. Using the blank recording chart (Figure 3.11):

- Complete the patient details using a fictitious date of birth and unit number.
- Record the admission observations on the chart.

Mr Brown returns to the ward from theatre at 02.00 hours having had an internal fixation of the fractures. You are responsible for observing his condition. His vital signs are recorded immediately following his return from theatre and then at 15-minute intervals. Record the following three sets of vital sign observations on the chart:

Set 1: temperature 35.7°C; pulse 94; blood pressure 112/58; respirations 12; oxygen saturations 96 per cent on 4 litres per minute (28 per cent oxygen).

Set 2: temperature 35.9°C; pulse 86; blood pressure 116/66; respirations 15; oxygen saturations 96 per cent on 4 litres per minute (28 per cent oxygen).

Set 3: temperature 36.8°C; pulse 79; blood pressure 128/74; respirations 20; oxygen saturations 92 per cent on 4 litres per minute (28 per cent oxygen).

The child

Jamie Buchan is a 14-month-old baby boy who has been admitted to the medical ward at the children's hospital on 10 November 2008 at 11.00 hours. He has a three-day history of respiratory distress and poor feeding, and has suspected bronchiolitis. On admission the following observations were noted: temperature 38.2°C; pulse 166; blood pressure 112/68; respirations 72; oxygen saturations 87 per cent in air; no audible wheeze; use of accessory muscles of respiration noted. Using the blank recording chart:

- Complete the patient details using a fictitious date of birth and unit number.
- Record the admission observations on the chart. Remember to complete the sections on wheeze and use of accessory muscles of respiration.

Due to Jamie's pyrexia he is given a dose of paracetamol. Due to his respiratory distress and low oxygen saturations he is commenced on 1 litre of oxygen via a set of nasal cannula. It is decided to monitor Jamie's observations every hour. Record the following three sets of observations on the chart:

Set 1: temperature 37.4°C; pulse 142; blood pressure 98/64; respirations 66; oxygen saturations 98 per cent on 1 litre of oxygen; no audible wheeze; use of accessory muscles of respiration.

Set 2: temperature 36.8°C; pulse 122; blood pressure 96/66; respirations 50; oxygen saturations 96 per cent on 1 litre of oxygen; no audible wheeze; use of accessory muscles of respiration.

Set 3: temperature 37.2°C; pulse 126; blood pressure 104/72; respirations 54; oxygen saturations 99 per cent on 1 litre of oxygen; no audible wheeze; use of accessory muscles of respiration.

Check whether you have completed the recording chart correctly by comparing it with the examples shown in Figures 3.1, 3.3, 3.5, 3.8 and 3.9.

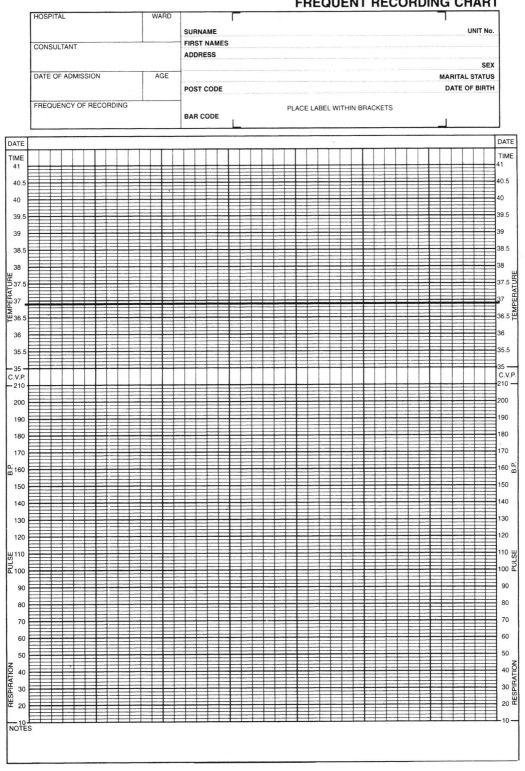

Figure 3.11 Blank recording chart

and local policies, all of which determine practice for the administration of medicines.

Activity 3.8

Visit the NMC website at www.nmc-uk.org/. Download and read **Standards for medicines management** (found under 'M' in the advice by topic section).

There are five fundamental questions that a nurse should consider before administering a medicine. These are sometimes referred to as the 'five Rs'.

1. **R**ight patient?
2. **R**ight medicine?
3. **R**ight dose?
4. **R**ight route?
5. **R**ight time?

If the nurse can answer all these questions in the affirmative, then medication errors should be avoided and patient safety will be maintained.

Identifying the correct patient

You must be aware of the potential for error in identifying the correct patient, particularly in a busy ward where you are nursing patients who have just recently been admitted and you have not yet had the time to get to know them. The use of the patient identity bracelet in such cases is invaluable, provided, of course, that the information on the bracelet is accurate, complete and attached to the correct patient.

Activity 3.9

Go to the Media Tool DVD, select **Case Studies** and then **Adult Health (Margaret)**, then watch the video clip **Margaret has an injection for pain** and then identify all the measures the nurse takes to determine that she is about to give the medication to the correct patient. Compare your answers to those at the end of the chapter.

Medicine prescription

It is the responsibility of the prescriber to ensure that statutory requirements, professional guidelines, national and local policies are adhered to in relation to the information recorded on the prescription. The medicine prescription must include information that determines the date the medicine was prescribed (start date of prescription), the name of the medicine, the dosage to be administered, the route of administration, the time/frequency it is to be administered and the full signature of the prescriber for each prescription. The prescription must also include the full name of the patient, age, date of birth and, if hospitalized, the patient's unit number. The patient's address is recorded on the prescription if they are not hospitalized.

The medicine dose must be prescribed using the metric system and the exact dose must be identified in metric terms and not in terms of the form the medicine presents – i.e. '100mg', *not* 'one tablet'. This avoids error when tablets are available in a variety of strengths.

Most importantly all the information recorded on the prescription must be legible, indelible and unambiguous, whether it be hand-written, typed or computer-generated. Any alterations to the prescription must be accurately recorded using the correct procedures and format determined by local policy. The prescription must meet all these criteria before the nurse can legally and safely administer the medicine. If the nurse has any queries at all about the prescription, then they must be clarified beyond doubt *before* the medicine is administered.

Selecting the correct medicine

Accurate and clear labelling of the medicine container is essential to facilitate the safe administration of medicines. The label will identify the following features of the medicine:

- Name
- Form
- Strength
- Expiry date
- Batch number

Depending on how the medicine is packaged, it is important that all packaging labels are checked – i.e.

inner packaging as well as outer packaging, to ensure that all the information matches accurately. Medicines must be prescribed using the approved (*generic*) name where possible. There may be some circumstances where the *brand* or *trade* name is used – for example, where the medicine consists of more than one active ingredient. Before selecting the medicine the nurse must check that it has not already been administered. This check can be made by reading the recording chart, which will state when the medicine was last administered. The nurse must check that the medicine label on the container selected from the trolley or cupboard matches with the medicine recorded on the prescription and that the medicine is within its expiry date. After removing the required dose from the container, the label and prescription should be compared once again before the container is returned to the cupboard or trolley.

After checking the identity of the patient and administering the medication, which includes witnessing that the patient has received and taken the medication, the nurse must record the information to indicate that the medicine has been administered. This information must be recorded immediately after administration, and must identify which medication was administered, at what time and who administered it. If, for any reason, the patient did not receive the prescribed medicine, a record of non-administration must be made. The format for such recording will be determined by local policy.

Activity 3.10

Go to the Media Tool DVD, select **Case Studies**, then **Child Health (Tom)**. Work through the sections on **Tom's pain assessment and analgesia**.

Use of abbreviations

The use of abbreviations in record keeping has already been mentioned earlier in the chapter (see page 29); however, it is worth referring to again, in relation to the administration of medicines.

There are certain abbreviations that are widely recognized and acceptable for use in records relating to the administration of medicines. These abbreviations principally relate to the dose of medicine and the route of administration. In relation to recording medicine dose, the abbreviation 'mg' is widely accepted as representing the term 'milligram'. It should be noted, however, that the term 'microgram' must not be abbreviated *at all* as there is a risk of confusion with the abbreviation 'mg'. With regard to route of administration, the abbreviation 'IM' is widely accepted as representing the term 'intramuscular' and the abbreviation 'TOP' as representing the term 'topical'. It should be noted, however, that the term 'oral' must not be abbreviated to 'O' as it may be confused with the number 'zero' in relation to dose of medication (Downie *et al.* 2003).

Controlled drugs

The same fundamental principles of medicine administration apply to those drugs classified under the Misuse of Drugs Act (1971) as *controlled drugs*. However, there are additional measures that must be taken in terms of record keeping. Legislation requires a register of controlled drugs to be kept. This register includes a running total of the stock amount of each controlled drug stored in the controlled drugs cupboard. Although the legislation exempts a charge nurse in charge of a ward, theatre or nursing home from maintaining a register for the administration of controlled drugs, local policy will always require this. In most areas local policy will require two people to be involved in the administration of a controlled drug, one of whom must be a registered nurse or registered doctor, and the other a 'checker'.

The nurse and drug checker ascertain that the stock balance corresponds with the last entry in the register. The nurse selects the medicine, replaces the remaining stock in the controlled drugs cupboard, secures the lock and records the new balance in the register along with the date, name of the patient and the dose to be administered. After the medicine has been administered and witnessed, the time of administration and the signatures of both nurse and checker are recorded in the register.

Record keeping and pressure ulcers

Record keeping does not just relate to the recording of vital signs, drug intake and patient progress, but to anything at all relevant to the patient. Comprehensive

Activity 3.11

Here are some revision questions for you to tackle on what you have learned so far. All the answers are contained in the previous sections of this chapter.

1. State the information that must be recorded on a prescription to enable the nurse to accurately identify the patient.

2. State the information that must be recorded on a prescription to enable the nurse to legally and safely administer the medicine to the patient.

and accurate record keeping is also an essential component of nursing care in relation to the prevention and management of pressure ulcers. As has been stated previously in this chapter, in the eyes of the law if nursing actions are not recorded in the patient's documentation, they simply did not happen. Many litigation cases, relating to deficient standards of care resulting in a failure to prevent pressure ulcers, cite poor record keeping as a contributing factor. The only way a nurse can legally prove that evidence-based practice was carried out is to ensure that the interventions are accurately recorded in the patient's nursing notes and that those records make specific reference to the best practice guidelines being used.

Risk assessment

Records must include information about the initial assessment of the patient's risk of developing pressure ulcers, and if trigger factors are identified, then the records must show that a formal assessment and subsequent reassessments have been carried out. Such records must include reference to any *risk assessment* tool that has been used and indicate that an appropriately trained member of staff carried out the risk assessment. You will find further information on risk assessment throughout this book.

Skin inspection

Records must identify how often skin inspections are carried out, including an explanation as to why any changes in the frequency of inspections has occurred.

It is important that pressure areas, identified as susceptible to breakdown in the patient's risk assessment, are a particular focus of the records. The results of the skin inspection must be clearly recorded along with the interventions taken (NICE 2001).

Activity 3.12

Go to the Media Tool DVD, select **Case Studies**, **Adult Health (Margaret)**, and watch the video clip **Nurse checks Margaret's skin**. Make a note of the information the nurse must record in Margaret's nursing notes after carrying out this aspect of nursing care. Then check the suggested answer at the end of the chapter.

Pressure-relieving devices and actions

A record must be kept of the date and time the patient is repositioned, including a description of the position they are placed in. This record should reflect the patient's specific needs as identified in their individual risk assessment. There must also be a record of any pressure-relieving devices used and the reason why specific devices have been selected – for example, an alternating pressure mattress. If there are any problems resourcing appropriate and fully functioning equipment, then such problems must also be documented in the nursing notes. A lack of appropriate equipment or deficient equipment is a failure of the organization and should be reported and noted in writing.

Patient compliance

In some cases the success of pressure ulcer prevention is, in part, dependent on the patient's willingness to comply with instructions – for example, concerning the use of certain pressure-relieving devices or advice related to repositioning. If a patient is unwilling to comply with advice, it inevitably results in difficulties for the nurse in both the implementation and maintenance of best practice guidelines relating to the prevention of pressure ulcers. In such instances the nurse must ensure that records reflect that the patient was provided with information on which to base their decision and was given a clear explanation of the potential consequences of their non-compliance.

Ulcer development

In the unfortunate event that a pressure ulcer develops, the nurse must record on which part of the body it is located, grade it according to depth, describe its appearance and size, describe any resulting pain and identify the presence or absence of infection (NICE 2005). The description of the pressure ulcer can be enhanced by the use of photographs or tracings. The record must clarify when the ulcer first developed, factors considered to have contributed to its development, frequency of reassessment and the rationale for that frequency. Such detail is required in order to select and record the appropriate wound management of the pressure ulcer, including making reference to the best practice guidelines utilized. If there is more than one pressure ulcer present, the record must clearly identify which ulcer is being referred to. Wound management must be recorded in detail, identifying the plan of care for the wound(s), type of dressing to be used and review dates. Please refer to Chapter 11 for further information on pressure ulcers.

Access to healthcare records, confidentiality and security

In this chapter, some of the issues surrounding what, when and where to record patient information have been discussed. The next stage is to ensure that you are also aware of the issues surrounding confidentiality, security and access to patient records.

As previously indicated, nursing has its own 'paperwork', on which many things are recorded, including shift evaluations, care plans, vital sign charts, clinical reviews, initial assessments and home visits. However, it must be remembered that, when discussing issues regarding access to records, confidentiality and security, a patient's records are defined in a much wider sense, and are deemed to include hospital notes (general, psychiatric or children's), general practitioner (GP) notes, health visitor notes and reviews by a community psychiatric nurses, among others.

A healthcare record can be electronic or hand written and will hold information about a person's health and any care they have required or received. This information can be in the form of clinical notes, correspondence from one party (patient or doctor) to another, and results of tests (including scans, X-ray films or blood tests) that have been made by or on behalf of a healthcare professional (DoH 2003).

These notes can be held by a variety of healthcare professionals. Patients do not just have one set of individual case notes that follow them wherever they go in terms of geography or healthcare service. For example, if a patient lived in Newcastle and was treated in his local hospital for a gastric ulcer but later moved to live in Glasgow, the information recorded while in Newcastle would not automatically be forwarded to his local hospital in Glasgow. In a similar way, even within the same NHS Board or Trust, a patient may have case files at the general hospital, with their GP, children's services, psychiatric hospital, dental services and/or maternity services.

Activity 3.13

Go to the Media Tool DVD, select **Case Studies**, then **Learning Disability (Alex)**. Read the **Alex case study** page and consider the implications – to both Alex and the healthcare professionals involved in his care management – of Alex's case notes being held in separate departments, before reading on.

Such a situation could lead to a breakdown in communication between healthcare professionals and might reduce the likelihood of Alex receiving optimal appropriate care. The use of integrated case notes would be useful in this situation, providing permission was given by the patient.

The use of integrated case notes (see Activity 3.13) has legal ramifications, and it is therefore useful to consider the legal aspects in relation to record keeping in healthcare in more detail.

Legislation

Confidentiality, security and access to records are governed by legislation not only from within the UK but also by the *European Convention on Human Rights*. The varied legislation has an impact on how patients can access information and how nurses must protect personal information recorded about their patients. However, this legislation is not specific to healthcare information. It has to be remembered when considering legislation that the UK does not have one blanket legal system – in fact, there are three: English (and Welsh) Law, Northern Irish Law and Scottish Law. Therefore not all Acts of Parliament passed by the government in Westminster are applicable to the UK as a whole.

Box 3.5 Summary of legislation

The primary legislation that concerns healthcare professionals is:

- Data Protection Act 1998.
- Freedom of Information Act 2000.
- Freedom of Information (Scotland) Act 2002.
- Human Rights Act 1998.

You should also be generally aware of the following legislation:

- Access to Health Records Act 1990: this deals with situations where someone is requesting access to a deceased person's health records. The person requesting access could be the personal representative or any other person who may have a claim resulting from the patient's death. These notes are normally kept for three years.
- Access to Medical Reports Act 1988: this allows the patient to see any medical reports written about them by a doctor. These medical reports are normally written for employment or insurance purposes.
- Computer Misuse Act 1990: this ensures that secure computer records cannot be accessed or amended by those without authorization. Contravening this act can lead to a prison sentence or monetary fine.

Data Protection Act 1998

The Data Protection Act (DPA) (1998) requires staff to manage and process personal information properly. Every single person's right to privacy must be protected and every single person has the right to access personal information stored about them.

Data protection legislation protects not only patients but employees within a particular organiza-

tion. Records held by NHS Boards or Trusts are subject to the DPA. This covers personal information recorded about patients, staff, students or research studies in terms of name, date of birth, address, medical history, religious beliefs, and Community Health Index (CHI) number – a unique number given to individual patients used by all Scottish healthcare providers.

There are eight principles set down within the DPA. These state that personal data shall be:

1. Obtained and processed fairly and lawfully and shall not be processed unless specific legal conditions are met.

2. Obtained only for one or more specified and lawful purposes, and not processed for any other purpose.

3. Adequate, relevant and not excessive.

4. Accurate and, where necessary, kept up to date.

5. Held for no longer than is necessary.

6. Processed in accordance with the rights of the data subject(s), including the general rights to access information held about them and, where appropriate, to correct or delete it.

7. Kept securely and safely, with appropriate measures to prevent unauthorized or unlawful processing of the data.

8. Only transferred to a country outside the European Economic Area if that country has an adequate level of protection for the personal data.

To be able to understand the Act better it is necessary to define some of the terminology used in relation to 'data':

- *Data:* the information that affects a person's privacy, in their personal or family life, business or professional capacity. This can take the form of paper records, computer records, personnel records, CCTV footage and medical/clinical records (including photographs, X-rays and any other images).
- *Personal data:* the information about a living person (including your opinion of the person) which could be used to identify them (name, address, full postcode, the first person to have a type of operation in a local area, etc.).

The DPA does not apply if the subject is dead (this is presumed if the subject would have been 100 years old at the time of the application). Nor does it apply if the information is already in the public domain, from publications or from open court. When an individual applies for access to information, an NHS Board or Trust is obliged to reply within 40 days; if this is not achieved, the Trust may be fined by the Information Commissioner's Office. The application must be submitted in written form either by letter, email or fax. If the applicant is not the data subject, there must be appropriate written permission from them, if applicable. The applicant must be informed that a fee will be charged. The applicant is not required to state why they wish to obtain the information.

Box 3.6 Web link – Data Protection Act 1998

The following website can be accessed for further reading on the DPA: http://www.ico.gov.uk/what_we_cover/data_protection.aspx.

The Caldicott Guardian

The Caldicott Guardian principle has been in place since 1997 following the publication of the *Report on the Review of Patient Identifiable Information*, undertaken by the Caldicott Committee for the Department of Health (Caldicott Committee 1997). The report was intended to increase awareness of what is required to ensure confidentiality, and recommended that a network of Caldicott Guardians be set up within the NHS to oversee access to patient identifiable information (Dimond 2005b).

The Caldicott Guardian should be seen as the gatekeeper for patient information held within a healthcare setting. The role of the Caldicott Guardian is usually undertaken by a senior clinician within an NHS Trust. While this is a mandatory requirement in England, Wales and Northern Ireland, within Scotland it is only advisory. This person is responsible for the protection of and uses of patient identifiable information by staff, and for developing and monitoring policies of interagency disclosure.

Freedom of Information Act 2000

The Freedom of Information Act (FoI) Act 2000 came into force on 1 January 2005 and covers the UK as a whole, although Scotland also has its own Freedom of Information (Scotland) (FoIS) Act 2002. These Acts aim to increase openness and accountability in government and across the public sector. They grant the right to access information held by public authorities.

A 'public authority' is described as any body, person or holder of any office listed in the FoI, along with all publicly owned companies. Some non-publicly owned companies volunteer to meet FoI requirements to ensure their openness and transparency. Examples of public authorities are government departments, the House of Commons, the House of Lords, the National Assembly for Wales, the Northern Ireland Assembly, local authorities, the police and the NHS (including opticians, pharmacists and dentists).

Requests for information should be in written form (including emails). The applicant does not need to be the subject of the information or be affected by knowing it, nor do they need to state why they want the information. If the information is about a third party or about an individual, the DPA will always take precedence over the FoI.

Public authorities are required to make public the type of information they hold. If information is not proactively made available, the authority is required to respond to specific requests for information. Any requests for information must be dealt with promptly and within a 20-day limit. The authority can request more details before responding if this aids the retrieval of appropriate information. Public authorities are required to provide information recorded both *before* as well as after the Act came into force – as far back as 100 years!

There are some exemptions that prevent information being published, and an authority is not obliged to comply with a request if such an exemption applies – for example, if the cost of retrieving the information exceeds the amount sent as set by the Fees Regulations, or if the information is not held. Exemptions are split into two categories: absolute and non-absolute. If the absolute exemption applies, the authority is not required to release the information. Absolute exemptions include areas of national security or confidential material. When a non-absolute exemption applies, the authority has to undertake a public interest test, to determine if the information should be released. Public authorities are not obliged to respond to repeated or vexatious requests. The Act favours release of information where possible, but when an exemption applies, the authority must write to the applicant to explain the situation and provide details of the appeals procedure. If the applicant is unhappy, they can refer the case to the Information Commissioner's Office.

The Information Commissioner's Office

The Information Commissioner's Office is an independent authority set up in the UK to promote access to official information and to protect personal information. It is sponsored by a government department and oversees the DPA and FoI for the UK.

The Information Commissioner's Office has three main areas of responsibility:

1. Educating and influencing: giving information, advice and producing good practice statements.
2. Resolving problems: reviewing eligible complaints from people who think their rights have been breached.
3. Enforcement: using legal sanctions against those who ignore or refuse to accept their obligations.

Box 3.7 Web link – Information Commissioner's Office

Further material about the Information Commissioner's Office can be accessed at: www.ico.gov.uk.

Freedom of Information (Scotland) Act 2002

The FoIS came into force on 1 January 2005, and has a similar aim to that of the FoI 2000. It applies to most of the public bodies in Scotland, but also to companies who are owned by a Scottish authority, for example, if on a contract. As with the FoI, exemptions are in place to prevent some information from being made known to the public, however, there are fewer exemptions than those applying to the FoI.

An applicant can appeal to the Scottish Information Commissioner for a review if they are unhappy with the

response they receive. The Scottish Commissioner can only review requests that are applicable under the FoIS. Requests made by those living in Scotland with regard to information from a non-devolved Scottish body are required to be processed under the FoI and are referred to the Information Commissioner in England.

The Scottish Information Commissioner

The Scottish Information Commissioner is a public official appointed by Her Majesty the Queen on the nomination of the Scottish government. The Commissioner is also a public authority and therefore under the same duty as all other Scottish public authorities to respond to requests for information that they hold. The Scottish Commissioner's decisions are legally enforceable. They can require an authority to give out previously withheld information and they may uphold the decision of an authority to withhold information, but in doing so they will have rigorously investigated that decision to ensure it is legal. As well as enforcing the Act, the Commissioner informs the public about their rights under freedom of information laws and promotes best practice to public authorities.

Box 3.8 Web link – Scottish Information Commissioner

Further information about the Scottish Information Commissioner can be accessed at: www.itspublicknowledge.info/home/scottishinformationcommissioner.asp.

Human Rights Act 1998

Another piece of British legislation that covers the rights of a person with regard to access to information stored about them is the Human Rights Act (HRA) 1998, which came into force in 2000 with the DPA. The European Convention on Human Rights, which is the source of the Act, is a treaty agreement from the Council of Europe. Within this legislation the people of the UK are given 16 fundamental rights and freedoms.

Two particular articles are relevant to accessing information. Article 8 states that:

Everyone has the right to respect for his private and family life, his home and his correspondence. There shall be no interference by a public authority with the exercise of this right except such as in accordance with the law and is necessary in a democratic society ... for the protection of the rights and freedom of others.

Article 10 states that:

Everyone has the right to freedom of expression. This right shall include freedom to hold opinions and to receive and impart information and ideas without interference by public authority and regardless of frontiers. The exercise of these freedoms, since it carries with it duties and responsibilities, may be subject to such formalities, conditions, restrictions or penalties as are prescribed by law and are necessary in a democratic society ... for preventing the disclosure of information received in confidence.

Under this Act, public authorities are prohibited from interfering with the release of information about a person unless in the interest of national security, public safety, prevention of crime or for the protection of the health of others.

Accessing health care records

Given the legislative nature of accessing information, it is easy to forget that there is a wider scope to accessing paper files, copied papers or electronic notes. Once a person has obtained access to the specific piece of information they have requested, they have the right to access that information in a format that is appropriate for them. Assistance may be required if the person accessing the information cannot read the information – for example, if the person is illiterate, blind, does not have English as their first language or does not understand medical terminology or abbreviations.

Confidentiality

The NMC code of professional conduct clearly states that 'You must respect people's right to confidentiality' (NMC 2008: 2). It then goes on to say that: 'You must ensure people are informed about how and why information is shared by those who will be providing their care' (NMC 2008: 2). Patient information can be used by many different healthcare professionals. For example, within an acute hospital setting the patient's records could be accessed by the medical staff, nursing staff, pharmacists, physiotherapists, occupational therapists and dieticians. The DPA 1998 gives a clear definition of who constitutes a 'health professional'. These include:

- registered medical practitioners;
- registered opticians;
- registered dentists;
- registered pharmaceutical chemists;
- registered nurses, midwives or health visitors;
- any person who is registered as a member of a profession which is included in the Professions Supplementary to Medicine Act 1960;
- clinical psychologists, child psychotherapists and speech therapists.

Sharing information with people not on the above list has to be guided by the patient's agreement. Within England, Wales and Northern Ireland, guidance is given by the Department of Health within its document, *Confidentiality, NHS Code of Practice* (DoH 2003). Within Scotland, guidance is usually received from human resource departments when staff sign an employment contract with an NHS Trust.

Staff within the NHS should not routinely share information about a patient's personal health with the patient's family or friends. If the patient is an adult who cannot make known or tell other people their wishes, the family can either apply to the court for guardianship or may have been given power of attorney prior to that time. If the patient is a child, the law is likely to allow the person with parental responsibility to see their records or discuss their care.

Confidential information within the healthcare environment is information given by a patient about themselves. This information is given on the premise that it will only be disclosed to others within the healthcare environment. It must be remembered that not every patient is capable of giving their consent. If a patient makes it clear that they object to information being disclosed about them, the NHS is bound to follow their wishes. If medical staff feel that this could harm the patient's health or someone else, they are still legally bound not to discuss it with family or friends.

Activity 3.14

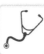

Take time to find out more about the legislation and guidance documents governing consent for the patients in your area of the UK with regard to mental health, children, vulnerable adults or adults with incapacity.

Security

Security of information can be an area of concern to patients and staff, especially as more information is now being sent electronically. The type of information that can be sent via email is an area that still requires an increased awareness among staff within the NHS, in particular, the use of non-identifiable information within the subject line of emails. Storage of emails should conform to the organization's corporate guidelines on how to keep such information safe.

Concern with regard to electronic data extends further than emails. Any personal information sent electronically should be encrypted, by using, for example, the email system *nhs.net*. Any database that stores information is a potential risk, and therefore databases should be held in a secure, password-protected format. There should also be a clear reason for the storage of information.

A further area of concern surrounds the safe and secure storage of case records. In this respect each NHS Trust is required to determine a local policy for not only the safe storage of healthcare records but the safe destruction of notes – when and where appropriate. The guidance documents for destruction and retention of case files are currently under review and differ between Scotland and the rest of the UK.

Integration of records

There are some basic points to remember regarding the integration of patient records:

- There should be promotion of partnership between patient and professional.
- There should be meaningful participation of patient and/or carer in the record keeping process.

- There should be effective communication between patient and professional.
- The purpose should be working towards a single, patient-held record which represents interprofessional and interagency working.

Patient and professional partnerships

The promotion of a partnership between the patient and the professional should be enhanced by the fact that patients have a legal right of access to their records, and it is becoming more common practice that the patient is involved in both the composition and holding of their records. However, it should be remembered that the healthcare organization has ultimate responsibility when it comes to the safe-keeping of patient-held records. Should a patient's confidentiality be breached as a result of the patient-held record falling into the wrong hands, the organization could be held responsible for such a breach.

The NMC advise that, wherever possible, the patient or their carer should participate in the record keeping process. This participation should be regarded as an equal partnership. Meaningful participation by the patient or their carer requires that records be documented using terminology that is understood by all involved, including the patient and carer (NMC 2007). Indeed, the concept of patient and professional partnerships is clearly echoed in the NMC code of conduct, which states: 'As a registered nurse, midwife or specialist community public health nurse, you must treat people as individuals and respect their dignity ... You must recognise and respect the contribution that people make to their own care and wellbeing' (NMC 2008b: 2).

Many patients value an active engagement in the decision-making processes relating to their care and treatment and wish to influence that care and treatment. Effective communication between professional and patient is required to ensure such engagement is meaningful. The patient needs to be well informed about their condition in order to make genuinely informed choices about their care and treatment. If the patient feels that the professional values their contribution to this partnership, then it could be argued that the patient is more likely to comply with their care and treatment options. However, it should be acknowledged that this level of involvement and information does not appeal to all patients and carers; in fact, it may be a great source of anxiety for some. Nurses and other health professionals need to be sensitive to cues from the patient and/or carer as to their willingness to engage in such a partnership.

Professional and organizational boundaries

The NMC also supports the use of a single record that can be accessed by all members of the healthcare team involved in the care and treatment of an individual for the purposes of recording such care and treatment. Central to the concept of using a single record is the fact that no one input is regarded as any more or less important than that of another professional, and all record keeping must be carried out in accordance with an approved local protocol (NMC 2007). To achieve such practice requires an understanding by all professionals of the role records play in their profession and a willingness to promote interprofessional/inter-agency collaboration, along with the optimal use of resources for the benefit of the patient.

The use of computer-held records can enhance communication across the healthcare professions and facilitate the success of a single record. Computer records should be easier to read than illegible hand-written records, take up less physical space and decrease the amount of duplication within the records.

Lifelong records

The participation of the patient in the decision-making processes about their care and treatment, the related record keeping and the integration of records across professional and organizational boundaries all lend themselves to the notion of a lifelong record that is held by the patient/carer or, in the case of children, by the parent/legal guardian. This concept is becoming increasingly accepted by professionals and patients alike, however, it is dependent on the patient's awareness of the purpose and importance of such a record, and therefore their willingness to keep it safe.

There are several advantages for the patient in keeping their own health record. It could be argued that the record is less likely to be mislaid if in the safe-keeping of the patient. It could also be argued that the patient may be more knowledgeable about their condition and care because of their ready access to the record. On the other hand, there are aspects of this practice that could be considered to be dis-advantageous to the patient: as previously suggested, a patient-held record may be a source of anxiety for some patients in terms of both the responsibility of keeping it safe and confidential, and in terms of its content.

A patient with a chronic condition managed for the most part outside a hospital setting, but who occasionally requires hospitalization either for the management of an acute episode of the condition or for respite care, is a strong candidate for a patient-held record. In such cases the relevant healthcare professionals would have easy access to records that are up to date and provide a full picture of all the care and treatment received by the patient, thus inevitably improving their ongoing care.

Activity 3.15

Go to the Media Tool DVD, select **Case Studies**, **Mental Health (Chris)**, then read the page **Introduction to Chris**. Consider the advantages and disadvantages of Chris holding a lifelong health record. Write your answers down and compare them to the ones at the end of the chapter.

Summary and key points

Record keeping is a vital and integral part of the nurse's role and not a task to be done at the end of a shift if there is time! This chapter has highlighted the importance of accurate record keeping. The basic principles of record keeping have been addressed and best record keeping practice has been shown for vital signs, administration of medicines and prevention and management of pressure ulcers. The issues of confidentiality, security and access have also been explored and addressed from a UK-wide perspective. Finally, the integration of records has been highlighted. The Media Tool DVD activities throughout the chapter will have helped you to link theory to practice. Before moving on, remember the following key points:

- Record keeping is an integral part of nursing care, it is not an optional extra.
- Competent record keeping reflects competent nursing practice.
- If it has not been recorded, in the eyes of the law, it did not happen.
- Confidentiality, security and access to records are all governed by legislation of which the nurse should have a working knowledge.

References

Boyle, B. (2003) Age-appropriate vital signs and blood pressure, in K. Barnes (ed.) *Paediatrics: A Clinical Guide for Nurse Practitioners*. Edinburgh: Elsevier Science.

British Hypertension Society (2006) *Fact File 01/2006 – Blood Pressure Measurement*, www.bhsoc.org/publications_leaflets.stm, accessed 14 January 2008.

Butler-Williams, C. Cantrill, C. and Maton, S. (2005) Increasing staff awareness of respiratory rate significance, *Nursing Times*, 101: 2727, 35–7.

Caldicott Committee (1997) *Report on the Review of Patient Identifiable Information.* London: DoH.

Childs, C. (2006) Temperature control, in M. Alexander *et al.* (eds) *Nursing Practice, Hospital and Home: The Adult,* 3rd edn. Edinburgh: Churchill Livingstone.

Davidson, K. and Barber, V. (2004) Electronic monitoring of patients in general wards, *Nursing Standard*, 18(49): 42–6.

Dimond, B. (2005a) Abbreviations: the need for legibility and accuracy in documentation, *British Journal of Nursing*, 14(12): 665–6.

Dimond, B. (2005b) *Legal Aspects of Nursing*, 4th edn. Harlow: Pearson Education.

DoH (Department of Health) (2003) *NHS Confidentiality Code of Practice*. London: The Stationery Office.

Downie, G. Mackenzie, J. and Williams, A. (2003) *Pharmacology and Medicines Management for Nurses*, 3rd edn. Edinburgh: Churchill Livingstone.

Hooper, V. and Andrews, J. (2006) Accuracy of non-invasive core temperature measurement in acutely ill adults: the state of the science, *Biological Research for Nursing*, 8(1): 24–34.

Lederer, R. (2000) *The Bride of Anguished English: A Bonanza of Bloopers, Blunders, Botches, and Boo-Boos*. New York: St Martin's Press.

NICE (National Institute for Health and Clinical Excellence) (2001) *Pressure Ulcer Risk Assessment and Prevention*. London: NICE.

NICE (National Institute for Health and Clinical Excellence) (2005) *The Management of Pressure Ulcers in Primary and Secondary Care*. London: NICE.

NMC (Nursing and Midwifery Council) (2003) *Professional Conduct Annual Report 2002–2003*. London: NMC.

NMC (Nursing and Midwifery Council) (2007) Advice sheet for record keeping, www.nmc-uk.org/aArticle.aspx?ArticleID=2777.

NMC (Nursing and Midwifery Council) (2008a) *Fitness to Practise: Annual Report, 1 April 2007 to 31 March 2008*. London: NMC.

NMC (Nursing and Midwifery Council) (2008b) *The Code, Standards of Conduct, Performance and Ethics for Nurses and Midwives*. London: Nursing and Midwifery Council.

Wood, C. (2003) The importance of good record-keeping for nurses, *Nursing Times*, 99(2): 26–7.

Zeitz, K. and McCutcheon, H. (2006) Observations and vital signs: ritual or vital for the monitoring of postoperative patients? *Applied Nursing Research*, 19(4): 204–11.

Answers

Activity 3.9

You will probably have identified that:

- The nurse checks information on the identity bracelet (full name, date of birth and unit number) with the doctor who is checking this information on the prescription sheet.
- Two persons are involved in the checking process: nurse and doctor.
- The nurse addresses the patient by her first name several times. Although this is not foolproof, if the patient protested that this was not her name, it would alert the nurse to a possible error.

Activity 3.12

Your answer should have included:

- Date and time of the skin inspection.
- An observation made of the skin – and a recording of whether it was healthy, its colour, whether it was intact and well perfused.
- The intervention used – use of glide sheet to prevent shearing and friction to the skin when repositioning Margaret.
- The position Margaret was placed and left comfortable in.
- The continuing frequency of skin inspections.

Activity 3.15

In your advantages section you will have probably identified that:

- records may be safer and less likely to be lost;
- Chris has ready access to his records;
- Chris may be more knowledgeable about his condition;
- continuity of Chris's care could be enhanced.

In your disadvantages section you may have noted that:

- responsibility for his records may be a source of worry for Chris;
- Chris may not want to hold his own records;
- Chris's confidentiality may be breached.

4

The care environment

Calbert H. Douglas, Mary R. Douglas and Karen Staniland

Chapter Contents

Learning objectives

The aim of this chapter is to explore the role of health professionals involved in patient care in relation to the built environments within which that care takes place and to emphasize good practice in meeting patients' needs within the care environment. Throughout the chapter we will be referring to the accompanying Media Tool DVD. Please watch the video clips as directed as these will reinforce your learning and expand upon the information given here. After reading this chapter and interacting with the Media Tool DVD you will be able to:

- Recognize the importance of creating a good first impression where the built care environment is welcoming, friendly and supportive.
- Identify factors relating to the need for easy and safe access to the care environment.
- Provide excellent customer care by being approachable, polite and responsive to people's needs in a timely and welcoming manner.
- Recognize the importance of always having a clean, well-maintained healthcare environment.
- Recognize the importance of ensuring that infection control precautions are in place and adhered to.
- Identify how a patient's personal environment is managed to meet individual needs and preferences.
- Support patients by the effective use of resources to maintain their independence in meeting their needs.

Introduction

This chapter focuses on aspects of the care environment identified in *The Essence of Care* (DoH 2003) benchmarks, such as good access, a welcoming atmosphere, supportive design, cleanliness, safety, personal space and control of infection which apply to all clinical settings including hospitals, health centres and GP practices. It will consider the elements that are important to patients and will identify actions that health professionals can take to make real improvements to patients' experience in healthcare environments.

The *healthcare environment* can be a very strange and frightening place for both patients and visitors. Every member of staff is responsible for creating a good first impression, despite the many difficulties that will be highlighted in this chapter. As a student nurse, you too are in an ideal situation to ensure that a patient's *personal environment* is safe and left in their control as much as possible. The care environment is a theme that can be identified throughout all the other chapters in this book, in that it must be configured so that patients and healthcare professionals can communicate, keep records, preserve the privacy, dignity and safety of patients, be able attend to patients' needs and, very importantly, use the correct equipment and furniture to ensure the prevention of pressure ulcers.

Despite major investment in NHS facilities since 2000, many hospitals are still situated within old buildings. Hosking and Haggard (1999), in describing the general appearance, interior design and environmental quality of hospitals and healthcare buildings, emphasize the important influence these can have on patients, staff and the public. Significant improvements have been made to hospital environments in recent years, but further work is necessary to meet patient and staff expectations.

In this chapter, discussions about the *built care environment* focus on institutional settings, because it is in these places that patients and their carers are less able to have influence on and control of their environment. However, the issues raised are relevant to all built healthcare environments, wherever care is provided.

First impressions: accessing the care environment

The design and provision of built healthcare facilities should be responsive to patients' needs and provide patient-friendly environments (Douglas and Douglas 2004). In 2000, the NHS Plan pointed to a major investment in NHS buildings to reshape healthcare provision in the UK (DoH 2000). Its vision was that these developments could achieve real benefits for patients and healthcare staff in meeting modern public expectations.

It is well recognized that the built healthcare environment can significantly influence the healing process and have a direct impact on patients' health outcomes – for example, through enhanced relaxation, enabling views of nature and creating a healing environment (Lawson and Phiri 2003; Ulrich *et al.* 2004; Douglas and Douglas 2005). Appropriately designed and managed healthcare environments can contribute to reducing the stress that patients encounter during their hospitalization period and directly help them in their personal recovery and recuperation (Ulrich 1984). Of course, as you are not directly involved in the design of wards, day rooms, clinics, reception areas and transitional spaces, your job is to provide healthcare which takes place in these environments. However, by understanding the importance of the correct management of the process of care in these environments, you can contribute to patients' experience of care and to their recovery from illness.

Activity 4.1

What do you believe 'built healthcare environments' and 'personal environment' mean? Write out your answers and check them with those at the end of the chapter.

A patient's initial perceptions of the healthcare environment are of immense significance, as they have a dramatic effect on their experiences, subsequent reactions, healing and recovery. The patient's journey begins with the trip from home to hospital, clinic or GP surgery. It also includes their movements during their stay in hospital and then the journey home. In their study of patients' perceptions of hospital environments, Douglas and Douglas (2005) reported that patients identified accessibility as a key element that influenced their views and perception of the care environment. They reported that the design and feel of the environment played an important role in the overall patient experience.

From home to healthcare

Patients may travel to a healthcare facility by car, taxi, public transport or ambulance, or walk to their local clinic or GP surgery. This variously involves travel, finding parking, finding the entrance, orientation once inside the building and the journey to the destination within the facility. Patients bring with them a set of requirements that are based on their personal respective health status – for example, impaired mobility, visual or physical impairment, psychological concerns such as a fear of confined spaces, and other biological, gender and ethnic concerns.

To assist patients and their families, nurses and all other healthcare professionals should ensure that wherever possible for all planned admissions or hospital visits, patients and their carers are provided in advance with clear, easy to understand information about the care environment. This will include how to travel to the facility, where to park (including any costs involved) and how to notify staff if they require assistance with mobility. Also, for those who may have a physical impairment, details of who to contact for accessing the building on their arrival.

Activity 4.2

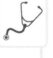

To gain a deeper understanding of the everyday access problems experienced by patients, at the commencement of your next clinical placement request a copy of the information that is given or sent to patients. Make your way from the car park or the bus stop to your clinical area, using the directions given in the information sheet. Repeat this exercise as if you were a patient confined to a wheelchair and identify the obstacles that hindered or impeded your progress.

Wayfinding

Each NHS organization will have systems in place to ensure that entrances are clearly signposted, well lit,

easily reached and welcoming to patients. In addition, where possible, a reception desk, help desk or help lines will be in place to assist people to navigate through the building. All signage and maps should be clear, consistent, colour coded and easy to understand.

It is of great importance that all staff are responsive, welcoming and ready to provide directions and assistance to people when they arrive. People arriving at hospital or a GP surgery may be experiencing emotional or psychological stress. This may mean that finding their way, which under normal situations would be considered routine, can become very complex and frightening.

Activity 4.3

As a reasonably healthy person and a member of staff, try and think back to your first ward experience. Did you have any difficulties finding your allocated ward? Was anybody you asked helpful and polite? Write out your answers so that you can reflect on how you felt. If you did experience difficulties, list some of these and then suggest improvements that might be made.

Activity 4.4

Next time you are in a hospital environment, check if there are any patient seats along the long corridors. Identify if they can be easily seen and are not obscured by trolleys or open doors. See how many are in use.

Wayfinding within a healthcare environment can also cause stress for patients and their families. Typically, hospitals are large, complex buildings. This means that in some instances an individual may be required to travel along long corridors and use lifts or stairways to get to their destination. Stress, due to disorientation, can express itself in anger, hostility, discomfort and even panic. Nursing and other healthcare staff working in reception areas should pay particular attention to checking what assistance patients invited to visit the facility may require. For example, a visually impaired person may need assistance in finding the desired route, an individual who has impaired hearing will need to be able to find their way without spoken directions, while an individual in a wheelchair needs to be able to access lifts and open doors along corridors. Some key points regarding wayfinding are identified in Box 4.1.

> ## Box 4.1 Key points for wayfinding
>
>
> - Give patients and their carers advance information about the care environment and how to access it.
> - Parking should be provided as near as possible to care areas.
> - Entrances should be clearly visible, well signposted, welcoming, accessible, and have a help desk or reception point in place to assist people in navigating through the facility.
> - All staff should be welcoming, responsive and willing to provide directions and assistance to people when they arrive.
> - Signage, maps and wayfinding information should be clear, consistent, logical and easy to understand.
> - The environment should be easy to move around, should encourage independence and provide assistance for those who require it.
> - All available resources should be used to provide good communication.
> - Areas should be available for rest and privacy, for patients, their visitors and their carers.
> - Facilities for refreshment should be available at all times.
> - Relevant health and safety issues should be assessed and systems in place to protect patients and staff.

A supportive care environment

A good healthcare environment matters to patients, carers and staff, and is a key element in the patient's experience. The care environment should feel welcoming, calm, safe, secure and reassuring. When appropriate, you should ensure that people are welcomed immediately into the clinical area. It is always polite, if possible, to acknowledge a new presence immediately and not continue a conversation with a colleague when a patient or visitor is waiting to speak to you.

> ## Activity 4.5
>
>
> Hopefully, as a student nurse, you should never be put in a position of having to deal with anxious or stressed patients. However, if you are involved or happen to witness this, it is far better to prevent situations getting out of control before they happen. Go to the Media Tool DVD, click on **Chapter Resources**, then **Chapter 5 Weblinks and Resources**, then **Activity 4.5**. Work through this activity and make notes on what you observe.

Customer care

Many hospital wards have bedside information packs which notify patients about issues such as visiting times, meal times, how to identify staff and the location of parking. Supplies of these packs should be kept within the care environment and offered to all patients and/or their carers as appropriate.

Patients and carers should receive optimum levels of customer care. Many large healthcare organizations have introduced a *housekeeper* role to ensure that a patient-focused approach is provided. The introduction of ward housekeepers in hospitals has improved the level of customer care for patients (NHS Estates 2003). The ward housekeeper supports the delivery of clinical care by releasing nursing time and ensures the ward is kept clean and safe by overseeing cleanliness standards. Housekeepers make the ward welcoming for patients and their visitors, and ensure that patients' food is tasty and well presented. The housekeeper liaises with nurses, dieticians, domestic and catering staff to make sure that the environment is as welcoming, comfortable and reassuring as possible (DoH 2007a).

Supportive environments

In the study by Douglas and Douglas (2005), patients identified the need for personal space, a homely welcoming atmosphere, a supportive environment, good physical design, access to external areas and provision of facilities for recreation and leisure as important to their well-being. In particular, they sought a welcoming space for themselves and their visitors. Patients reported that they wanted a sense of connection with the outdoors via windows, courtyards and balconies, to give them a sense of normality. While you cannot directly influence these aspects of the environment in which you work, an awareness of them will enable you to improve your level of professional care.

Teamwork is important and the full clinical team should demonstrate a good working relationship. Patients put their trust in professionals to provide and maintain a supportive environment for them and their visiting family and friends. It is vitally important that they are supported by properly skilled, competent and capable healthcare professionals and nursing staff. As a team member, each nurse should seek out opportunities to maintain and enhance that supportive environment.

The Healthcare Commission (England's healthcare watchdog) checks to ensure that services are meeting set standards and promotes improvement in the quality of healthcare and public health in England. The Health Inspectorate Wales (HIW) is responsible for inspection and investigation of NHS bodies and the independent sector in Wales. Scotland has its own body, called NHS Quality Improvement Scotland, and reviews of quality are undertaken by the Regulation and Quality Improvement Authority (RQIA) in Northern Ireland.

The Healthcare Commission stresses that hospital wards should have quiet and private spaces available to patients to cater for spiritual needs and confidential consultation. It also emphasizes that particular attention should be paid to end-of-life care and care for patients with dementia. Standard C20b of the Healthcare Commission Standards states: 'Healthcare services are provided in environments which promote effective care and optimise health outcomes by being supportive of patient privacy and confidentiality'

> **Box 4.2 Web links – Healthcare Commission**
>
>
>
> Further information on the work of the Healthcare Commission can be found at www.healthcarecommission.org.uk/homepage.cfm, and www.healthcarecommission.org.uk/aboutus.cfm.

> **Box 4.3 Web link – the King's Fund**
>
> You can find out more about the work of the King's Fund in improving healthcare design at www.kingsfund.org.uk.

(Commission for Healthcare Audit and Inspection 2005).

Despite increasing awareness of the positive impact that the environment can have on health, many healthcare environments remain in need of improvement and redesign. To address this need the King's Fund charity set up the 'Enhancing the Environment' programme' in 2000. The programme has subsequently been rolled out and has led to many examples of local improvements to healthcare environments across England. Each project has involved nurse-led teams in partnership with service users, arts coordinators, estates staff and managers interested in improving the care environment.

Environments for older people

A personal healthcare environment that is clean and supports privacy and confidentiality is a key issue for older people. In particular, older people want to have private space for their own personal needs and for private consultation with medical staff and consultants. Healthcare professionals need to make the needs of vulnerable people a high priority and recognize the personal, cultural and spiritual needs of these patients, so as to create an environment which empowers older people to be able to express their views if services are not meeting acceptable levels.

End-of-life care

The King's Fund announced in December 2007 that an additional £1 million would be allocated to transform the physical environment in hospitals and hospices for those who are dying, and their relatives. The intention is that improvements to the physical environment will also be accompanied by changes and improvements in the way that care and support are offered to patients and their families.

Care homes

In 2007, recognizing the importance to people living in care homes of having an environment they are happy with, the Department of Health allocated funds as part of the 'Dignity in Care' programme towards refurbishment of care homes across England. The types of improvements covered included: replacing worn carpets to reduce the risk of falls; upgrading bedrooms and bathrooms; improving gardens and outside spaces; providing greater privacy; and providing information technology that would benefit older residents, including access to the internet and email.

Mental health environments

With recent developments in the care of mentally ill people, inpatient hospital facilities now generally offer care and treatment for acute phases of mental illness in contrast to the more traditional long-term 'asylum' model (Curtis *et al.* 2007). In this setting, it is particularly important for healthcare professionals to recognize that the hospital environment and the care that is provided should respect personal preferences and the cultural and religious needs of patients. This applies even in those situations where a patient has been detained in hospital against their will.

Curtis *et al.* (2007) reported that hospital design is important for patient well-being because it has a bearing on perceived levels of respect and empowerment for people with mental illness. They recommended that healthcare professionals caring for patients with mental illness should provide a sense of privacy and the comfort of a homely environment, a relaxed atmosphere for normal everyday living and a feeling of refuge or protective space.

Activity 4.6

Go to the Media Tool DVD, select **Case Studies**, then **Mental Health (Chris)**, then **Chris arrives on the mental health ward**, and watch the two admission video clips of good and bad practice. Complete the activities on the Media Tool DVD after watching the two clips.

Children and adolescents

The National Service Framework (NSF) standard for children specifies that they should be treated in accommodation that meets their needs for privacy and is also appropriate to their age and level of development. According to the NSF, segregation according to age is of more importance to adolescents than segregation by gender. Adolescents in particular have reported that they want to be with other patients of similar age. In addition, they want to be able to choose whether to be in single- or mixed-sex environments.

Activity 4.7

Go to the Media Tool DVD, select **Case Studies**, then **Child Health (Tom)** and watch the **Introduction to Tom** video clip. Identify how the environment has been adapted to meet Tom's psychological needs and note your findings. You will find our response to this at the end of the chapter.

To conclude this section, some key points in relation to a good healthcare environment are identified in Box 4.4.

A supportive physical environment

Over the last two decades, the quality of the physical care environment has become an established factor in defining quality healthcare services. Research in the USA and the UK has confirmed that the environment of care has a direct effect on medical outcomes and patient and staff satisfaction. For example, there is now clear evidence that well-designed and well-maintained health care environments can positively influence health outcomes such as quicker recovery from surgery, reduced need for strong pain medication, and reduced anxiety and confusion (Lawson and Phiri 2003; Ulrich *et al.* 2004; Rothberg *et al.* 2005). Conversely, there is also evidence that links poor design and poorly maintained environments with negative outcomes – for example, increased anxiety, greater need for analgesia, sleeplessness and higher rates of delirium (Rubin *et al.* 1998).

Hospital patients' perceptions of the ward environ-

Box 4.4 A good healthcare environment

- A good first impression is essential.
- The built healthcare environment should be welcoming, friendly and supportive.
- People should be welcomed immediately on arrival and familiarized with their surroundings.
- Staff should provide excellent customer care including being approachable, polite and responsive to people's needs in a timely and willing manner.
- Staff should always introduce themselves to patients and their visitors and family on initial contact with them.
- Staff should always be visible, well presented and easy to identify.
- There should be a culture of teamwork and support evidenced through teamwork and good relationships across teams.
- Patients and carers should be supported to be as independent as possible in meeting their daily needs.
- Staff should instil confidence and security by being skilled, competent and able to do their job.

Noise

Noise is an ever-present problem in most healthcare environments. It can be generated by monitoring devices, TVs, pagers, telephones, patient buzzers and other patients in close proximity. As noted by Mazer (2003: 1), 'at any given time in most hospitals anywhere in the world, noise levels may exceed those recommended or be inappropriate to the objectives and needs of patients and staff'.

Sudden, sharp, loud or continuous droning noises can directly contribute to increased use of painkillers, panic and heightened anxiety, loss of sleep, confusion and distress. Examples could include the dropping of a bedpan or other heavy object, poorly maintained monitoring equipment that has a loud hum or small talk by nursing staff and other visiting friends and relatives. The problem becomes further magnified during night hours. In the Douglas and Douglas (2004) study, patients reported being kept awake by noise, which included staff talking to one another, the opening and closing of doors, telephones ringing and noise from other patients. As a nurse you can actively seek ways to reduce ambient noise levels in patient areas, and should be aware of your responsibility for maintaining an appropriate sound environment.

ment are influenced by factors that affect their normal lifestyle. For example, being able to eat and sleep, feeling secure or insecure, the amount of privacy that the environment allows them, and to what degree they are able to control their environment (Douglas and Douglas 2005). A 'good' environment will be affected by the level and type of noise, the lighting, the temperature, the colour scheme, and the nature and availability of personal storage space.

Activity 4.8

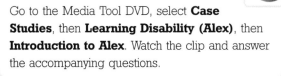

Go to the Media Tool DVD, select **Case Studies**, then **Learning Disability (Alex)**, then **Introduction to Alex**. Watch the clip and answer the accompanying questions.

Activity 4.9

List five simple things that you could do to prevent avoidable noise in your clinical environment, and then compare them to the list at the end of the chapter.

Light

Numerous studies conducted on the effect of daylight and windowless environments have confirmed the major benefits that bright light, particularly daylight, brings to people (LaGarce 2002; Ulrich *et al.* 2004; Walch *et al.* 2005). Windows, in addition to providing a source of light, also expose people to natural daylight and help them to connect with their surroundings. This provides them with essential information on the local social environment and maintains a sense of normality. Contact with the outside world provides information on what the weather is like, what time of day or night it is, and even who is passing by outside. In applying this knowledge to the built healthcare environment, benefits from access to natural daylight for hospital inpatients have been shown to include alleviating symptoms of Alzheimer's disease, reducing the required length of hospital stay for patients who are depressed, and quicker and improved recovery from surgery (Ulrich 1984; Beauchemin and Hays 1998).

Similarly, in a recent study of medical centre outpatients' perceptions of the physical environment in waiting areas in Taiwan, Tsai *et al.* (2007) found that outpatients who visited in the morning were more satisfied with the physical environment than those who visited in the afternoon. The researchers reported that in the outpatient department, overall lighting was brighter in the morning and slightly reduced in the afternoon, and that this appeared to indirectly affect patients' perceptions of the environment as a whole. They concluded that the facility should continuously maintain the lighting system in all waiting areas.

The overall conclusion from available research is that people with access to natural light feel more positive and recover more rapidly from illness than those who do not have such access.

Healthcare staff can influence this aspect of care by ensuring, where possible, that furniture and beds are positioned so that patients can experience good lighting and can see out through a window. This is particularly important for those confined to bed or for patients who need to remain in hospital for more than a few days. Window areas should be kept clear and clean so that the maximum amount of daylight can penetrate the wards and clinical areas. This will be of benefit both to patients and healthcare staff.

Colour

Many healthcare architects and providers, including the Department of Health, have demonstrated some degree of recognition and acceptance that appropriate use of colour can make a significant contribution to patients' well-being. There are nevertheless contentions concerning the role of colour in patients' healthcare outcomes. Tolfe *et al.* (2004) undertook a critical review of the literature on the use of colour to identify supportable design implications. They found that the influence of colour on emotional states and behaviour is unsubstantiated by current research.

However, Dalke and Matheson (2007) provide evidence that colour, and impressions of colour, can affect the experience and performance of people in certain environments.

Cooper *et al.* (1989) found that painting bedroom doors in bright primary and secondary colours, and other areas in pale colours, helped patients who had dementia find places such as their bedrooms more easily. Colour can also be used on the outside of healthcare buildings to assist patients and visitors with orientation, access, navigation and wayfinding.

To conclude this section, some good practice indicators related to a supportive physical environment are identified in Box 4.5.

Box 4.5 Good practice in relation supportive physical environment

- Create a good first impression by maintaining a tidy and well-maintained care environment.
- Use lighting and colour to support a therapeutic and healing environment.
- Keep the area uncluttered, stain-free and in good repair.
- Promote the use of natural daylight.

A clean environment

Cleanliness is a major concern for patients, their visitors and families. In particular, hospital-acquired infections are a constant and growing problem. Patients rightly expect hospitals and other care environments to be clean, tidy and welcoming. A clean care environment gives a good initial impression and can give patients and carers confidence in the overall level of care they can expect. The current NHS approach is to be open about the importance of the issue of cleanliness by:

- giving patients knowledge to empower them to demand the highest standards of hygiene;
- giving matrons and ward nurses practical advice and power to maintain high standards;
- putting inspection processes in place to measure progress;
- learning from examples of best practice, research and technology from the UK and abroad to tackle

the increasing problem of infection prevention and control.

National standards

National standards of cleanliness were first published by the NHS in 2001. These were revised in August 2003 and again in December 2004. The specifications apply to hospitals and acute, mental health or primary care Trust communities. The principles apply equally to all other care environments. Every NHS Trust is required to develop action plans to improve their hospitals, and there is now an annual system of assessment and monitoring of cleanliness in place.

> ### Box 4.6 Web link – national specifications for cleanliness
>
> These standards have now been updated in *The National Specifications for Cleanliness in the NHS: A Framework for Setting and Measuring Performance Outcomes* (NPSA 2007). For further information, go to www.npsa.nhs.uk/patientsafety/ improvingpatientsafety/cleaning-and-nutrition/ national-specifications-of-cleanliness/.

Roles and responsibilities

The key to a successful clean care environment is a sense of healthcare team ownership of cleaning and infection control and a recognition that keeping the environment clean is everyone's responsibility. In NHS hospitals, matrons, ward managers and facilities staff work together to plan and agree a cleaning routine. Matrons have overall responsibility for monitoring standards and generally do weekly or more frequent rounds with domestic supervisors and housekeepers. However, all healthcare staff should promote the principles of a clean environment at all times and nurses, who are present on the ward at all times, can act as the coordinators of this.

Cleaning activity as well as cleanliness should be *visible*. Patients should be involved in the monitoring and reporting of standards of cleanliness. In July 2004, the government released a document entitled *Towards Cleaner Hospitals and Lower Rates of Infection* (DoH

2004a). This in turn led to the development of the 'Matrons' Charter', which has ten key commitments (see Box 4.7).

> ### Box 4.7 The ten key commitments of the Matrons' Charter
>
> 1. Keeping the NHS clean is everyone's responsibility.
> 2. The patient environment will be well maintained, clean and safe.
> 3. Matrons will establish a cleanliness culture across their units.
> 4. Cleaning staff will be recognized for the important work they do. Matrons will make sure they feel part of the ward team.
> 5. Specific roles and responsibilities for cleaning will be clear.
> 6. Cleaning routines will be clear, agreed and well publicized.
> 7. Patients will have a part to play in monitoring and reporting on standards of cleanliness.
> 8. All staff working in healthcare will receive education in infection control.
> 9. Nurses and infection control teams will be involved in drawing up cleaning contracts, and matrons have authority and power to withhold payment.
> 10. Sufficient resources will be dedicated to keeping hospitals clean.
>
> The full document can be found online at www.dh.gov.uk/en/Publicationsandstatistics/ Publications/PublicationsPolicyAndGuidance/ DH_4091506.

The Matrons' Charter sets out clear recommendations to improve cleanliness in hospitals, including creating strong cleaning teams, making roles and responsibilities for cleaning clear, identifying how patients' views can be heard and setting up a direct line for patients to contact domestic services.

To build on the Matrons' Charter and as part of an ongoing campaign to improve hospital cleanliness, from May 2008 additional matrons have been appointed to acute care settings. Their role will focus in particular on:

- providing a clean environment for care;
- ensuring best practice in infection control;
- improving clinical care standards;
- treating patients with dignity and respect.

Patient Environment Action Teams (PEATs)

The PEAT programme was established in 2000. Every inpatient facility in England with more than ten beds is assessed annually and given a rating on a scale from 'excellent' to 'unacceptable'. The PEAT assessment team comprises nurses, matrons, catering and domestic managers, medics, service managers, direct- ors, dieticians and estate managers. The team also includes patients, patient representation or members of the public. PEAT data for all Trusts are published annually by the National Patient Safety Agency (NPSA).

Box 4.8 Web link – PEATs

National PEAT scores can be found at http://www.npsa.nhs.uk/corporate/news/peat-results/.

To achieve high PEAT scores means that a hospital must focus on cleanliness 24 hours a day, every day of the year. Achieving an 'excellent' PEAT rating will demonstrate to patients and staff that cleanliness is a very high priority for that organization. National PEAT scores between 2004 and 2007 are shown in Table 4.1.

Clearly, cleanliness in general practice is just as

Table 4.1 National PEAT scores for 'patient environment', 2004–7

Patient environment: hospital rates (%)

	2004	2005	2006	2007
Excellent	10.00	10.3	14.2	14.3
Good	38.5	44.8	49.8	48.9
Acceptable	49.2	40.1	31.1	34.8
Poor	2.0	4.6	4.8	1.6
Unacceptable	0.3	0.2	0.2	0.5

Source: www.npsa.nhs.uk

important as in hospitals, and the web link below will provide a good guide to this topic.

Box 4.9 Web link – infection control for general practice

Detailed guidance on infection control for general practice is available from: www.thenvqman.co.uk/Documents/goodpracticeinfectioncontrol.pdf

In 2007, to respond to concerns about the care environment, NHS Lothian introduced a system of monitoring cleanliness in all acute hospitals using teams of patients and staff mirroring the concept of PEAT teams in England and Wales.

Hand hygiene

Hand hygiene is the single most important thing that healthcare staff can do to reduce the spread of disease. Hand hygiene must be seen as a key priority by every single healthcare professional from porter to consultant.

Activity 4.10

Go to the Media Tool DVD, select **Skill Sets**, then **Infection Control and Hygiene**, then **Handwashing and Universal Infection Control Precautions** and work through this section, paying particular attention to the hand-washing technique. It will be useful at this stage to refer to Chapter 8 on personal and oral hygiene as well.

Following this, select **Case Studies, Adult Health (Margaret)**, then **Nurse checks Margaret's skin**. Watch the video clip and answer the questions afterwards.

In 2004, the NPSA launched the 'cleanyourhands' campaign across England and Wales. This campaign provides practical support to help healthcare organ- izations fight infection. It also involves education and development of an organizational culture where indi- viduals take personal responsibility for the delivery of safe, clean care. Staff are prompted to clean their hands at the critical time and place, that is, where and when patient care is being provided.

The importance of hand hygiene for every member of staff involved in healthcare cannot be over-emphasized. Healthcare associated infection (HCAI) is estimated to cost the NHS at least £1 billion annually and cause at least 5000 deaths (ONS 2005). Many of these infections are preventable. Tackling HCAI is a global issue and the NPSA supports the World Health Organization's (WHO) 'Global Patient Safety Challenge: Clean Care is Safer Care' initiative. Since its launch, the 'cleanyourhands' campaign has been adopted by all NHS Trusts in England and Wales and is to be extended to primary care, mental health, community and ambulance environments as well as care homes and hospices.

Box 4.10 Web link – hand washing

A good resource for more information on hand washing is the www.npsa.nhs.uk/cleanyourhands website, which contains best practice guidance, resources, background information and research study results to support the maintenance of cleanliness in NHS healthcare environments.

The key initiatives aimed at improving NHS cleanliness during the years 2000–7 are identified in Box 4.11.

Despite reports year on year from the NPSA of improved rates of cleanliness in hospitals, patients and visitors are increasingly concerned about the risk of acquiring infections when they visit or are admitted. This may be due in part to high levels of coverage in the media of methicillin resistant Staphylococcus aureus (MRSA) and other 'super bugs' rather than any actual deterioration in cleanliness levels. However, standards still remain below optimal levels of cleanliness and all staff must strive to provide excellence in this area.

Good practice indicators related to maintaining a clean environment are identified in Box 4.12.

Infection control

Cleanliness is closely linked to *infection control* but there are important distinctions. Cleanliness contributes to the *control* of infection, but *prevention* of

---

Box 4.11 Key initiatives to improve NHS cleanliness (2000–7)

- National investment of £68 million to improving cleanliness since 2000.
- Annual PEAT visits since 2000.
- NHS Trust director to oversee cleanliness.
- National cleaning standards for hospitals (2001).
- Over £14 million invested in ward housekeepers.
- Publication of *Winning Ways – Working Together to Reduce Healthcare Associated Infections* (Chief Medical Officer 2003).
- Publication of the *NHS Healthcare Cleaning Manual* (NHS Estates 2004).
- Publication of *Towards Cleaner Hospitals and Lower Rates of Infection: A Summary of Action* (DoH 2004a).
- Publication of the *Matrons' Charter* (DoH 2004b).
- NPSA 'cleanyourhands' campaign (2004).
- Publication of *The National Specifications for Cleanliness in the NHS: A Framework for Setting and Measuring Performance Outcomes* (NPSA 2007).
- Introduction of 'Deep Clean' teams (2007).

---

infection requires more than cleanliness. Key legislation relating to the control of infection includes:

- *A Strategy for Workplace Health and Safety in Great Britain to 2010 and Beyond* (Health and Safety Commission 2004).
- *Control of Substances Hazardous to Health* (Health and Safety Commission 2002).
- *Safe Management of Healthcare Waste* (Health and Safety Commission 2006).

These regulations are incorporated into the policies and guidelines of all health organizations to support staff in establishing and maintaining a safe care environment. Nurses and all health workers must be aware of the need to follow infection control procedures at all times.

When on placement, you should constantly assess your working environment to identify any potential

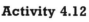

Box 4.12 Good practice indicators related to maintaining a clean environment

- Internal and external areas should be clean with no avoidable unwanted odours.
- Flexible cleaning arrangements should be in place to meet the needs of patients.
- Adequate hand-washing facilities should always be available.
- Regular cleaning and waste management routines should be in place which meet national standards.
- All areas should be checked for cleanliness on a regular basis and any faults acted upon immediately.
- The national colour code for cleaning equipment should be in place.
- Cleaning equipment should be readily available and stored appropriately.
- The area should meet PEAT requirements.
- Regular audits of levels of cleanliness should take place, staff should be aware of the findings and these findings must be acted upon.
- Patients should be encouraged to raise any concerns about cleanliness and request action be taken.
- Systems should be in place to deal with any spillages and emergency clearance 24 hours a day.

Activity 4.11

Go to the Media Tool DVD, select **Case Studies**, **Child Health (Tom)**, then scroll down the page **Tom is transferred to the ward** to the **Safety and risk management** section. Work through the question there.

safety risks to patients or staff and inform managers of any risks that you recognize. Safe infection control practice is also paramount to the provision of quality safe care.

Activity 4.12

Go to the Media Tool DVD, select **Case Studies**, **Mental Health (Chris)**, then **Chris is moved to the Medical Emergency Unit**. Scroll down to the **risk assessment** section and revise the background on risk of harm to self and risk of harm to others. Local guidelines on these areas may vary. See if you can locate your local guidelines.

Control of hazardous substances, spillages and disposal of hospital waste

The Control of Substances Hazardous to Health (COSHH) regulations first came into force in 1988 and have been regularly updated since, most recently in 2002. The purpose is to ensure that employees systematically undertake risk assessments of all *hazardous substances*. Each organization will have clear policies concerning the use of cleaning materials and the management of spillages. Potential hazards exist when handling devices. For example, a nurse can come into contact on a daily basis with items such as needles, scalpels, stitch cutters or even glass ampoules. The main potential hazards which can result from a sharp injury are hepatitis B, hepatitis C and HIV. It is vitally important that when using any sharp devices the nurse takes action to reduce the risk of potential injury by following instructions for safe use of the device and by disposing of it safely after use, following any workplace policies and procedures.

Some procedures are known to carry a higher potential risk of injury than others. These include venepuncture, cannulation and injection. When undertaking any of these procedures the nurse should always ensure that handling of equipment is kept to a minimum, needles are not broken or bent before use, needles are never re-sheathed and all sharps that have been used are disposed of in a designated container at the point of use (RCN 2005).

Every healthcare workplace will have written policies on all aspects of waste disposal including special waste, segregation of waste and audit trails. A system of colour coding to identify segregation of waste exists and is shown in Box 4.13.

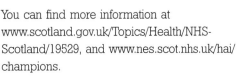

Box 4.13 Colour-code system for the segregation of waste

- Yellow bags for infectious waste – incineration.
- Orange bags for infectious waste –alternative treatment.
- Black bags for household waste.
- Special bins for glass and aerosols.
- Colour-coded bins for pharmaceutical or cytotoxic waste.

Box 4.14 Web link – Cleanliness Champions Programme

You can find more information at www.scotland.gov.uk/Topics/Health/NHS-Scotland/19529, and www.nes.scot.nhs.uk/hai/champions.

For information on policies in Wales, see www.wales.nhs.uk.

Activity 4.13
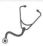

At the beginning of your next clinical placement, request a copy of the infection control policy. Read the document and identify what action you should take to dispose of used sharps safely.

Activity 4.14

Go to the Media Tool DVD, select **Case studies**, **Child Health (Tom)**, then **Tom is painting and then gets ready for lunch**. Watch the video clip and answer the question. What important aspects of infection control are being demonstrated by the nurse? Then watch the clip on personal hygiene and infection control and observe what actions the nurse takes to minimize the risk of cross-infection.

See our suggested answer at the end of the chapter.

The general principles of infection control are summed up in Box 4.15.

Box 4.15 General principles of infection control

- Achieving optimal hand hygiene.
- Using personal protective equipment.
- Safe handling and disposal of sharps.
- Safe handling and disposal of clinical waste.
- Managing blood and bodily fluids.
- Decontaminating equipment.
- Achieving and maintaining a clean clinical environment.
- Appropriate use of indwelling devices.
- Managing accidents.
- Good communication with other healthcare workers, patients and visitors.
- Training/education.

(Source: RCN 2005)

The Cleanliness Champions Programme

In Scotland, the Scottish Ministerial Healthcare Association Infection Task Force was established in 2003. The Task Force comprises membership from the healthcare sector and members of the public. Its message of 'clean healthcare environment, clean hands, clean instruments' applies across all healthcare boundaries. NHS Education Scotland has developed the Cleanliness Champions Programme for all staff working within the NHS in that country, details of which can be found in Box 4.14.

Uniforms and workwear

The possibility of transmitting infection via uniforms is an important issue for employers, staff and patients. The Department of Health has put together a document on the wearing and laundry of uniforms, entitled *Uniform and Work-wear Policy* (DOH 2007b) (see Box 4.16). This document outlines existing legal requirements along with evidence-based findings from two wide-ranging literature reviews carried out by Thames Valley University, plus further research conducted by University College London Hospitals NHS Trust. Based on the literature reviews and empirical evidence, a set of good practice examples has been devised, which can be used by organizations to compile uniform policy. Examples of accepted good practice based on informal common sense rather than scientific evidence are also identified.

> ### Box 4.16 Web link – uniforms andwork wear
>
> The full report by the Department of Health can be found at www.dh.gov.uk/en/Publicationsand statistics/Publications/PublicationsPolicy AndGuidance/DH_078433.

Although from the evidence base it seems unlikely that uniforms are a significant source of cross-infection, the way that staff dress does send messages to patients and the public.

Further information on infection prevention and control can be found in the Royal College of Nursing document *Good Practice in Infection Prevention and Control – Guidance for Nursing Staff* (RCN 2005). Some key good practice indicators related to infection control are identified in Box 4.17.

Activity 4.15

When you are next in a clinical area, observe how many healthcare professionals are wearing their uniforms correctly. Check for unnecessary jewellery, wristwatches, or non-uniform cardigans, tights and shoes. List any potential risk to patients from what you have observed – for example, scratching from a wristwatch when moving and handling, or the possibility of confused patients grabbing dangling chains worn around the neck.

Activity 4.16

1 What do you think is meant by *personal protective equipment* (PPE)?

2 When would you use PPE?

Write down your answers and include them in your portfolio. Then check them against our response at the end of the chapter.

> ### Box 4.17 Key good practice indicators related to infection control
>
> - Patients, carers and visitors should be informed of what they should expect to see and do in relation to infection control measures and should be empowered to challenge staff where there are poor hygiene practices.
> - Patients should be informed about why specific infection control precautions are taken.
> - A policy should be in place to ensure that people are informed if they have a healthcare acquired infection.
> - Staff should clean their hands between tasks and patient care.
> - Equipment should be cleaned appropriately between use by different patients.
> - Staff should wear personal protective equipment (PPE) as appropriate.
> - An infection control and visitors policy should be in place and regularly reviewed.
> - Systems should be in place to replace mattresses, covers, baby-changing mats, and other equipment as necessary.
> - Systems should be in place to manage any outbreak of infection.
> - Audits of infection control precautions and practices should be completed regularly.
> - Staff should receive regular education in relation to infection control.
> - The infection control team should be involved in the design of new NHS buildings to minimize the risk of infection and cross-infection.

The personal healthcare environment

Evidence base

Several recent studies in the UK have sought to discover what patients find important about their care environment and how nurses and other healthcare staff can enhance that environment. Patients consistently report that they want to have control of their personal environment. For example, in the study by Douglas and Douglas (2005), acute hospital inpatients reported that they wanted to have a sense of control over their own activity. Patients interviewed explained that they wanted to be able to move around the ward area, open and close curtains, control lights and temperature and access external areas of the building. These findings are supported by a previous study by Lawson and Phiri (2003) which also reported on the importance of increasing patients' personal control and how supporting them to take responsibility for aspects of their care can reduce helplessness and improve other outcomes.

More recently, Curtis *et al.* (2007) explored patients' views of the environment in modern mental healthcare facilities and reported that what was especially important was 'a hospital design which helps retain and develop skills for independent living, and provides sustainable connections to the wider community' (Curtis *et al.* 2007: 617).

Control of the environment

Control of our immediate environment is something that we take for granted. Not having this control leads to feelings of frustration and dissatisfaction. At the simplest level, patients want to be able to reach the light switch so that they can turn their light on and off. You should always check to ensure that patients have access to a switch to control their lights whether they are in bed or sitting in a chair beside their bed.

Patients would like to be able to open and close their bedside curtains without having to call the nurse to assist them. However, even today, most patients are not able to open and close their curtains unless they are able to walk around the bed themselves to do this. Too often, the healthcare professional opens and closes bedside curtains at their own preference without seeking and adhering to the wishes of the person who is confined to bed. Until self-opening and closing

facilities are made available to all patients, you can assist by asking patients how they want their curtains positioned (open, closed or partly open), and can ensure that their wishes are followed. This is all about preserving the patient's privacy and dignity. Remember this when you read Chapter 5 of this book.

Patients also want to be able to regulate the temperature and to turn their television or radio on and off. Not being able to control these simple environmental functions causes much frustration and stress and can significantly affect a patient's perception of their whole hospital stay.

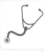

Activity 4.17

Next time you are on the ward look around at the general environment for patients. How much privacy and dignity is afforded to patients? How much control do they have over their own environment?

Researchers in Canada and the USA have identified how 'healing' environments shorten patients post-operative recovery period and help them to return to a good state of mental and physical health. As far back as 1979, Ulrich suggested that stress was a major obstacle to healing and that the well-being and recovery of patients were directly related to the physical environment of the hospital and its healthcare facilities. Ulrich's (1997) study on supportive design for healthcare environments suggests that hospitals should take steps to enhance the features of patients' surroundings to hold their attention and interest without creating further difficulties that can add to their fatigue and distress.

As part of a project supported by the Picker Institute, Fowler *et al.* (1999) carried out a study of consumer perceptions of healthcare environments to determine what mattered to patients. This study found that patients cared and were concerned about the nature of the physical environment around them – in particular, they wanted care environments to facilitate connections to staff and carers that were conducive to a sense of well-being and provided connections to the outside world.

In general, then, we can see that all these studies contribute clear evidence that the care environment influences the healing process and has a direct impact on patients' health outcomes.

Surroundings and furnishings

Furniture and its positioning play an important role in supporting a healing care environment. Well-designed furniture and ambient surroundings can potentially influence patients' behaviour and well-being. A careful balance of colour, furniture, style and function can contribute to meeting individuals' needs and preferences.

Safety

Patient falls account for almost two-fifths of the total patient safety incidents reported to the NPSA. A recent report entitled *Slips, Trips and Falls* (NPSA 2008) identified how many everyday aspects of the care environment can have an impact on the risk of falls and injury for patients. These include the type of floor surface, the level and type of lighting and the design of doors and handrails. By being better informed and aware of these elements and taking action where possible, nurses can assist patients to avoid preventable falls.

Activity 4.18

Go to the Media Tool DVD, select **Skill Sets**, **Risk and Comfort**, then **Falls risk assessment**, **Bed rail assessment**. Read through these and try and identify any potential risks to patients on your ward.

Furniture

Furniture and its positioning can affect patient mood, independence and behaviour. This is particularly true for mental health units and care of the elderly units, where patients may display challenging or confused behaviour. For example, at the Maudsley Hospital in London, nursing staff found that on average patients were pulling down up to seven pairs of cubicle/window

curtains per week (Urch 2007). These curtains were often unusable as a result, and had to be replaced. Following consultation, it was decided to trial disposable curtains made from material that does not rip. These new curtains offer complete patient privacy and can be changed in a few minutes. They offer a warm look in a choice of colours and since installation none have been pulled down by patients. This provides a clear demonstration that a cosy, clean, fresh environment can have a dramatically positive impact on patient well-being.

Activity 4.19

Next time you are on the ward look around at the furniture. Is it all necessary and in use? Is it clean, in good repair and able to be moved easily as required? Does the positioning of the furniture enable you to have a good working space when you are attending to patients?

Finally, some key practice guidance can be found in Box 4.18.

Box 4.18 Key good practice indicators related to linen and furnishings

- Patients should receive care in well-maintained environments where linen and furnishings are designed and provided to meet their personal needs.
- Furnishings should be adequately maintained to prevent slips, trips and falls.
- The layout of beds and other furniture should be organized and located in positions where people can maintain the maximum level of independence possible and in ways that facilitate social interaction.
- Patients' preferences should be sought and their involvement secured when planning refurbishment and redesign of facilities.

Summary and key points

This chapter has explored the importance of the built healthcare environment and the role of health professionals involved in patient care within such environments. The chapter has also identified the role of all healthcare professionals in contributing to the patient experience through the provision of a welcoming, responsive culture.

It is important to remember the following:

- A healthcare facility should be responsive to patients' needs and provide a friendly environment.
- The importance of maintaining clean and infection-free facilities.
- The importance of ensuring that patients' personal environment meets their individual needs and preferences.
- The importance of the effective use of resources to assist people to maintain their independence.

References

Beauchemin, K.M. and Hays, P. (1998) Dying in the dark: sunshine, gender and outcomes in myocardial infarction, *Journal of the Royal Society of Medicine*, 91: 352–4.

Chief Medical Officer (2003) *Winning Ways: Working Together to Reduce Healthcare Associated Infection in England*. London: DoH.

Commission for Healthcare Audit and Inspection (2005) *Healthcare Commission Inspection Guide*, www.healthcarecommission.org.uk/homepage.cfm.

Cooper, B. Mohide, A. and Gilbert, S. (1989) Testing the use of colour, *Dimensions in Health Service*, 66: 22–6.

Curtis, S. Gesler, G. Fabian, K. Francis, S. and Priebe, S. (2007) Therapeutic landscapes in hospital design: a qualitative assessment by staff and service users of the design of a new mental health inpatient unit, *Environment and Planning C: Government and Policy*, 25(6): 591–610.

Dalke, H. and Matheson, M. (2007) *Colour Design Schemes for Long-term Healthcare Environments*. Kingston upon Thames: Arts & Humanities Research Council.

DoH (Department of Health) (2000) *The NHS Plan: A Plan for Investment and Reform*, Cm 4818-1. London: HMSO.

DoH (Department of Health) (2003) *The Essence of Care: Patient-focused Benchmarking for Health Care Practitioners*. London: The Stationery Office.

DoH (Department of Health) (2004a) *Towards Cleaner Hospitals and Lower Rates of Infection: A Summary of Action*. London: DoH.

DoH (Department of Health) (2004b) *Matrons' Charter: An Action Plan for Cleaner Hospitals*. London: DoH.

DoH (Department of Health) (2007a) *Assessing the Successes and Impact of the Ward Housekeeper Role: Summary Report*. London: DoH.

DoH (Department of Health) (2007b) *Uniform and Work-wear Policy*. London: DoH.

Douglas, C.H. and Douglas, M.R. (2004) Patient-friendly hospital environments: exploring the patients' perspective, *Health Expectations*, 7: 61–73.

Douglas, C.H. and Douglas, M.R. (2005) Patient-centred improvements in health-care built environments: perspectives and design indicators, *Health Expectations*, 8: 264–76.

Fowler, E. MacRae, S. Stern, A. Harrison, T. Gerteis, M. Walker, J. Edgeman-Levitan, S. and Ruga, W. (1999) The built environment as a component of quality care: understanding and including the patient's perspective, *The Joint Commission on Accreditation of Healthcare Organisations*, 25(7): 352–62.

Health and Safety Commission (2002) *The Control of Substances Hazardous to Health: Regulations*, 4th edn. Sudbury: HSE Books.

Health and Safety Commission (2004) *A Strategy for Workplace Health and Safety in Great Britain to 2010 and Beyond*. London: HSE.

Health and Safety Commission (2006) *Environment and Sustainability: Health Technical Memorandum 07-01. Safe Management of Healthcare Waste*. London. The Stationery Office.

Hosking, S. and Haggard, L. (1999) *Healing the Hospital Environment: Design, Management and Maintenance of Healthcare Premises*. London: E&FN Spon.

LaGarce, M. (2002) Control of environmental lighting and its effects on behaviours of the Alzheimer's type, *Journal of Interior Design*, 28(2): 15–25.

Lawson, B. and Phiri, M. (2003) *The Architectural Healthcare Environment and its Effect on Patient Health Outcomes*. London:The Stationery Office.

Mazer S.E. (2003) 'Quiet please. healing in progress', *Hospital Development HD Magazine*, January.

NHS Estates (2003) *Improving the Patient Experience: Ward Housekeepers Contributing to Care*. London: DoH.

NHS Estates (2004) *The NHS Healthcare Cleaning Manual*. London: DoH.

NPSA (National Patient Safety Agency) (2004) 'Cleanyourhands' campaign. London: NPSA.

NPSA (National Patient Safety Agency) (2007) *The National Specifications for Cleanliness in the NHS: A Framework for Setting and Measuring Performance Outcomes*, London: NPSA, www.npsa.nhs.uk/site/media/documents/ 2859_NPSA_Cleaning_spec.pdf, accessed 22 February 2008.

NPSA (National Patient Safety Agency) (2008) *Slips, Trips and Falls in Hospital*. London: NPSA, www.npsa.nhs.uk/site/media/ documents/2786_PSO_Falls_WEB_x.f.pdf, accessed 22 February 2008.

ONS (Office for National Statistics) (2005) Deaths involving MRSA, England and Wales, 1993–2003, *Health Statistics Quarterly*, 25 (Spring).

RCN (Royal College of Nursing) (2005) *Good Practice in Infection Prevention and Control – Guidance for Nursing Staff*. London: RCN.

Rothberg, M. Abraham V. Lindenauer, P. and Rose, D. (2005) Improving nurse-to-patient staffing ratios as a cost-effective safety intervention, *Medical Care,* 43: 785–91.

Rubin, H.R. Owens, A.J. and Golden, G. (1998) *An Investigation to Determine Whether the Built Environment Affects Patients' Medical Outcomes*. Martinez, CA: The Centre for Health Design.

Tolfe R.B. Schwartz, B. Yoon, S-Y. and Max-Royale, A. (2004) *Color in Healthcare Environments: A Critical Review of the Literature*. Coalition for Health Environments Research (CHER).

Tsai, C.Y. Wang, M.C. Liao, W.T. Lu, J.H. Sun, P.H. Lin, B.Y. and Breen, G.M. (2007) Hospital outpatient perceptions of the physical environment of waiting areas: the role of patient characteristics on atmospherics in one academic medical center, *BMC Health Services Research*, 7, www.biomedcentral.com/1472-6963/7/198.

Ulrich, R.S. (1979) Visual landscapes and psychological well-being, *Landscape Research*, 4(1): 17–23.

Ulrich, R.S. (1984) View through a window may influence recovery from surgery, *Science*, 224: 420–1.

Ulrich, R.S. (1997) A theory of supportive design for healthcare facilities, *Journal of Healthcare Design*, 9: 3–7.

Ulrich, R.S. Zimring, C. Joseph, A. Quan, X. and Choudhary, R. (2004) *The Role of the Physical Environment in the Hospital of the 21st Century: A Once-in-a-lifetime Opportunity.* Concord, CA: The Center for Health Design.

Urch, A. (2007) Infection control: curtain credentials, *HD Hospital Development*, May.

Walch, J.M. Rabin, B.S. Day, R. Williams, J.N. Choi, K. and Kang, J.D. (2005) The effect of sunlight on post-operative analgesic medication usage: a prospective study of spinal surgery patients, *Psychosomatic Medicine,* 67(1): 156–63.

Answers

Activity 4.1

A built healthcare environment is any area where care takes place.

A personal environment is the immediate area surrounding the patient. For example, the hospital bed space, a consulting room, a patient's home or any treatment or clinic area.

Activity 4.7

Tom has a TV, video, toys, posters, his own clothes, colourful surroundings, a balloon, his own cup and a blanket, all of which will contribute to his sense of security and well-being.

Activity 4.9

Your list may have included closing doors, staff using a separate lounge area for breaks, avoidance of conversations directly outside patients' rooms or near bedsides on the ward, the use of sound-absorbing materials where possible (for example, non-metal chart holders), modification of patient call systems, and, where patients are well enough, the provision of personal headphones and a library of music CDs.

Activity 4.14

The nurse is wearing a blue apron, the table is cleaned and Tom's hands are washed.

Activity 4.16

1 PPE includes the use of aprons, gloves, goggles, visors or masks. In specialist areas such as theatre, it can sometimes also include footwear and hats (RCN 2005).
2 PPE is used in any situation where there is a risk to the nurse or the patient from cross-infection. In some instances it may be required for contact with hazardous pharmaceuticals or chemicals.

5

Privacy and dignity

Helen Iggulden and Ruth Chadwick

Chapter Contents

Learning objectives

The aim of this chapter is to explore the nurse's role in supporting patients' privacy and dignity. Throughout the chapter we will refer to the accompanying Media Tool DVD. Please watch the video clips as directed as these will reinforce your learning. After reading this chapter and interacting with the DVD you will be able to:

- Understand how attitudes and interpersonal behaviour styles develop.
- Identify how one's personal world and personal identity influence the experience of dignity.
- Explain the significance of a patient's personal space.
- Differentiate between communicating *with* and communicating *at*.
- Utilize the principles of patient confidentiality and balance these with interprofessional working.
- Apply the meaning of privacy, dignity and modesty to the healthcare setting.
- Identify the importance of risk assessment to ensure dignity.

Introduction

Over the last 20 years concern for a patient's privacy and dignity in the healthcare setting has grown. The Human Rights Act (1998a) has given patients using healthcare services more power to assert their human and ethical rights, and their right to *privacy*. Many nursing activities covered in the other chapters within this book, such as washing a person's body, assisting them to meet their nutritional and elimination needs and asking them questions to assess their care needs, involve a clear understanding of the principles of privacy and *dignity*.

Human rights are tied to the laws, customs and religions of the time, and the culture within which we live. The promotion and protection of human rights has been a major concern of the United Nations since 1945 when it was resolved that the human horrors of the Second World War should never happen again, and the General Assembly declared that respect for human rights and human dignity is the foundation of freedom, justice and peace in the world.

Legislation in most countries now protects human privacy and dignity and provides protection from discrimination on the grounds of race, colour, disability, gender and creed. This chapter will help you to understand how you can carry out your nursing skills in a multicultural society, in a way that incorporates both privacy and dignity.

Background

In 2003, the Department of Health produced *Building on the Best: Choice, Responsiveness and Equity in the NHS*. This document addresses recurring themes:

- All of us, not just some affluent middle classes, want the opportunity to share in decisions about our health and healthcare.

- We want the right information at the right time and most suited to our needs as possible.
- Our health needs are personal and we would like services to be shaped around our needs.

The document has several goals including the following:

- to give patients more say in how they are treated;
- to increase access to a wider range of services in *primary care*;
- to increase choice about how, where and when patients get medication;
- to give more choice in booking appointments;
- to give greater choice over care at the end of life;
- to ensure choices are available to everyone, including the most disadvantaged and marginalized groups.

An editorial response from Grandison-Markey (2005) suggests that many professionals still have a strong perception that users should be subservient to

---

Box 5.1 Legislation relating to human rights

Race Relations Act 1976 (amended 2000) makes it unlawful to discriminate on racial grounds. The Act defines 'racial grounds' as being colour, race, nationality or ethnic or national origins. The Act also makes *victimization* and *harassment* illegal. This includes verbal or physical bullying, jokes or excluding people because of race or sex.

Human Rights Act 1998a makes it unlawful for public bodies to act in a way that is incompatible with the articles of the European Convention on Human Rights. The Act can be accessed via www.opsi.gov.uk/ACTS/acts1998/ukpga_19980042_en_3#sch1, and comprises:

Article 2 Right to life
Article 3 Prohibition of torture and inhuman treatment
Article 4 Right to freedom from slavery and forced labour
Article 5 Right to liberty and security of person
Article 6 Right to a fair trial
Article 7 No punishment without law
Article 8 Right to respect for privacy in a person's private life, family life, home life and correspondence
Article 9 Freedom of thought, conscience and religion
Article 10 Right to freedom of expression
Article 11 Freedom of assembly and association
Article 12 Right to marry and found a family
Article 14 Prohibition of discrimination on the grounds of sex, race, colour, language, religion, political or other opinion, national or social origin, association with a national minority, property, birth or other status

them. She suggests that professionals need to rectify their own ignorance and prejudices and to understand how *stereotypes* and misunderstandings can arise. In addition, Woogara (2005) found that most practitioners had little or no awareness of the importance of the Human Rights Act, or indeed any of the documents regarding the privacy of patients, although newly-qualified staff showed greater knowledge. Box 5.1 lists the key points in the human rights legislation.

The Data Protection Act 1998 also has implications for healthcare professionals. Box 5.2 covers the key points of this Act.

Scenario 5.1

You have been working on your first clinical placement and a friend tells you that her aunt has been admitted to the ward you are working on. She asks you to look in the medical notes and tell her what is wrong with her aunt, and what treatment she is receiving. Which aspects of the law would you be breaching if you agreed to do this? Check your answer with that given at the end of the chapter.

Box 5.2 The Data Protection Act

The Data Protection Act 1998 declares that all records about clients are seen as data, whether electronic or paper. Individuals are given rights which include:

- the right to know what information is held about them and to see and correct the information if necessary;
- the right to refuse to provide information;
- the right that data should be accurate and up to date;
- the right that information should be kept no longer than necessary;
- the right for the data to be used only for the specific purpose for which it was collected;
- the right to *confidentiality* – that the information should not be accessible to unauthorized people or other parties without the *consent* of the individual to whom it refers.

Professionals always need to be conscious of these legal requirements, and even as a student you are bound by them (NMC 2002) and by your professional code of conduct (NMC 2008).

Attitudes and behaviour

It is possible to obey the letter of the law but to do so in a manner or with an *attitude* that conveys contempt or disrespect. Attitudes have a significant impact on our behaviour and what it conveys to others. In a healthcare setting a therapeutic attitude conveys to patients a feeling that they matter all the time. *The Essence of Care* (DoH 2003b) indicates that patients respond pri-

marily to a nurse's attitude and non-verbal behaviour, such as body language.

Activity 5.1

Go to the Media Tool DVD, click on **Skills Sets**, then **Observations**, to bring you to **Temperature taking** and watch the video clip, **Nurse takes and records TPR BP, good practice**. How does the nurse's non-verbal behaviour convey respect? Check the suggested answer at the end of the chapter.

Good practice guidelines (DoH 2004b) also draw attention to the needs of vulnerable and minority groups and the need for partnerships that support the promotion of good attitudes.

Activity 5.2

Go to the Media Tool DVD, select, **Learning Disability (Alex)**, then watch the video clip **The nurses demonstrate bad practice**.

Do you think their behaviour makes Alex feel that he matters? What aspects of human rights legislation are being breached here? Write down your answers and add them to your portfolio. Then look at our suggestion at the end of the chapter.

Unfortunately, nurses can sometimes demonstrate discourteous behaviour towards vulnerable patients, such as those with a *learning disability* or *dementia* that results in several breaches of human rights. This is probably not deliberate, but a result of unconscious attitudes. Their verbal and non-verbal behaviour can indicate *paternalistic* attitudes and the desire to 'take over' a person's life. This attitude can also sometimes be seen directed towards other groups – older adults, for example, or children. Some indicators of a paternalistic, disrespectful attitude are shown in the following list relating to Alex's case study:

- Walking into a person's room without knocking (breach of Article 8 – in care, the room is a person's temporary home).
- Introducing visitors to the room rather than the person (breach of Article 8).
- Sitting on a patient's bed without asking permission to do so (breach of Article 8).
- Standing over a patient and talking about them as if they are not there.
- Not introducing yourself by name.
- Not asking a person about how they are feeling.
- Attempting to remove their personal belongings from them without asking permission (e.g. the nurse tries to take Alex's bottle of soft drink from his hand and scolds him – breach of Article 3).
- Taking control of a person's life (e.g. 'We are going to have to control what you eat. We're going to have to tell you what you can and can't have' – breach of Articles 5 and 9).

Autonomy and children

In caring for a child you need to know how to meet their needs for *autonomy* and how to respect their dignity. An example of how to do this is demonstrated in the following activity.

Activity 5.3

Go to the Media Tool DVD, **Case Studies, Tom**, and watch the video clip **Tom is painting and then has his lunch**.

List the ways in which the nurse respects Tom's privacy and dignity.

There are further ways that she could have improved upon her behaviour. Think about how she could have further enhanced Tom's privacy and dignity. Compare your lists to our suggested answer at the end of the chapter.

What do we really mean by 'attitude'?

Although 'attitude' is a word we use every day, social psychologists have devoted a whole field of study to it, since it forms a very important part of people's social worlds. An attitude is the state of mind of an individual towards an object. The object can be a person, a physical object or something more abstract such as a 'hospital' or an 'illness'. Hence, a patient's attitude towards a nurse or towards their illness, or the fact that they are in hospital, is an important element to consider. It is a learned predisposition to think, feel and behave towards a person or an object in 'a particular way'. 'Attitude' therefore means the feelings and cognitions that determine whether we respond in a favourable or an unfavourable manner to a person, object or idea.

Our attitudes allow us to organize and make sense of the world. They provide us with clues about why people behave as they do and help us summarize experience. Attitudes also help us to maintain our *self-esteem* and foster a positive sense of ourselves as individuals. Not only that, they serve as 'glue' that bonds us and helps us to develop group and social identity and status. For example, when you need to take a patient to the toilet, or you need to feed them because they are unable to feed themselves, it is important to take into account their attitude towards needing that assistance. Many patients in this situation may express their dismay or anger at what they see as 'being like a child again'.

Activity 5.4

Go to the Media Tool DVD, select **Skills Sets, Nutritional Intake**, then **Assisting patients to eat poor practice–How not to feed a patient**, and scroll down to watch the clip **Lyn's reactions to being fed by Jayne**. This clip clearly demonstrates how much patients are disheartened by negative attitudes.

How do attitudes develop?

We are not born with attitudes. We develop them through experiencing the physical and social world and on the basis of whether we find that experience pleasant or unpleasant. So, we may develop a negative attitude towards a certain type of food such as meat because we do not like it or because we have an allergy to it. Or we might believe that eating animals is wrong or we might have grown up in a vegetarian community.

The attitudes that we develop through experience are influenced in several ways (Erwin 2001):

1. *Informational influences.* You will develop your nursing skills based on information that you get from textbooks, journal articles, hospital policies and practice guidelines.

2. *Person to person.* In other words, family, friends and colleagues. You will already have been influenced by family and friends and you will also be influenced by course colleagues, tutors, mentors in practice, other qualified nurses, healthcare assistants and the multidisciplinary team.

3. *Mass media.* TV, books, newspapers, internet. You may be influenced by healthcare reports, documentaries and the websites you visit on the internet.

4. *Direct experience.*
   a) Traumatic experiences. For example, if you make a mistake in practice, such as nearly giving some medication to the wrong patient; this can profoundly affect your attitude towards carrying out the correct procedure so that you *never* make that mistake again.
   b) Positive experiences. For example, if a patient thanks you for your patience and understanding when helping them to eat, you are more likely to develop a positive attitude to the experience of feeding patients.
   c) Exposure. On your clinical placements you will see a variety of attitudes to both patients and to members of the healthcare team.
   d) Direct interaction. Your attitudes can be directly influenced by someone discussing your attitude with you.

5. *Social comparison and consensual validation.* You will probably notice that each placement has its own culture and that people have different attitudes toward aspects of care. A mental health placement will have a very different 'feel' to it compared with a special care baby unit.

6. *Heredity.* You may have inborn elements that make you tend towards positive or negative attitudes.

Activity 5.5

Think about your own attitudes to the following: work, sport, shopping, school, hospital, injections, patients, relatives, children, elderly people, Chinese people, teenagers, mental illness.

What do you think has influenced the development of your attitudes? There are no real right or wrong answers, but make a note of your thoughts and add them to your portfolio.

Woogara's (2005) ethnographic study involving observation and interviews with patients and staff found the following:

Patients did not feel that they mattered all the time. Certain behaviours by professionals were institutionally driven. Patients were routinely woken before 6 am and their sleep pattern was disturbed by professionals. Many activities, for example the completion of patients' vital signs, administration of morning medication and making certain groups of patients sit by their beds ready for breakfast, had to be completed before the arrival of the morning shift. Throughout the day, care of the patients was constantly interrupted by professionals no matter what the patient was doing at the time.

(Woogara 2005: 35)

By such actions, patients' needs for privacy and some solitude were not respected (Westin 1967). Although ward routines have certain benefits for professionals, sometimes we develop 'blind spots' through a habituation process that often makes us perform daily activities without reflection (Berger and Luckmann 1966; Menzies 1988).

Habituation

Habituation describes the process by which people respond less with the repetition of a *stimulus*, simply because they have got used to it. Common examples include the screening out of background noise such as the fridge, or becoming used to the feel of your clothes as you wear them.

Often, in situations where patients have a negative experience of their value in the care setting, nurses have routinized and stereotyped their work to the extent that, rather than holding an actively negative attitude to their patient, they simply no longer notice the behaviour or the responses it elicits. Woogara (2005) points out that this routinized behaviour actively prevents the achievement of the first privacy and dignity benchmark factor for good practice: that people feel they matter *all the time*.

Activity 5.6

Go to the Media Tool DVD, select **Skills Sets**, **Nutritional Intake**, then **Assisting patients to eat poor practice**, and scroll down to watch the clip **How not to feed a patient!**

- Which of the following words describes the nurse's attitude towards her patient? Patient, impatient, kind, unkind, compassionate, uncompassionate, respectful, disrespectful.
- Which of these words do you think describes the nurse's attitude towards the act of feeding her patient? Positive, negative.
- How much do you think is due to attitude, how much to habituation and how much to other stress-producing factors (e.g. shortage of staff)?

Our suggested answers are given at the end of the chapter.

Recognizing examples of good practice

Conveying a respectful and mindful attitude is achieved by a subtle blend of verbal and non-verbal behaviour, and the cultural conventions of common courtesy.

Activity 5.7

Go to the Media Tool DVD, select **Case Studies**, **Learning Disability (Alex)**, then **The nurses visiting Alex demonstrate good practice**, and watch the clip. What courtesies facilitate a respectful approach and a dignified discussion? See the end of the chapter for a suggested answer.

Identity and the personal world

Another important aspect of dignity is the extent to which the care setting and the care that patients receive take into account a patient's individual values, beliefs and personal relationships. Achieving respect for a patient's sense of personal identity is possible in an environment that values an individual's needs, respects their choices and understands diversity. *The Essence of Care* (DoH 2003b) uses the term 'personal world' to describe this: 'To look at a patient holistically, not only have they got physical needs, but social, spiritual and emotional needs, and they live in the context of who they are, their family, their lifestyle. All of that is going to affect how they respond to the illness they have' (p. 3).

Box 5.3 shows some terms which you might find useful in thinking and talking about what 'personal

---

Box 5.3 Our sense of self

- *Self-concept* (Who am I?) is our sense of identity, based on a set of beliefs that we have about ourselves. Personal identity is the combination of roles and group categories to which we belong and the personal meanings and significances they have for us, along with the traits and behaviours we use to describe ourselves. Self-concept is concerned with our beliefs and cognitions.
- *Self-schema* relates to more specific personality dimensions – such as independence, aggression and sociability – that make up our self-concept. People with a well-developed self-schema in relation to independence will be distressed in situations where their independence is threatened.
- *Self-awareness* is a state in which our attention is focused on our self.
- *Self-esteem* is our feelings of positive and negative self-evaluation.
- *Self-efficacy* is the learned expectation about whether we are capable of carrying out a behaviour or producing a desired outcome in a particular situation.
- *Self-perception* is when we judge our own dispositions, emotions and attitudes by our own behaviour.

world' and 'personal identity' mean. All of these ideas are involved in how we view and evaluate ourselves. Our self-presentation strategies, or impression management, is the way in which we attempt to create positive impressions regarding ourselves. We do this by monitoring ourselves in situations and to a greater or lesser extent regulating our behaviour to meet the demands of the situation or the expectations of others. The purpose may be either to please others or to confirm our own view of ourselves.

What is a stereotype?

Personal world and identity are the beliefs that we have about ourselves. These may not always be matched by how others see us because they might be 'pigeon-holing' or *stereotyping* us. Stereotyping is an over-generalized, inaccurate set of beliefs and expectations about a group and its members. People can be stereotyped according to gender, race, sexual orientation, nationality, class or role, among other things. Stereotyping is often used in jokes and cartoons which may be regarded as hurtful and tasteless. Stereotyping has no place in a patient-centred care system.

What is prejudice?

Prejudice is a usually negative preconceived judgement of a group and its members. It usually indicates a negative attitude towards something. Prejudice is often expressed as a stereotyping attitude. It has no place in a patient-centred health care system and it cannot support a reasoned and clinically sound approach to care planning or care delivery.

What is discrimination?

Discrimination is a negative behaviour, arising from prejudicial attitudes and stereotyping actions taken towards members of a group because of their membership of that group. Discrimination is illegal, as stated in Article 14 of the Human Rights Act 1998, which prohibits discrimination on the grounds of sex, race, colour, language, religion, political or other opinion, national or social origin, association with a national minority, property, birth or other status including age.

Activity 5.8

Go to the Media Tool DVD, select **Case Studies** and access the following clips: **Adult Health (Margaret)**, **Margaret arrives in hospital**, **Margaret and her husband in A+E**; **Child Health (Tom)**, **Introduction to Tom**; **Mental Health (Chris)**, **Chris to A&E**.

In each of these cases the nurse is careful to introduce herself by name, to establish rapport by asking questions in a respectful and friendly manner, and to take some time to develop a therapeutic relationship. Notice how the nurse strikes up a rapport with Tom by greeting him by his name and asking him if he slept OK. She follows this up immediately by telling him her name and describing to him exactly what she is about to do. This approach helps to create a relaxed atmosphere between the nurse and Tom and respects his individuality.

Stereotyping, prejudice and older people

Several studies (e.g. Cooper and Coleman 2001; Calnan *et al.* 2003) indicate that the dignity needs of older patients are often unmet. Prejudice against people purely on the grounds of age has been countered by both legal and policy changes which have successfully challenged overt discrimination, but ageist attitudes remain a serious issue (Social Care Institute for Excellence 2006).

In 2006, the Department of Health launched the 'Dignity in Care' campaign, which is aimed at eliminating such lack of respect (see Box 5.4).

Jacelon (2003) showed that older people in acute care used active strategies to manage their own dignity and to judge the amount of respect with which they were being treated. An earlier study by Jacelon *et al.* (2001) identified three phases in hospitalization through which older people's personal worlds and identities were threatened:

● *Phase 1, stabilization,* describes how they lost a sense of personal identity as hospital gowns, lack of privacy and the attention of a lot of people to their bodies catapulted them from their normal lifestyle. However, anxieties about their health and relief at

- Ensure your care is person-centred and not service- or task-centred.
- Ask people how they would like to be addressed and respect their wishes.
- Include time to talk as part of your care plan.
- Involve people in planning their own care.
- Ensure people have all the information they need and in a form that they can understand.
- Acknowledge the importance of social and family networks in well-being.

getting help often diminished the immediate impact of the loss of dignity. Patients in this phase actively introspect – one participant said: 'Your attitude towards the staff makes a big difference with respect to the way the staff treat you. You need to have a positive attitude toward the staff so that they treat you positively as well' (paraphrased from Jacelon *et al.* 2001: 80). Participants also indicated how they managed their 'image' and dignity, often by selecting what information they provided to the hospital staff.

- *Phase 2, re-establishing.* As the acute stage resolved, participants indicated a change in focus from their health to their self-identity and personal world. They told stories that recalled memories, particularly related to successes and influence on others. This had the effect of reminding both patients and staff of their worth and dignity. They also asked staff about their families and hobbies in order to establish a relationship that wasn't just nurse–patient.
- *Phase 3, normalization.* As the promise of discharge home emerged, participants felt greater dignity at the returning autonomy, improved health and gained resilience. They accepted this latter stage of hospitalization by thinking about times in their lives when they had survived difficult situations.

It is not only older people who may experience discriminatory or prejudicial attitudes. Patients who attempt suicide often experience the initial encounter at the hospital as difficult and are very sensitive to the attitudes and behaviours of the healthcare staff.

Negative attitudes can contribute to a powerful sense of shame, making it difficult to accept and benefit from psychiatric care (Wiklander *et al.* 2003).

Personal boundaries and space

We have to modify our sense of personal boundaries and personal space considerably when we enter healthcare. As a species we are highly territorial, but we are rarely aware of it until that space is violated.

Personal space and personal territory

The difference between personal space and personal territory is that personal space accompanies the individual while territory is stationary. Most patients assume that their bed and the space around it are their territory, including the bedside table and locker. However, Woogara (2005) found that this physical space and territory were largely determined by staff. Sitting on the patient's bed without his or her consent was a frequent occurrence, by both doctors and nurses. It was also common for staff to access a patient's personal belongings either in or on the lockers without seeking permission.

It is part of the care teams' responsibility to ensure that they do not violate temporary territory and personal space themselves, and that they are considerate and discreet in assisting patients to carry out activities that would usually be carried out independently and privately. You may wish to refer to Chapter 4 for further information.

Activity 5.9

Think about the practical skills that you will carry out on the ward – for example, taking someone's temperature, feeding them, passing a urinary catheter, administering an injection, administering suppositories. Identify how many of these actions involve entering the patient's *personal* space and how many will take place in a person's *intimate* space.

Activity 5.10

Go to the Media Tool DVD, select **Case Studies**, then **Child Health (Tom)** and watch the video clip **Tom brushes his teeth**.

Notice how during this activity both Tom's mum and the nurse operate within Tom's intimate space. He is cooperative with their requests and he does not seem to mind when the nurse tries on his toy glasses, but she didn't ask his permission to do so. Not every child will respond as graciously as Tom, but even so just observe how he holds on to the glasses in the immediate following frames. Personal space is particularly important when children are restricted to bed, as Tom is, because of the treatment required to manage his fractured femur. In Tom's situation virtually every encounter with those caring for him is a violation of his personal space. He cannot get away, so carers must be considerate in their engagement with him.

Now watch the video clips **Tom has his observations done** and **Tom has his pain relief**. What strategy of Tom's do you observe that may be helping him with his need for personal space? Write out your answers and add them to your portfolio. Then look at our suggested answer at the end of the chapter.

Illness and personal space

People are anxious and fearful when they are ill. Their intimate personal space is available to complete strangers for important clinical reasons which most people accept as inevitable. You need to be aware that this intrusion to personal space should only ever be made with informed consent and only for that intervention for which the consent has been given. Interestingly, the hospital ward round, by doctors, nurses and students, has been identified as an avoidable violation of personal space and personal boundaries.

Indignity

In a study by Walsh and Kowanko (2002), one patient experienced a loss of dignity when her body was used as an example to medical students: 'I had a catheter placed in my toilet area, if you know what I mean. I didn't really like having seven strangers that I didn't know from a bar of soap standing there and looking at my private bit' (Walsh and Kowanko 2002: 148). She went on to say, 'I thought that was a bit crude. I mean, you'd think they'd have dummies and stuff to do that . . . I don't think anyone would like to be used as an example.'

She is of course absolutely right and the unwarranted intrusion on her personal space can be seen as an act of aggression as well as a breach of Article 8 of the Human Rights Act. As a student it would be difficult for you to intervene in preventing this intrusion of space by the doctors ward round, however, it would be

worth discussing a situation such as this with your mentor.

Professional boundaries

The *therapeutic relationship* that you develop with patients is an important part of their individualized care. Personal warmth and a caring attitude are significant elements in this, as long as they remain at the level of human compassion. The NMC code of conduct (2008: 4) states that, 'You must maintain clear professional boundaries', and this principle encourages good judgement about the needs of the patient and meeting those needs through effective team planning.

Violations of professional boundaries can include:

- getting involved in a patient's personal affairs;
- buying or selling a patient's personal items;
- becoming involved in their lives as a friend or romantically.

These are violations because they tend to focus on the needs of, or the gain to, the nurse rather than the patient.

Communication and courtesy

Courteous communication with colleagues and patients conveys respect. *The Essence of Care* (DoH 2003b) makes the following distinctions regarding communication:

- *Communicated at*: talked at, talked over, unwarranted assumptions made regarding the patient's level of understanding.
- *Communicated with*: listened to, individual needs and views taken into account, respected as a person. Communication between patient and nurse demonstrates caring and concern and is at the correct pace and level.

Courtesy in healthcare settings involves not only the common social courtesies, but also making sure that your communication takes into account all your patient's needs. You can assess whether patients are experiencing a courteous encounter with you by their

Scenario 5.2

A 41-year-old Polish lady has been admitted to the endoscopy unit for a colonoscopy. She can speak some social English, but is accompanied by her teenage son who can speak both Polish and English. She looks withdrawn and talks to her son in Polish, and he says that she keeps telling him to go and that she can manage. What action would you take if the son did as his mother requested and left her alone in the hospital? See the end of the chapter for a suggestion.

Activity 5.11

Go to the Media Tool DVD, select **Skill Sets**, **Observations**, and then **Temperature-taking – bad practice**. What features of this scenario indicate that this patient is being talked *at*, rather than communicated *with*? Check your answers with the sample answer at the end of the chapter.
Now go to **Skill Sets**, **Observations**, **Taking temperature – good practice**, then read the following commentary.

Here the same nurse demonstrates good practice in communicating with patients. She introduces herself by name. She explains fully, using words that the patient will understand, what she is going to do and any temporary discomfort the patient may feel while the blood pressure is being recorded. She makes good eye contact with the patient and waits for a response, such as head nodding or verbal indicators that she understands. She draws attention to the equipment she is using, giving the patient the opportunity to ask questions, which she does. The nurse has clearly established a rapport in which the patient feels comfortable to ask questions. She chats with the patient and supports her during the discomfort of having her blood pressure taken. She gives the patient feedback on the results of her observations with indications of whether they are normal or not, and if not what the explanation might be. The nurse is right in the patient's intimate personal space. Her communication strategies are clearly aimed at constantly checking consent and maintaining the patient's dignity through respectful interactions.

Activity 5.12

Go to the Media Tool DVD, select **Case Studies, Tom** and watch the video clip **Tom has his pain relief**. This very brief clip illustrates several important points:

- The nurse *talks with* Tom.
- She is *seeking his view* of his pain rather than assuming she knows best.
- She uses a child-appropriate pain scoring chart which *helps Tom's understanding*.
- She *explains why* it is appropriate for him to have some pain relief.
- She offers Tom a choice as to the mode of medication and *accepts his request*.

In summary, the nurse communicates with Tom in a way which respects his individuality and is mindful of his age and stage of development.

verbal and non-verbal responses. It is important to adapt information to meet their individual needs and also keep an accurate record of the communications that take place. You need to ensure they have access to translation and interpretation services if they need them. See Chapter 2 for more information.

Confidentiality of patient information

The care that you deliver and record is only part of the total care that the patient receives. Sometimes information has to be shared with other members of the interdisciplinary team. This information is shared in several ways: at handover, during ward rounds, by referrals, across the telephone and in patients' records.

The Data Protection Act 1998 has a number of implications for how information is shared (Birrell *et al.* 2006). The right to confidentiality means that information should not be accessible to unauthorized people or other parties without the consent of the individual. Interdisciplinary working means that members of the team must share and coordinate care.

The NMC code (2008: 5) states that, 'you must keep your colleagues informed when you are sharing the care of others'. While many healthcare professionals would never discuss patients in public places either in or out of the hospital, confidentiality of information is more difficult to achieve in the wards where all that separates one bed from the next is a curtain.

Rylance (1999) found that dignity, privacy and confidentiality were poorly respected on children's wards and more than four-fifths of parents reported overhearing confidential information from 'ward rounds'. The ward rounds were made up of between one and eight people, sometimes more. Their structure varied according to the consultant leading the round. Some preferred a business round away from patients, followed by a bedside review; others conducted full discussion round the bedside. Rylance concluded that 'breaches of confidentiality and privacy and lack of respect for patients' dignity seemed primarily to be problems of attitude, behaviour and lack of thought' (p. 304).

Woogara (2005) notes that the present format of ward rounds by both nurses and doctors is one of the main vehicles of breaching the information privacy of patients. He consequently suggests that mobile patients be seen in designated quiet places.

Promoting privacy, dignity and modesty

There are several quite simple ways in which you can promote a patient's privacy and dignity and protect their modesty. To begin with, Box 5.5 defines the meaning of these three terms.

Box 5.5 Some definitions

Privacy –freedom from intrusion
Dignity – being worthy of respect
Modesty – not being embarrassed

A study by Walsh and Kowanko (2002) found that very similar ideas were held by patients and nurses in terms of their perceptions of dignity. These are outlined in Box 5.6.

Box 5.6 Perceptions of dignity

The staff perspective:

- Privacy of the body
- Private space
- Consideration of emotions
- Giving time
- The patient as a person
- The body as an object
- Showing respect
- Giving control
- Advocacy

The patients' perspective:

- Being exposed
- Having time
- Being rushed
- Time to decide
- Being seen as a person
- The body as an object
- Being acknowledged
- Consideration
- Discretion

Some simple measures that can protect patients from unwanted public view include:

- using curtains, screens, walls, clothes and covers;

- giving patients who cannot wear their own clothes appropriate garments that protect their modesty;
- providing facilities for patients to have access to their own clothes;
- providing the opportunity for patients to have a private telephone conversation;
- making sure that patients who are moving for investigations or transfer have adequate warm, protective and modest coverings.

A common observation in all the literature is the inadequacy of a curtain to ensure privacy. Curtains should be drawn fully to prevent embarrassing exposure of the patient to the gaze of others. There should be a culture on the ward that peeping through the curtains is not acceptable. You need to be aware that although the patient is not visible to others, conversations can easily be heard.

For this reason it is preferable whenever possible to help patients with their activities of living in the privacy of the bathroom or lavatory. (You may wish to refer to Chapter 8 on personal and oral hygiene for more information.) Every patient should have access to an area for bathing, showering and going to the lavatory that is clean and private. Some patients may need the assistance of nursing staff to achieve this and other ward staff should respect their privacy.

In one study (Walsh and Kowanko 2002), a nurse in charge of the shift explained that because the ward was short-staffed, she had to help with bathing patients. There was a constant stream of nurses walking into the bathroom to ask her questions, thus compromising her patient's modesty and dignity. The nurses would not have dreamt of walking into the bathroom like that in their own homes.

It can also be very embarrassing to use the commode by the bedside. Wherever possible, you should help anyone who is unable to use the lavatory unassisted by taking them there in a wheelchair, or helping them to use the commode in the privacy of the lavatory.

Clothing and dignity

There is also a strong culture in hospitals for all patients to identify themselves by wearing pyjamas, nightdresses or hospital gowns. The reasons for this are unclear, except for those who are acutely ill or are undergoing investigations or active treatment. In many phases of hospital care it is entirely appropriate for patients to wear their own clothes. If the hospital needs to provide a gown or night garments, these gowns should provide the patient with suitable dignity and close completely at the back.

Activity 5.13

Go to the Media Tool DVD, select **Case Studies, Child Health (Tom)** and watch the video clip **Tom needs a bedpan**. What does the nurse do to minimize Tom's embarrassment, and protect his modesty and dignity? Note your response before reading on. There is a suggested answer at the end of the chapter.

Now consider what you have just watched and considered in relation to the findings of Walsh and Kowanko (2002) outlined at the start of this section.

Contributing to patients' privacy and dignity

Developing practical skills and good techniques is an important aspect of your pre-registration experiences. In addition to practical competence in procedural skills, patients see your *time* as an integral part of being treated with dignity (Walsh and Kowanko 2002). A number of patients mentioned being rushed as compromising their dignity. They appreciated nurses who took the time to forewarn them of things that were about to happen. Patients also wanted nurses to recognize their innate individuality rather than being treated as a collection of human tissue. This includes acknowledging and greeting patients courteously, being considerate and anticipating a patient's needs, being discreet and using small talk to reduce embarrassment.

Activity 5.14

Go to the Media Tool DVD, select **Case Studies, Learning Disability (Alex)** and watch the video clip **Interview with Alex**.

What were Alex's views on how courteously he was treated? Compare your answer with the sample one at the end of the chapter.

The availability of an area for complete privacy for patients is not something that as a student you can provide yourself, but you need to be aware of how the need for complete privacy can be met. For example:

- you can create privacy in a patient's home;
- you can make patients aware of the availability of a 'quiet' and/or private space;
- you can ensure private areas are available;
- you can help patients to get to private areas such as a quiet room, gardens or a prayer room.

Privacy and risk

Sometimes an identified clinical risk means that patients may not be safe in complete privacy. Risk of self-harm is a good example. Chapter 6 covers this area more fully and discusses several levels of observation if a patient is at risk of harm to themselves or others. Possible harm includes suicide, self-harm, aggression and violence or an inability to maintain their safety. In acute general hospitals, risk can include falls, development of pressure ulcers, deterioration of medical condition, and life- and limb-threatening conditions. In child health, risk includes accidents if unsupervised during play or therapeutic activities, falls or ingestion of noxious substances.

Box 5.7 Events and incidents

A *near miss* is a potential for harm or error which is intercepted and which results in no harm to the patient. Lessons can be learned to improve patient care.

An *incident* is an event that has caused harm, or has the potential to harm a patient or visitor, that involves malfunction, loss of equipment or property, and also applies to any event that may lead to a complaint.

An *adverse event* is an unintended injury or complication, which results in disability, death or prolonged hospital stay and is caused by healthcare management rather than the disease process.

What is clinical risk?

Clinical risk is an avoidable increase in the probability of harm occurring to a patient. Events or incidents occur in daily practice that could affect the quality of patient care. Sometimes this can lead to harm; sometimes harm is avoided and is classed as a 'near miss'. When there is an incident, many factors relating to the

Scenario 5.3

You are working in a six-bedded ward as a first year student. Several things could happen which patients might ask you about, for example:

- when the patient in the next bed deteriorates and is moved to the intensive care unit;
- what is wrong with the patient opposite, when he keeps throwing off the bedclothes, clambering out of bed and falling?;
- a complaint that another patient is making about an alleged drug error.

What would your response be? Consider this before reading on.

You may have thought about the following. Complete privacy on a ward is difficult to achieve and confidentiality is sometimes breached by professionals inadvertently while on the ward. Also, the patients themselves may discuss certain things among themselves which as a nurse you are not able to engage in. However, in these circumstances you need to develop a professional attitude towards confidentiality and privacy. If the patient in the next bed has been moved, is restless or wandering, or you know they are making a complaint, you have no need to enlarge on this. You could explain to the patient, kindly, that because of confidentiality you are unable to disclose any further details, just as you would if it was information about them. If you are concerned that this patient may be worrying because they have a similar condition or fear, ask a senior colleague to speak to the patient about their concerns.

system, the environment and the individuals are involved. Clinical risk management provides a structured process of protocols and assessments to improve patient safety and prevent near misses, incidents and adverse events. Box 5.7 lists a range of events and incidents.

Clinical risk management

The aims of risk management are to reduce the frequency of adverse events and harm to patients, to reduce the chance of a claim being made and to control the cost of claims that are made. Risk management is the systematic process of identifying, evaluating and addressing potential and actual risk, through a well-designed programme that prevents, controls and minimizes risk exposure.

It is usual for near misses, incidents and adverse events to be reported as part of ongoing clinical risk management. However, any involvement of patients and clients in this process should be done in private without breaching confidentiality.

Restlessness and risk

In making an assessment of actual and potential risk of injury or falls in restless, confused or wandering patients, you need to take into account local policies, guidelines and protocols in relation to risk assessment. For example, there is now a requirement to complete and document a risk assessment in relation to the use of bed rails and the Medical Devices Agency (2001) have produced guidelines on bed rail use.

Activity 5.15

Go to the Media Tool DVD, select **Chapter Resources**, then **Privacy and Dignity** and work through the activities in each subsection. They draw attention to aspects of privacy and dignity in many of the clips in other sections of the DVD.

Summary and key points

This chapter has explored the role of privacy and dignity in delivering daily practical care. Remember that patients may have reasonable concerns for their privacy, dignity and modesty in all the activities of living, particularly washing and dressing, and meeting elimination needs. Privacy and dignity needs can be met using a sensitive balance of features of the environment, space, solitude, company, quiet, choices, good dining arrangements and protection from intrusion. All patients need access to a private space at some time where they can balance their needs for solitude and company and quietness and conversation.

It is important to remember the following key points:

● Stereotyping is irrational and leads to prejudice and discriminatory behaviours. Don't make assumptions about your patient based on their age, colour, gender, sexual orientation or creed.
● Personal space is an individual and cultural thing and you need be fully aware that your nursing role takes you right into a patient's personal space. Nurses develop skills in verbal introductions and using appropriate body language when approaching a patient.
● When giving practical care, check with the patient that they are comfortable with the care and that you have their consent.
● When seeking consent or negotiating care, make sure you are communicating 'with' and not 'at' patients. Be courteous to patients and staff.
● Remember how much a patient can pick up about your attitude from your non-verbal behaviour.

- Never divulge details of patients to anyone outside the clinical context and take care that clinical information cannot be overheard.
- Share clinical information (with the patient's consent) with other members of the interdisciplinary team to ensure good quality care.
- Whenever possible and appropriate, encourage patients to dress in their own clothes.

References

Berger, P. and Luckman, T. (1966) *The Social Construction of Reality: A Treatise in the Sociology of Knowledge*. New York: Doubleday.

Birrell, J, Thomas, D. and Alban Jones, C. (2006) Promoting privacy and dignity for older patients in hospital, *Nursing Standard*, 20(18): 41–6.

Calnan, M. Woolhead, G. and Dieppe, P. (2003) Older people: courtesy entitles, *Health Service Journal*, 113(5843): 30–1.

Cooper, S.A. and Coleman, P.G. (2001) Caring for the older person: an exploration of perceptions using personal construct theory, *Age and Aging*, 30(5): 399–402.

Department of Health (2003a) *Building on the Best: Choice, Responsiveness and Equity in the NHS*. London: HMSO.

DoH (Department of Health) (2003b) *The Essence of Care: Patient-focused Benchmarking for Health Care Practitioners*. London: The Stationery Office.

DoH (Department of Health) (2004) Benchmark for privacy and dignity, in *The Essence of Care: Patient-focused Benchmarking for Health Care Practitioners*. London: The Stationery Office.

DoH (Department of Health) (2006) *Dignity in Care*, www.dh.gov.uk/en/SocialCare/Socialcarereform/Dignityincare/index.htm, accessed 6 May 2008.

Erwin, P. (2001) *Attitudes and Persuasion*. London: Routledge.

Grandison-Markey, C. (2005) Choose the best editorial, *Multicultural Nursing*, www.nursing-standard.co.uk/multicultural/editorial.asp, accessed 22 February 2008.

Jacelon, C.S. (2003) The dignity of elders in an acute care hospital, *Qualitative Health Research*, 13: 543.

Jacelon, C.S. Conelly, T.W. Brown, R. Proulx, K. and Vo, T. (2001) A concept analysis of dignity for older adults, *Journal of Advanced Nursing*, 48: 76–83.

Medical Devices Agency (2001) *Advice on the Safe Use of Bed Rails*. London: MDA.

Menzies, I. (1988) *Containing Anxiety in Institutions: Selected Essays*, Volume 1. London: Free Association Books.

NMC (Nursing and Midwifery Council) (2002) An NMC guide for students of nursing and midwifery, www.nmc-uk.org/aFrameDisplay.aspx?DocumentID=1896, accessed 6 May 2008.

NMC (Nursing and Midwifery Council) (2008) *The Code, Standards of Conduct, Performance and Ethics for Nurses and Midwives*. London: Nursing and Midwifery Council.

Rylance, G. (1999) Privacy, dignity and confidentiality, *British Medical Journal*, 318: 301.

Social Care Institute for Excellence (2006) *Practice guide 09: dignity in care*, www.scie.org.uk/publications/practiceguides/practiceguide09, accessed 19 February 2008.

Walsh, K. and Kowanko, I. (2002) Nurses' and patients' perceptions of dignity, *International Journal of Nursing Practice*, 8: 143–51.

Westin, A. (1967) *Privacy and Freedom*. New York: The Bodley Head.

Wiklander, M. Samuellsson, M. and Asberg, M. (2003) Shame reactions after suicide attempt, *Scandinavian Journal of Caring Sciences*, 17(3): 293–300.

Woogara, J. (2005) Patients' rights to privacy and dignity in the NHS, *Nursing Standard*, 19(18): 33–7.

Answers

Scenario 5.1

The Data Protection Act stipulates:

- The right for data to be used only for the specific purpose for which it was collected.
- The right to confidentiality (see also Article 8 of the Human Rights Act).

Scenario 5.2

Your answer should include that if this is her wish, then an interpreter should be present to ensure informed consent. The interpreter will also need to be present after the investigation to explain the findings and to make sure she understands what she must do when she gets home.

Activity 5.1

Your answer might include that the nurse takes her time, she explains to the patient what she is doing, and she uses a non-hurried pace of speech and a gentle touch.

Activity 5.2

The behaviour clearly does not make Alex feel he matters. Article 10 is being breached. What is being demonstrated in the attitude towards Alex in this bad practice clip is a paternalistic, patronizing attitude and a lack of respect for his privacy and dignity.

Activity 5.3

Your answer should have included the following points related to the Human Rights Act:

- The nurse approaches Tom, and calls him by his name. She advises him what she is going to do (Article 8 – this is Tom's temporary home).
- The nurse looks with interest at what Tom is doing (Articles 8, 9 and 10).
- The nurse asks, 'Shall we clear away these paints?' rather than just taking over and imposing this action on Tom (Articles 8 and 10).
- The nurse appreciates the significance of what Tom is doing and so respects him as an individual as she knows he will soon be 10 (Article 8).
- She starts to clear away the paint pots by replacing the lids and asks Tom if he has finished with a particular colour before removing it (Articles 8, 9 and 10).
- The nurse does not rush Tom; she waits for him to indicate that he had finished what he wanted to do (Articles 8, 9 and 10).
- She offers to put his picture somewhere to dry, so giving value to his efforts (Article 10).
- She responds positively to Tom's request to return to the painting (Articles 8, 9 and 10).
- She recognizes that intervention is required to rectify the temporary deterioration of Tom's immediate environment with respect to the paint he was using, in order to facilitate Tom's consumption of his dinner in a pleasant, clean physical environment (Article 8).
- She also pays attention to Tom's personal hygiene needs (Article 8).
- She is content to let Tom assist in the cleaning activities both of the table and his hands (Article 10).
- She brings his dinner to him presented appropriately, and encourages him to try the food (Article 8).
- Although she has to say no to Tom's preferred choice of drink, she successfully steers him to a more suitable drink by modifying its mode of presentation and offering him a choice of flavours, so enhancing Tom's participation and esteem (Article 10).

Your answer should have included any or all of the following:

- She could have introduced herself by name, although it is subsequently apparent that Tom does know her (Article 8).
- She could have asked him how he was feeling (Article 9).
- She could have asked if he had finished with all of the colours before removing them (Article 10).
- She could have asked what Tom would like for his dinner, although her response would be constrained by what was available (Articles 9 and 10).
- She could have offered Tom a choice from what was available (Article 9 and 10).
- She could have stayed with Tom to encourage him to eat his meal (Article 10).
- She could have removed the skin from the chicken like his mum did when she arrived (Article 10).

Activity 5.6

- The following words describe the nurse's attitude towards her patient: unkind, uncompassionate and impatient.
- 'Negative' describes the nurse's attitude towards the act of feeding her patient.
- Whatever has influenced the development of this attitude, it is not acceptable.

Activity 5.7

Your answer may have included any of the following:

- They knock on Alex's door.
- They ask if it is OK to come in, just as they would if it were his house.
- They introduce themselves by name and shake his hand.
- They ask permission to sit down and the discussion is carried out with all seated at the eye level.
- They ask Alex questions to help elicit his understanding and views on his diabetes.
- They negotiate with him when would be a suitable time to come and visit him again.

Activity 5.10

Tom's headphones may just be helping him to escape from his immediate surroundings and giving him space where only he can go.

Activity 5.11

The following features indicate that this patient is being talked *at*, rather than communicated *with*:

- The patient is awoken rudely and the nurse tells her what she is going to do. She does not ask and therefore does not have the patient's consent.
- There is no eye contact between the nurse and the patient. The nurse is only interested in the readings on the machine.
- The nurse speaks very quickly and does not check that the patient has understood her. She rushes the patient and indicates clearly her impatience and exasperation.
- She does not offer any assistance or support when the patient coughs, she restrains the patient and ignores the discomfort the blood pressure cuff is causing her.

The nurse here is in breach of several aspects of the NMC code:

- As a registered nurse, midwife or specialist community public health nurse you must respect the patient or client as an individual.
- As a registered nurse, midwife or specialist community public health nurse you must obtain consent before you give any treatment or care.
- As a registered nurse, midwife or specialist community public health nurse you must maintain your professional knowledge and competence.

Activity 5.13

The nurse responds swiftly to Tom's request, dealing with it with no fuss and using language with which he is familiar and that he understands. In this way she minimizes his potential embarrassment. She also protects his modesty by drawing the curtains around his bed. You will also note that Tom is wearing day clothes, not pyjamas, and that the nurse encourages him to help her to help him by getting him to use the monkey pole while she places the bedpan beneath him, but without rushing him. At no time in this clip is Tom exposed in any way. A strategically-placed blanket protects his modesty throughout this intervention. The nurse shows her consideration for Tom as she leaves him in peace to allow him some privacy while letting him know that she is still accessible to him if he needs help. When Tom's mum arrives, the nurse tells her what is happening but neither the nurse nor his mum go behind the curtains until Tom says he is 'done'. His mum assists in the necessary bottom-wiping process, still with the blanket in place. The nurse removes the bedpan and then returns to the bedside to offer Tom the opportunity to wash his hands and so complete this particular elimination and personal hygiene experience.

Activity 5.14

Alex clearly identifies that in the first demonstration the nurses did not recognize his individuality or greet him courteously; they were inconsiderate and did not anticipate his needs. In the second demonstration Alex said he felt more dignified because the nurses involved him in the discussions and actively sought his views.

Safety of patients with mental health needs

Elizabeth Collier and Seán Welsh

6

Chapter Contents

Learning objectives

The aim of this chapter is to describe and discuss issues relating to the safety of clients with mental health needs in acute mental health and general hospital settings. Throughout the chapter we will be referring to the accompanying Media Tool DVD. Please watch the video clips as directed as these will reinforce your learning. After reading this chapter and interacting with the DVD you will be able to:

- Discuss issues of stigma and discrimination for people with mental health problems.
- Reflect on your approaches to meeting people's mental health needs in general hospital environments as well as mental health environments.
- Develop an understanding of self-harming behaviours.
- Describe the process of risk assessment.
- Identify skills relevant for managing aggression.
- Recognize the effect of street drugs on mental health.
- Discuss different ways of understanding mental ill health.
- Identify information, support materials and resources.

Introduction

An understanding of the concepts of mental health and mental ill health is important for nurses working in any setting. We know that if people feel emotionally and mentally supported, they will get better more quickly, and as Prince *et al.* (2007) state, there is 'no health without mental health'.

Mental health and mental ill health

Mental health exists on a continuum and has been defined as 'a state of well-being in which every individual realises his or her own potential, can cope with the normal stresses of life, can work productively and fruitfully, and is able to make a contribution to her or his community' (WHO 2007). It influences our thoughts and refers to our *emotional experiences*, *feelings* and *perceptions*, as well as our capacity to learn, to communicate and to form, maintain and end relationships.

Life stresses affect our mental health and our ability to cope with change, transition and life events (Scottish Executive 2005). Consider divorce, for example. While this is very stressful, people may cope with support from friends, counselling or mediation. If, however, during this process there is a death in the family, a prospect of homelessness or children have school difficulties as a result of the break-up, then the person is less likely to have the personal emotional resources to deal with all of this at the same time. They may have what some people call a 'nervous breakdown'. This term is commonly used in everyday life outside professional settings to refer to any emotional or mental health crisis. It is not a psychiatric or medical term.

Fed up or depressed?

Sometimes people may refer to themselves as 'depressed' in order to describe their feelings of low mood. This could be mistakenly confused with a clinical diagnosis of depression where low mood is only one symptom. The diagnosis of depression has clearly defined characteristics and symptoms, as defined by the WHO (1992). Possible symptoms are summarized in Box 6.1.

Clinical depression can be classified according to severity and is treated based on that severity. Consider how a person might respond to such a diagnosis. Some people may experience what is happening to them as a spiritual crisis. Marwaha and Livingstone (2002) illustrate this in the context of African-Caribbean perspectives of mental illness, where an older adult with *psychosis* and depression thought help from a spiritual leader was more appropriate.

Box 6.1 Symptoms people may experience if they are clinically depressed

Mood (affective)
Sadness
Hopelessness
Anxiety
Irritability
Agitation (most common in older adults)
Reduced energy
Inability to feel enjoyment
Loss or absence of interest in anything

Biological
Reduced appetite
Loss of weight
Variation of mood at different times of day (diurnal variation)
Sleep disturbances
Decreased sexual interest (libido)
Cessation of menstruation (amenorrhoea)

Cognitive (thinking)
Reduced concentration
Reduced attention
Ideas of guilt
Ideas of worthlessness
Reduced self-esteem
Psychotic symptoms
Suicidal thoughts

Behavioural
Neglect of personal appearance
Neglect of personal hygiene
Self-harm

Cultural aspects

Cultural distinctions are extremely important when considering these issues as they may not 'fit' with western ideas of health, and the way our mental health services are organized reflects this. There are many questions about why the proportion of black people in mental health services differs from people of other ethnic backgrounds (Commission for Health Care Audit and Inspection 2007). Sashidharan (2001) examines this issue and indicates that the overall experience of mental health services by black and South Asian people in the UK (and also Irish people) remains largely negative and aversive to the extent that black and South Asian people are disadvantaged in every single aspect of modern mental healthcare.

Many of the arguments are framed around whether practitioners misinterpret 'symptoms' and behaviours of people from differing cultures. In addition, western ideas of medicine have tended to separate physical health from mental health, whereas this has not happened in the same way in eastern cultures that tend towards more holistic understandings of health.

Activity 6.1

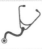

Read the MIND booklet on *Understanding Mental Illness* at www.mind.org.uk/Information/Booklets/Understanding/Understanding+mental+illness.htm. Think about how the information may apply to people from differing cultures.

Background theories

There are a number of different theoretical perspectives that help us understand mental ill health. Some examples of these can be seen in Box 6.2. These theoretical approaches have been derived from thinking related to sociology, psychology and neurobiology. There is not a single theoretical explanation for mental ill health, since well-being exists on a continuum in which many factors come into play.

Stress vulnerability theory and schizophrenia

Schizophrenia is a psychiatric diagnosis or classification that is commonly described as being linked with *stress*. A stress-vulnerability model by Zubin and

Box 6.2 Examples of different theories of mental illness

- Psychodynamic
- Biomedical
- Cognitive-behavioural
- Behavioural
- Stress vulnerability
- Learned behaviour
- Social construction

Activity 6.2

Go to the Media Tool DVD, select **Case Studies, Mental Health (Chris)** and read the **Introduction to Chris**. Then go to **Chapter Resources**, select **Mental Health Needs – Weblinks and Activities** and then work through Activity 6.2, **Shirley asks for her blood results – poor nursing response**.

Where would you place these patients on a continuum from poor to good mental health? Do you think they would agree?

Activity 6.3

Go to the Media Tool DVD, select **Chapter Resources** and then **Mental Health Needs Weblinks and Activities** and then work through Activity 6.3. This will give you an overview of the way mental health can be classified, theoretically explained and treated.

Spring (1977) explains the symptoms of schizophrenia as the effect of environmental stresses on the 'vulnerable' individual. The model suggests that each person has unique biological, psychological and social elements which include strengths and vulnerabilities for dealing with stress. It assumes that external and/or internal stressors can potentially elicit a crisis in *all* humans, and how a person deals with these *stressors* and *triggers* affects whether they maintain their *psychological equilibrium*, or experience psychological deterioration. So what are these 'vulnerability factors'? They include:

- basic information processing difficulties;
- biological factors;
- not taking prescribed medication;
- social skills difficulties;
- environmental stressors (such as substance misuse and social stressors, for example, unsettling life events, or a hostile or critical family environment).

The distress caused by the symptoms themselves is linked to the patient's own ways of coping with them. Falloon and Talbot (1981) studied the coping strategies employed by people who experienced *auditory hallucinations* and concluded that those who had a range of strategies available to them coped better with their voices. Tarrier (1987), however, when considering a broader range of psychotic symptoms, suggested that patients who applied a consistent strategy had the most successful results.

Anxiety as a mental health problem

In *anxiety*-provoking circumstances, the feelings and symptoms of anxiety can be helpful and are not normally problematic. However, if anxiety is prolonged and interferes with a person's everyday life, it may be considered a mental health problem. A person with a severe anxiety disorder can experience a lack of many of the positive features of mental health, as described by the WHO (2007).

Anxiety is a psychological state that has physical effects, and treatments will often treat the physical symptoms which assist in reducing the psychological

effects. The link here between biological and mental state is clear.

Despite your feelings and mental state, there are biological explanations for many of these symptoms, as shown in Box 6.3. When reacting to anxiety-provoking situations, the body initiates a reaction, which in turn triggers a range of physical systems in readiness to stand and fight, or alternatively to run away from the perceived threat. This is known as the 'fight or flight' response and it is the hormone adrenalin which produces it.

Box 6.3 Biological explanations of anxiety reactions

- Blood flow is redirected from digestive organs to your 'fighting muscles', making you feel sick or creating the feeling of 'butterflies' in your stomach.
- Body systems slow down – for example, there is decreased saliva output which induces the feeling of a dry mouth.

Self-harm

Self-injury is a behaviour, not a diagnosis, and people who experience mental ill health of any kind may find themselves thinking about self-harm. Self-harm commonly includes frequent overdoses, cutting and other high-risk behaviours.

Box 6.4 Possible explanations for self-harm (Kinsella and Kinsella 2006)

- To take control – for example, control over your own body after abuse.
- To release tension – for example, as relief from anger and frustration.
- As a means of communication – non-verbal communication of distress when there are no alternatives or *it feels as if* there are no alternatives.
- Stimulation – release of desired endorphins through pain.
- Negative body image – self-punishment reinforces negative feelings about oneself.

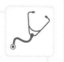

Activity 6.4

When you feel exceptionally anxious, for example, before an exam or interview, how do you feel?

You may have listed some of the following: feeling sick; shaking; diarrhoea; 'butterflies' in your stomach; dry mouth; increased heart rate; palpitations; heavy, rapid or difficult breathing; difficulty concentrating; feeling tired; feeling irritable; problems sleeping; sweating; tension and pains; dizziness; fainting; indigestion.

Cognitive-behavioural therapy

Cognitive-behavioural therapy (CBT) postulates a link between thoughts, feelings and behaviours where challenges to thought processes can change feelings and thus behaviour, or challenges to behaviour can then change thoughts and emotions. The approach is used in therapy to help people manage stress and grief, deal with worry and cope with psychosis. CBT is relatively quick and therefore not as expensive as some of the alternatives.

Substance misuse and addiction

Substance misuse can be considered a form of self-harm. The occurrence of a substance misuse problem, such as the misuse of alcohol and/or other substances including illegal drugs, solvents and over-the-counter medicines, and mental illness in the same patient at the same time is often referred to as a *dual diagnosis*. A person with substance misuse problems is three to six times more likely to have an additional mental health problem and vice versa (Regier *et al.* 1990). Menezes *et al.* (1996) found in a study of patients with a psychotic illness that 36 per cent also had substance misuse problems.

Patients with a dual diagnosis often have very complex needs and are frequently among the most socially excluded. Many of the negative outcomes are related to mental illness and substance misuse, such as an increased incidence of relapse in mental ill health, physical ill health (including sexually transmitted diseases) and substance dependency, demoralization, disengagement from services, non-concordance with treatment, repeated hospitalizations, suicide, violent behaviour, repeated imprisonment, homelessness and early mortality.

It is not always clear whether the substance misuse or the episode of mental illness is the primary diagnosis because substance misuse and mental illness can compound each other. There is also potential for confusion in terms of symptomology since signs and symptoms of mental illness may be mimicked by those of intoxication and withdrawal, and vice versa, potentially leading to misdiagnosis (Cohen 1995).

There is some debate (Smith 2002; Wenger *et al.* 2003; Hickman *et al.* 2007) about whether an addiction to cannabis can develop. There is also a growing body of evidence that links the use of cannabis with the development of schizophrenia (Smit *et al.* 2004; Macleod 2007). One argument is that cannabis triggers schizophrenia in vulnerable individuals.

In some cases, drug-induced psychosis can occur only when the drug is used. The assessment of Chris on the Media Tool DVD, when he arrives in A&E, is complicated by his psychosis. First, he has been consuming cannabis and, second, psychotic-type symptoms can occur when a person has taken an overdose of paracetamol, which he is thought to have done.

Activity 6.5

Think about the effect that drugs can have on mental health. Go to the Media Tool DVD, click on **Case Studies**, **Mental Health (Chris)**, then **Chris is discharged**, and view the slides about heroin and crack cocaine. Reflect on your own attitudes and knowledge.

Sociological issues

From a sociological point of view, there are a number of issues that are both the result of developing understanding of mental ill health over time and the influence of these changes in shaping future attitudes. These are indicated in Box 6.5.

Box 6.5 Sociological influences on mental health

- Decriminalization of suicide in 1961. However, the phrase 'committing suicide' remains, indicating a crime is being committed and hence perpetuating stigma.
- Decriminalization of homosexuality in 1967.
- Removal of homosexuality from psychiatric classification in 1973.
- Removal of epilepsy from psychiatric classification in the 1970s.

Attitudes towards mental health

Current attitudes towards mental illness can appear contrary. On the one hand, stigmatizing language is used in the media and in everyday life, such as the 'Bonkers Bruno' headlines in *The Sun* newspaper in 2006, when the boxer Frank Bruno was admitted to a mental health unit diagnosed with bipolar disorder, and *The Sun* apologized for their headline after a critical backlash. There have been a number of high profile 'celebrity' people who have disclosed their mental ill health and the use of 'rehabilitation' appears to be an acceptable place for 'celebrities' to go.

However, developments within mental healthcare include challenges to societal attitudes to disability and *labelling*. People with severe mental health problems can feel quite disabled by their experiences and can qualify for disability benefits. But it is not always helpful to think of mentally ill people as disabled (Sayce 2000). Current concepts of 'recovery' encourage people to view mentally unwell people in terms of their personal development and progress through life, where the challenge of mental ill health may be one of the life experiences they need to make sense of. The focus is not on 'symptoms' but on aspirations and life goals in the context of people's own lives (Repper and Perkins 2003).

Given the wide range of attitudes, beliefs, values and theories about mental ill health, some of which are discussed here, it is arguably reflected in service provision that there is an attempt to operate within a bio-psychosocial approach to care, where a multi-disciplinary team considers the biological, psychological and social aspects of a person's needs. Activity 6.6 examines some of the ideas outlined above and looks at how bio-psychosocial issues are all relevant when considering the help someone experiencing mental ill health may need.

The general care setting

All the issues outlined so far are relevant for nurses working in any healthcare setting. The examples provided on the Media Tool DVD are about people with specific mental health problems and may be considered complex. It is important that fundamental skills related to respect and human dignity are not overlooked by busy practitioners.

Familiarity with the technical complexities of healthcare work may prevent practitioners from stepping back from their practice and reflecting on how they are perceived or the effects that their behaviour

Activity 6.6

Consider the following behaviours:

- Getting drunk every night and during the day.
- Having sex with acquaintances.
- Having the TV and the radio on very loud most of the time.
- Preoccupation with religion to the exclusion of all else.
- Being argumentative and falling out with family and friends.
- Being consistently late for work.

What would you think if someone you knew began to behave like this? If you found out that this person was hearing abusive voices and they were trying to drown them out with other noise and self-medicate with alcohol, would this change your opinion?

What do you think the social consequences of these behaviours might be? Check your answer to this question with the answer at the end of the chapter.

has on patients, relatives and visitors. The National Collaborating Centre for Mental Health has suggested that professional responses are often negative and lacking in empathy (NCMH 2004).

Helping patients adjust to the hospital environment

When people are admitted to hospital, they are likely to be experiencing anxiety both about their state of health and also in relation to an unknown, unfamiliar and often frightening environment. It is easy to forget this when you are very familiar with your working environment. Consider Activity 6.7.

It will now be useful to consider Chris's mental health in relation to his physical environment.

Now add to the scenario outlined above the fact that the reason for attending hospital is because you were in such mental anguish that you tried to kill yourself. Or that you had tried to kill yourself because voices told you to, voices you did not like, voices that tormented you and controlled you, and voices that you are afraid of. You are worried about going to hospital because you have read about some people having bad experiences where staff have been dismissive, rude and unkind.

Activity 6.7

Have you ever been on holiday in an unfamiliar country and felt uncomfortable, self-conscious or awkward because you did not know the language, customs or way in which you are expected to behave? For example, when ordering a drink, do you go up to the bar, request and pay for it, or do you sit down and wait for someone to come and take your order? Do you go and pay at the bar, or do you ask the waiter for a bill? Will they be offended if you leave a tip or if you don't leave a tip?

You may recognize some of these feelings from your initial attendance at your first clinical placement. You may have subsequently learned some of the language, customs and etiquette and perhaps you also have some sense of what you can expect next time.

Compare your experiences with a patient arriving at a hospital for the first time; the patient is unlikely to have your knowledge to draw upon and in addition to the emotions already identified you can also factor in that they are probably frightened, ill and distressed.

If you were this patient, what do you think would help you feel better? Your answer may include the following:

- If people say 'hello', smile and introduce themselves.
- If people acknowledge you if you look a little lost.
- If people offer to help you find out what you need to do.
- If people explain the environment and what you can expect to happen next.
- If people make time for you and show you respect.
- If staff demonstrate competence.

Activity 6.8

Go to the Media Tool DVD, select **Case Studies**, **Mental Health (Chris)**, **Chris is told about the mental health ward**. You will see that some issues have been listed in relation to Chris's mental health and his physical environment. These are context-specific, but the principles are the same as those considered in this chapter. If his communication needs are addressed, this will also meet some of his mental health needs as he will feel more secure. Potentially everything you do as a nurse will have an effect on a patient's mental health – for example, whether they feel insignificant and dismissed (adding to any distress) because you are not listening to their concerns, or in control because you have taken the time to explain information and procedures to them.

If as a patient you experience the actions listed in Chris's case study, you might feel more secure, safer, more relaxed and less stressed as your feelings of anxiety settle down.

Although there may be some differences in the physical environment, purpose and philosophy of different hospital settings, there are many similarities including, for example, the responsibility for infection control, prevention of falls and pressure ulcers, and meeting the safety needs of people whose perceptions render them at risk if unsupervised. In hospital settings the ward orientation should include the physical layout of the ward, the ward routine, a description of the roles and responsibilities of the ward staff and the members of the interdisciplinary team, and any other specific information such as visiting times, mealtimes and hand-washing precautions. Wherever possible the relatives and/or carers should be included and questions encouraged. Chapter 2 will help you to communicate the necessary information, which should be available in an appropriate language or in Braille and be a combination of words and pictures to enhance understanding. If these are not available, a nurse should spend time with the patient ensuring the information is understood. It may be necessary to use an interpreter and further support may be needed from another resource. When the orientation process is complete, it should be recorded in the clinical notes as indicated in Chapter 3.

Activity 6.9

Go to the Media Tool DVD, select **Case Studies**, **Mental Health (Chris)**, **Chris arrives on the mental health ward**, and have a look at both the good and bad practice clips of Chris arriving on the mental health ward. Then complete the exercises. The scenario equally applies to a patient arriving at a general hospital ward.

Now go back to when Chris arrives at casualty, and watch the media clip of the nurse explaining what's going to happen. How do you think her approach might affect Chris's understanding of what is happening? Think about the verbal and non-verbal language she uses.

Check your response with our suggestions at the end of the chapter.

Another complicating factor in communicating with Chris is that he believes that the X Men told him to take the paracetamol. How would you respond to him if he spoke to you about this?

Now look at the **Mental Health (Chris) – Introduction to Chris – Key points lectures**. This will give you some ideas. Write out your answers and add them to your portfolio.

Activity 6.10

List the resource materials that you think might help Chris and other patients to be better orientated to a general hospital ward or an acute mental health setting. Check your answer with that at the end of the chapter.

Risk assessment

In most hospital settings nurses carry out a 'risk assessment' as a routine part of every admission. Risks include falls (a bed rail assessment may be necessary), pressure sores and risks related to orientation, mood, confusion, mobility, pain and discomfort. 'Orientation' for the patient includes negotiating any interventions deemed necessary to prevent risk or harm. Assessment of risk for a mental health patient includes the aforementioned risk assessment and also a risk assessment of harm to self and others.

Activity 6.11

Go to the Media Tool DVD, select **Skill Sets**, **Risk and Comfort**, then **Falls risk assessment**, **Bed rail assessment**. Read through these and try and identify any potential risks to patients on your ward.

Risk of harm to self

Caring for people who harm themselves can be a source of anxiety for staff, particularly when trying to assess the risk patients may pose to themselves. The reality is that none of us can read minds and our assessments may reflect our own anxieties, rather than any justifiable reasoning that the person is at risk of harming themselves. One of the main considerations in attempting to conduct an assessment of risk to self is the intentions of the person who has harmed themselves. They may be able to state quite clearly that they intended to end their life. Or they may tell you that harming themselves helps them cope with severe emotional distress, and that is in fact what keeps them *alive* (Rayner and Warner 2003).

Activity 6.12

What are some of the behaviours that people commonly engage in to help them cope with stress?

Your answer might include drinking alcohol, taking drugs, exercise and comfort eating.

What are the risks and benefits of each of these behaviours? Compare your thoughts to the sample answer at the end of the chapter.

The risks you identified in the exercise above probably pinpointed the fact that such behaviours can themselves cause harm to a person and yet people often continue to behave in the same way, despite knowing the harm that they can do. Thinking of self-harm in this way normalizes it. This removes the *stigma* that many people attach to what may be viewed as more extreme forms of self-injury, such as overdose or cutting arms and legs with razorblades. The action of cutting oneself in this way is sometimes described as a relief in relation to emotional distress and the only thing that made sense at that particular moment, but equally it may be followed by feelings of shame (Rayner et al. 2005). The negative after-effects do not stop a person seeking that same relief time after time, in the same way that someone who frequently gets drunk to alleviate stress (even though they know they will feel awful the next day) does not cease engaging in excessive drinking.

It is tempting at times to make assumptions about the level of risk associated with a particular diagnosis. This is not necessarily helpful and it is therefore important to understand individual mental health needs before discussing risk assessment.

Activity 6.13

Consider your own attitudes to self-injury and suicide and note them down. Examine what you have just written. How do you think that your attitudes would affect the way you would care for someone who has self-injured or tried to kill themselves?

What support do you think you need in order to understand and work with people effectively in such situations? Make a note of your answer and then check our suggestion at the end of the chapter.

People will experience 'symptoms' differently and they will be personal, but there are some general issues which may help in your risk assessment. Much work has been done in recent years to develop tools that can assist practitioners to assess whether someone is high risk or low risk. A number of characteristics have been found to be more common indicators for risk assessment.

First, for attempted suicide, whether the person has tried to kill themselves before. This may indicate that this person is able to consider suicide as a possible solution to their problems. Second, whether anyone in their family has killed themselves or tried to kill themselves, as this may indicate that they have learnt that it is a possible solution to their problems – i.e. it is an option (Hill 1995). If either of these is the case, then this information needs to be carefully recorded.

Vigilant and systematic records are the best way of organizing such information so that all risks are considered (see Chapter 3). For Chris it is likely that his particular psychotic symptoms, substance use and personal attitudes/feelings to these are the significant issues in his risk assessment. As a young man he is also in a high-risk group. He can probably be considered medium to high risk of self-harm on admission to A&E, but by the time he arrives at the mental health unit this has probably reduced to medium risk given that he is making positive choices about receiving help and his drug consumption has been nil for the time he has been at the hospital.

Assessment

Activity 6.14

Go to the Media Tool DVD. Select **Case Studies**, then **Mental Health (Chris)**, then **Chris is moved to the medical emergency unit**. Is there anything you would add to this assessment or do you think it identifies all the issues from the information available?

Risk assessment tools often appear to rely on largely quantitative (measurable) information, although clinical records will often contain more qualitative (in-depth) information – that is, including what the person is thinking, feeling, expressing, and their behaviour. One issue that has been consistently found in the research is that more suicides occur within a short time of discharge from hospital or a visit to the GP (DoH 2002). Appleby (2001) found that 23 per cent of people who killed themselves did so within three months of being discharged from hospital.

For reasons such as this, policies relating to *community psychiatric nurses* (CPNs) often state a follow-up visit time limit of one week following discharge from psychiatric units. For staff working in general hospital settings, informing the patient's CPN if they have one, and/or their GP, is essential and can contribute to the person's risk management.

Cattell and Jolley (1995) found that specialist services were seeing less than 25 per cent of older people with depression in the community who later went on

Box 6.6 Older adults and depression

- There is a high prevalence of mental ill health in older people in general hospital wards, possibly as high as 60 per cent (RCP 2005).
- High numbers of people with depression in general hospitals are not recognized or diagnosed (DoH 2001).
- Depression is implicated in most suicides (Cattell and Jolley 1995).
- Recognizing and treating depression in general hospitals will contribute to reducing the suicide rate for older people (DoH 2001).

to kill themselves, and nurses working in general settings may be in a good position to identify such people. Box 6.6 examines the issue of older adults and depression.

Young men between the ages of 15 and 24 are believed to have the highest suicide rate, and this accounts for 20 per cent of all deaths in this age group (MIND 2004). However, in England and Wales, males aged 65 and over accounted for 375 (11.4 per cent) of all suicides in 2003.

Chris falls into the young men category. Shafii (1989) states that there appears to be a reluctance to acknowledge suicidal feelings in the very young and this reluctance infiltrates youth suicide statistics. Box 6.7 identifies the other key groups at risk of suicide.

Box 6.7 High-risk groups

- Young men (aged 18–24)
- Young Asian women
- Farmers
- Doctors and nurses
- Prisoners

Risk assessments often try to identify 'protective' factors – i.e. issues and/beliefs of individual people that may prevent them from making the decision to commit suicide. Some religious denominations consider suicide to be a sin; however, this does not mean that people belonging to such religious groups do not kill themselves. It has been suggested that all that this

Activity 6.15

The use of alcohol or drugs is also implicated in suicide risk. What help is available in your local NHS Trust for supporting staff using alcohol or drugs in stressful environments? Make a note of your findings in your portfolio.

does is protect people from talking about it and if this is the case then they are potentially *more* at risk (Pritchard and Baldwin 2000). The best source of information is to ask the individual person.

Box 6.8 Web links

You will be able to find some useful web links for outside user agencies in the **Chapter Resources Mental Health Needs** section of the Media Tool DVD.

Risk of harm to others

This has the same complexity as assessment of harm to self. It is arguably more contentious as it involves harm to other people. The reporting of serious crime committed by someone who has a psychiatric diagnosis tends to be quite subjective in the media. This could relate to society's need to label 'perverse' or extreme behaviours as nothing to do with them. Even when a person does not have a psychiatric diagnosis but, for example, murders someone, people want to call them a 'psycho' or label that person as a 'nutter'. This has implications for how society learns and experiences such extremes of behaviour, and serious implications for those people who do not engage in criminal behaviour, but who *do* have a psychiatric diagnosis.

Misunderstanding and fear fuelled by media reporting may shape attitudes to people who are mentally ill. It is a consistent finding that we are more likely to be killed by someone in our own family or someone we know than by a stranger, and that people diagnosed with mental illness are a small minority of such cases (NPSA 2006). For the rare, but sensationalized, stories of mentally ill people who have attacked someone, it would not be unsurprising to learn that they have been given a diagnosis of paranoid schizophrenia or dissocial personality disorder.

Paranoid schizophrenia is a type of schizophrenia that is characterized by paranoid beliefs and dominated by the presence of paranoid symptoms such as *delusions* of persecution or jealousy, and threatening auditory hallucinations such as hearing voices (Puri 1995). For example, a person may believe that people are after them, that they are going to be killed and consequently that any subsequent acts of violence will be in self-defence. Or, the stressful and distressing experience of hearing voices telling the person what to do and goading them can result in a person 'acting' this out.

Dissocial personality disorder is characterized by irresponsible and antisocial behaviour, callous unconcern for others, disregard for social norms and obligations, incapacity to maintain enduring relationships, a low threshold for anger and frustration, and an incapacity to feel guilt or learn from being punished (Puri 1995).

In contrast, 'borderline personality disorder' is a diagnosis often given to people who self-harm by cutting themselves. These people are internalizing any anger by attacking themselves rather than attacking other people. Risk cannot be determined by diagnosis, however. It is important to understand a person's experience and thinking, as this will provide insight into their mental state and current reasoning.

Attempting to determine the risk a person poses to other people is a contentious issue. However, assessing risk to other people is taken very seriously and there is an attempt to constantly develop our understanding as to how this can be done. As with assessment of risk to others, the history of behaviour is one of the most important factors in this assessment. If someone has been violent in the past, they are more likely to be violent in the future.

Normal or abnormal emotions?

One problem that people with mental illness diagnosis often complain of is that of not being allowed to experience normal emotion. Whenever they get angry, people dismiss it as a 'symptom' rather than a justifiable expression of anger. For this reason it important to consider the environment where any aggression happens, and its context, in order to attempt to assess the risk. Box 6.9 provides a link to a helpful document.

Box 6.9 Web link – NMC guidance

The NMC has guidance on 'The recognition, prevention and therapeutic management of violence in mental health care' at the following link: www.nmc-uk.org/aFrameDisplay.aspx?DocumentID=664.

Scenario 6.1

Consider a relative who gets a call to say that their child has been involved in a serious road traffic accident and has been taken to hospital in an ambulance. They will most likely grab the car keys, race to the hospital in a state of high anxiety and stress and, if unable to find a parking space, will be in extreme distress, may abandon the car and rush in, shouting for information. They have no capacity to calm down and there is a potential for aggression here. To ask them to calm down and stop shouting is more likely to exacerbate their agitation. They may feel you are not listening.

Activity 6.16

Go to the Media Tool DVD, select **Chapter Resources** and then **Mental Health Needs Weblinks and Activities** and then work through Activity 6.16. Notice how the poor nursing response clip portrays Shirley being aroused to anger and the fact that the behaviour the nurse engages in contributes to an escalation of the situation. Note how a situation can be prevented before it arises. In the second clip showing a good nursing response you can see how, with support from the nurse Joanne, Shirley remains calm.

Understanding the precipitating factors does not mean you condone violence or aggression, but it does mean that you can arm yourself against being at the receiving end through your own skills rather than reacting emotionally.

Scenario 6.2

How might you respond to the situation described in Scenario 6.1 in a way that is most likely to reduce the risk of aggression?

Go to the Media Tool DVD, select **Chapter Resources** and then **Mental Health Needs Weblinks and Activities** and then work through Key Points lecture in Scenario 6.2. Which of the skills noted in the slides would you apply to the scenario above?

If the relative in Scenario 6.1 returned to their car to find it clamped, they would likely feel extremely angry, which in turn could increase the risk of aggression. Box 6.10 provides a link concerning 'zero tolerance' policy in healthcare.

Box 6.10 Department of Health zero tolerance policy

The NHS has a zero tolerance policy with regard to aggressive behaviour which can be viewed via the following link: www.dh.gov.uk/en/ Publicationsandstatistics/Lettersandcirculars/ Dearcolleagueletters/DH_4002937

Although clearly staff can expect to work free of the risk of assault, it remains important to reflect on the implications of a policy of zero tolerance. There is a danger that an expectation of zero tolerance develops an environment and culture that do not try to be skilful in managing the potential of violence in a way that prevents such behaviour.

It could be argued that an immediate punitive reaction of zero tolerance is *more likely* to exacerbate and inflame the situation and result in conflict. In contrast, sympathy, engagement and empathy on the part of the staff (which patients and relatives should be able to expect) may be more effective in certain circumstances.

Useful sources for risk assessment

As the guidelines from the Scottish Executive (2002) state, a single source of information should not be relied upon. Team meetings are a useful forum to discuss risk assessment and collate information. Knowledge of a client's history, social context and significant events should be ascertained, including sharing of information and liaison between general and mental health settings.

Risk assessment is an ongoing and changeable entity and can alter within minutes. Each decision may require a new assessment relating to the specific circumstances. It is also important to consider how staff are supported in their management of such difficult circumstances. Clinical supervision may be one way that this is done, but there should also be an opportunity in team meetings to debrief. Box 6.11 provides information about where staff can access help.

Box 6.11 Web links

You can find some useful links to domestic violence help lines, anger management and victim support, together with other relevant areas in the **Chapter Resources Mental Health Needs** on the Media Tool DVD.

Observation versus privacy

Observation, in the context of mental health issues, usually relates to observing people to ensure they remain safe. This is a risk management strategy. People whose safety may be at risk, or who may be at risk of compromising other people's safety, may need to be observed more closely. There is an inconsistent understanding of 'close observation' and different settings may have their own definitions and classifications. In 1999, the Department of Health published the *Standing Nursing and Midwifery Advisory Committee (SNMAC) Practice Guidance: Safe and Supportive Observation of Patients at Risk*. It states that: 'Observation is not simply a custodial activity. It is also an opportunity for the nurse to interact in a therapeutic way with the patient on a one-to-one basis' (DoH 1999: 2). It also states that:

'Observing a patient who is deeply distressed and potentially suicidal is one of the most difficult and demanding tasks that a nurse can undertake. Observation calls for empathy and engagement, combined with readiness to act. Whereas most nursing interventions are intended to help patients achieve their own goals, observation is deliberately designed to frustrate the patient's aims. Consequently, patients who are being observed may be very angry with staff, or may experience the process as custodial and dehumanising.'

(DoH 1999: 2)

It is this potentially dehumanizing experience that is of the most concern when attempting to balance privacy with a safe environment. If this is how a person feels, then it is not a psychologically safe environment, only a physically safe one. The attempt to stop suicide or harm to others is a compelling rationale for taking such action and if a risk assessment indicates high risk, then not implementing the observation policy would be difficult to justify and may be considered negligent. It is in this context that staff need to develop skills to minimize psychological harm.

Box 6.12 Levels of observation

The SNMAC recommends four levels of observation. These are explained in more detail in the **Chapter Resources** and then **Mental Health Needs Weblinks and Activities** and then Box 6.12:

- Level I: general observation
- Level II: intermittent observation
- Level III: within eyesight
- Level IV: within arm's length

Local policy should always be checked for local interpretations of observation policy. Level IV is the most invasive level of observation and means that the observer would have to stay with the person at all times including when they visit the toilet. Attempts to be sympathetic and negotiating, for example, waiting outside the toilet, could result in a suicide attempt being made while in the toilet. It is important to remember the reasoning behind the decision to implement Level IV in the first place. Policies generally state that the least restrictive option should be utilized, so this level of observation would not necessarily be a first choice. It depends on the risk assessment. Normally, a nurse would 'special' (language indicating Level IV observation) a patient for an hour and a rota system would be in place. During this time the nurse should try to engage with the patient in a therapeutic way. This might include being silent.

Respect for privacy in such circumstances is very difficult and it is important for staff to address this, particularly as MIND (2006) found that 17 per cent of inpatients felt they had never been treated with respect by staff. Respect is likely to be communicated through the attitude and manner in which the nurse undertakes the observation. For example, appearing indifferent and reading a paper while sitting by a patient lying on a bed could be disrespectful and harmful. The nurse who acknowledges that these are difficult circumstances and outlines what exactly the patient can expect, and responds to their concerns, is demonstrating respect.

Normally, student nurses would not undertake or be expected to undertake this role *unsupervised*. If they are involved, this involvement should be informed by their learning objectives and they should be supervised by a qualified practitioner. Different universities will have their own policy on this, so please check your local guidance.

Gender is also an important issue in relation to maintaining the dignity of a patient. A female patient, for example, who needs the toilet, should not be accompanied by a male nurse who is observing. For this time, a female observer should be found, and of course a male observer for men. Further information concerning privacy and dignity can be found in Chapter 5 of this book.

It may be that decisions about using the least restrictive observation method are informed by the environment in which those decisions are being made. For example, an environment that has a ligature point audit may be safer than one which hasn't. Access to and means of suicide need to be considered – for instance, opening windows, glass, hanging opportunities, safe storage of drugs and other harmful products, and effective administration of drugs.

Managing risk

The risk management issues that have been identified in the previous sections should be considered relevant for meeting patients' safety needs. Managing risk involves making decisions about what to do with the information gained from the risk assessment. If admission to a mental health assessment unit is necessary, decisions about levels of observation will have to be made.

Activity 6.17

Take at look at the illustration of the decision-making process on the Media Tool DVD, under **Chapter Resources** and then **Mental Health Needs Weblinks and Activities** and then **Activity 6.17**.

The safety and security concerns of patients may be quite different from those of staff. For example, bullying and harassment have been recognized as a problem on mixed-sex acute mental health wards (MIND 2006). The Government has been responsive to some of these issues and single-gender wards are an expectation. However, this does not mean that different genders cannot mix on a unit and such problems be eradicated. It is important for clients to feel able to express their needs, be able to inform staff of any problems that occur and expect some action and support – for example, challenging any racist comments by patients or visitors.

Maintaining physical safety on a general hospital ward is particularly problematic when the option to lock the doors is not available – this can be particularly pertinent for patients suffering from *Alzheimer's disease*. The best approach in these circumstances is to try to understand more about the person and their experience of their illness, including how it can be managed. People with dementing illness can maintain a capacity to make many of their own decisions and the main principle in making this judgement is that the greater the seriousness of the decision, the greater the capacity required. Consider the issues raised in Activity 6.18.

It is also important to consider how staff may misinterpret behaviours or speech, and to make reference to the context in which any assessment takes place – for example, different personal cultural issues, family dynamics or value systems. If someone seems para-

Activity 6.18

Ask yourself the following questions:

- What is the person's current capacity to make a particular decision?
- Do they have an infection? If so, has it been treated, as infections can cause worsening of the symptoms of confusion.
- Could they be dehydrated? Dehydration can cause confusion and in some instances hallucinations.
- Have they taken any medication or combinations of medications? These may be toxic. Remember that ageing means higher sensitivity to drugs.

Connect with the person. Talk to them kindly, explain things, repeat yourself, ask questions, remain calm, try to interpret their communication and don't assume it is nonsensical. In addition it is important to discuss with the patient and the carer what helpful actions can be taken – for example, use of notices, picture signs and familiar things.

noid, it is important not to passively assume they have a mental health issue and analyse possible explanations for their behaviour.

Activity 6.19

What do you think the effect of the following may be on a person's mental state?

- Sensory deprivation
- Exhaustion
- Foreign environment
- Illiteracy
- Drugs
- Physical disease

These conditions are likely to have an effect on paranoia; this does *not necessarily* mean that someone has a mental illness.

Psychological safety may be affected by the trust that a patient feels able to place in staff. This trust will be informed by how staff communicate their attitudes. As noted earlier in the chapter, MIND (2006) found low levels of respect communicated from staff to patients. Box 6.13 provides two useful web links.

Box 6.13 Web links

Psychological safety is as important as physical safety and the MNC has a guidance document entitled 'Registrant/client relationships and the prevention of abuse' which will be of interest to you and can be accessed here: www.nmc-uk.org/ aFrameDisplay.aspx?DocumentID=3294.

The NMC also provides guidance for students, which can be found at: www.nmc-uk.org/ aFrameDisplay.aspx?DocumentID=1896.

Scenario 6.3

James has vascular dementia which has only recently been diagnosed. He finds that he keeps forgetting names and words which is very embarrassing. He has been admitted for investigations of chest pain. James is easily confused, and being in an unfamiliar environment exacerbates this for him. He keeps forgetting why he is there and packs his bag to return home. He has been found leaving the ward on a number of occasions.

After discussion with James and his family the nurses and relatives write notes explaining where he is and why, and when he should be going home. They put these notes in different places: in his pockets, in his drawers, in the pockets of other clothes and jackets in his wardrobe, and on top of his holdall. Each time James comes to pack his bag, he is reminded that he needs to stay in hospital. He is also provided with a calendar so that he can see when his discharge date is planned. His family and the nurses reinforce the use of the notes each time they interact with James.

Scenario 6.4

What do you think about the following scenarios?

Tracey and Dave are addicted to heroin. They are unemployed and shoplifting as a way to raise money. Their three children are on the Social Services at-risk register and they have been in and out of foster care. Today, Tracey and Dave are incapable of looking after their children. The 8-year-old is trying to prepare some food for her siblings.

Ursula is a student nurse in a group of 15 students. She is a practising Muslim. She is feeling bullied by one of the group, Joe, who seems to have the support of others in the group. She is feeling isolated, anxious and upset. The group arrange to meet in a pub despite knowing that Ursula is unable to attend due to her religious beliefs.

James attends an Evangelical Christian church where he, with others in the congregation, speaks in tongues. He always carries his Bible with him and sees it as his duty to inform everyone he meets of God's word. This has resulted in people verbally abusing him.

Now imagine you are Tracey or Dave. What do you think and feel about your situation? What are your hopes and fears for the future?

Now imagine you are Joe. How do you feel about what is happening to Ursula?

Imagine you are James. How do you think it feels to be ridiculed and dismissed?

Can you identify any of your own values that you would be concerned that other people should understand and respect if you were in a dependent position in hospital?

Box 6.14 Web links – useful websites for further study

Royal College of Psychiatrists www.rcpych.ac.uk

Mental Health Charity www.mind.org.uk

Mental Health Foundation www.mentalhealth.org.uk

Alzheimer's Society www.alzheimers.org.uk

RCN Mental Health Zone www.rcn.org.uk/mentalhealth

Age Concern www.ace.org.uk

Hearing Voices Network. http://www.hearing-voices.org/

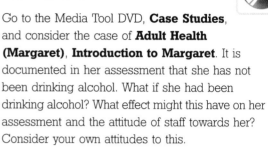

Activity 6.20

Go to the Media Tool DVD, **Case Studies**, and consider the case of **Adult Health (Margaret)**, **Introduction to Margaret**. It is documented in her assessment that she has not been drinking alcohol. What if she had been drinking alcohol? What effect might this have on her assessment and the attitude of staff towards her? Consider your own attitudes to this.

Summary and key points

This chapter has introduced you to many complex issues concerning mental health and ill health. One of the main challenges for you in your practice may be to learn that as a nurse in a particular speciality all aspects of a person's health are your responsibility. A person with mental health problems whose primary needs are physical can expect to have all their needs met in a general hospital environment. In the same way, a person with physical health problems whose primary need is a mental health problem can expect their physical health to be addressed within a mental health environment (DoH 2005).

To be able to meet these challenges, your education in mental and physical health issues is of equal importance. It is vital that you ensure you learn from experience, and as a student you can be expected to record what you have learned in a reflective diary. The following key points are important for you to remember. You can expect:

- to be encouraged to question practice;
- to be able to challenge poor practice;
- to know who to make a complaint to;
- to be involved in debriefing after serious incidents;
- to reflect on significant events;
- to receive support in your educational environment and in practice placements;
- to be able to access student support services in your university;
- to be able to access specific support for people from ethnic or other minority groups.

Remember: there is no health without mental health!

References

Appleby, L. (2001) *Safety First: Five Year Report of the National Confidential Inquiry into Suicide and Homicide by People with Mental Illness.* London: DoH.

Cattell, H. and Jolley, D.J. (1995) One hundred cases of suicide in elderly people, *British Journal of Psychiatry,* 166: 451–7.

Cohen, I.S. (1995) Over-diagnosis of schizophrenia: the role of alcohol and drug misuse, *The Lancet,* 346: 1541–2.

Commission for Health Care Audit and Inspection (2007) Count me in 2007: Results of the 2007 national census of inpatients in mental health and learning disability services in England and Wales, www.healthcarecommission.org.uk/_db/_documents/Count_me_in-2007.pdf, accessed 27 February 2008.

DoH (Department of Health) (1999) *Standing Nursing and Midwifery Advisory Committee (SNMAC) Practice Guidance: Safe and Supportive Observation of Patients at Risk,* www.dh.gov.uk/en/Publicationsandstatistics/Publications/PublicationsPolicyAndGuidance/DH_4007583, accessed 27 February 2008.

DoH (Department of Health) (2001) *National Service Framework for Older People.* London: DoH.

DoH (Department of Health) (2002) *National Suicide Prevention Strategy for England.* London: DoH.

DoH (Department of Health) (2005) *Meeting the Physical Needs of Individuals with Mental Health Problems and the Mental Health Needs of Individuals Cared for in General Health Sectors: Advice from the Standing Nursing and Midwifery Advisory Committee (SNMAC),* www.dh.gov.uk/en/Publicationsandstatistics/Publications/PublicationsPolicyAndGuidance/DH_4120771, accessed 27 February 2008.

Falloon, I.R.H. and Talbot, R.E. (1981) Persistent auditory hallucination: coping mechanisms and implications for management, *Psychological Medicine,* 11(2): 329–39.

Gough, K. and Hawkins, A. (2000) Staff attitudes to self-harm and its management in a forensic psychiatric service, *British Journal of Forensic Practice,* 2: 22–8.

Hickman, M. Vickerman, P. Macleod, J. Primary Care, University of Birmingham, Kirkbride, J. and Jones, P.B. (2007) Cannabis and schizophrenia: model projections of the impact of the rise in cannabis use on historical and future trends in schizophrenia in England and Wales, *Addiction,* 102: 597–606.

Hill, K. (1995) *The Long Sleep: Young People and Suicide.* London: Virago.

Huband, N. and Tantam, D. (1999) Clinical management of women who self-wound: a survey of mental health professionals' preferred strategies, *Journal of Mental Health,* 8: 473–87.

Jeffery, D. and Warm, A. (2002) A study of service providers' understanding of deliberate self-harm, *Journal of Mental Health,* 11: 3.

Kinsella, C. and Kinsella, C. (2006) *Introducing Mental Health: A Practical Guide.* London: Jessica Kingsley.

Macleod, J. (2007) Cannabis use and psychosis: the origins and implications of an association, *Advances in Psychiatric Treatment,* 13: 400–11.

Marwaha, S. and Livingstone, G. (2002) Stigma, racism, or choice. Why do depressed ethnic elders avoid psychiatrists? *Journal of Affective Disorders,* 72: 257–65.

Menezes, P.R. Johnson, S. Thornicroft, G. Marshall, J. Prosser, D. Bebbington, P. and Kuipers, E. (1996) Drug and alcohol problems among individuals with severe mental illness in south London, *British Journal of Psychiatry,* 168: 612–19.

MIND (2004) Suicide fact sheet, www.mind.org.uk/Information/Factsheets/Suicide/#_ftn19#_ftn19, accessed 27 February 2008.

MIND (2006) Ward watch report, www.mind.org.uk/News+policy+and+campaigns/Campaigns/Ward+Watch/Minds+Ward+Watch+report+key+findings.htm, accessed 27 February 2008.

NCMH (National Collaborating Centre for Mental Health) (2004) *Self-harm: The Short-term Physical and Psychological Management and Secondary Prevention of Self-harm in Primary and Secondary Care.* Leicester/London: British Psychological Society & Royal College of Psychiatrists.

Oliver, C. Hall, S. Hales, J. and Head, D. (1996) Self-injurious behaviour and people with intellectual disabilities: assessing the behavioural knowledge and causal explanations of care staff, *Journal of Applied Research in Intellectual Disabilities,* 9: 229–39.

Prince, M. Patel, V. Saxena, S. Maj, M. Maselko J. Phillips, M.R. and Rahman, A. (2007) No health without mental health, *The Lancet,* 370(9590): 859–77.

Pritchard, C. and Baldwin, D. (2000) Effects of age and gender on elderly suicide rates in Catholic and Orthodox countries: an inadvertent neglect? *International Journal of Geriatric Psychiatry,* 15(10): 904–10.

Puri, B.K. (1995) *Pocket Essential of Psychiatry.* London: WB Saunders.

Rayner, G. Allen, S. and Johnson, M. (2005) Counter-transference and self-injury: a cognitive behavioural cycle, *Journal of Advanced Nursing,* 50(1):12–19.

Rayner, G. and Warner, G. (2003) Self-harming behaviour from lay perception to clinical practice, *Counselling Psychology Quarterly,* 16(4): 305–29.

RCP (Royal College of Psychiatrists) (2005) *Who Cares Wins: Guidelines for the Development of Liaison Mental Health Services for Older People.* London: RCP.

Regier, D.A. Farmer, M.E. Rae, D.S. Locke, B.Z. Keith, S.J. Judd, L.L. and Goodwin, F.K. (1990) Co-morbidity of mental disorders with alcohol and other drug abuse: Results from the Epidemiologic Catchment Area (ECA) Study, *Journal of the American Medical Association,* 264: 2511–18.

Repper, J. and Perkins, R. (2003) *Social Inclusion and Recovery: A Model for Mental Health Practice.* London: Baillière Tindall.

Sashidharan, S.P. (2001) Institutional racism in British psychiatry, *Psychiatric Bulletin,* 25: 244–7.

Sayce, L. (2000) *From Psychiatric Patient to Citizen: Overcoming Discrimination and Social Exclusion.* Basingstoke: Macmillan.

Scottish Executive (2002) Engaging people: observation of people with acute mental health problems, good practice statement, www.scotland.gov.uk/Resource/Doc/46951/0013967.pdf, annexes at www.scotland.gov.uk/Publications/2002/08/15296/10454#b15, accessed 27 February 2008.

Scottish Executive (2005) *National Programme for Improving Mental Health and Well-being: Addressing Mental Health Inequalities in Scotland – Equal Minds.* Edinburgh: Scottish Executive.

Shafii, M. (1989) Completed suicide in children and adolescents: methods of psychological autopsy, in C.R. Pfeffer (ed.) S*uicide Among Youth: Perspectives on Risk and Prevention.* Washington, DC: American Psychiatric Press.

Smit, F. Bolier, L. and Cuijpers, P. (2004) Cannabis use and the risk of later schizophrenia: a review, *Addiction,* 99: 425–30.

Smith, N.T. (2002) A review of the published literature into

cannabis withdrawal symptoms in human users, *Addiction,* 97: 621–32.

Tarrier, N. (1987) An investigation of residual psychotic symptoms in discharged schizophrenic patients, *British Journal of Clinical Psychology,* 26: 141–3.

Wenger, T. Moldrich, G. and Furst, S. (2003) Neuromorphological background of cannabis addiction, *Brain Research Bulletin,* 61: 125–8.

WHO (World Health Organization) (1992) *The International Classification of Diseases, Tenth Revision (ICD-10): Clinical Descriptions and Diagnostic Guidelines.* Geneva: WHO.

WHO (World Health Organization) (2007) What is mental health? Online questions and answers, www.who.int/features/qa/62/en/index.html.

Zubin, J. and Spring, B. (1977) Vulnerability – a new view of schizophrenia, *Journal of Abnormal Psychology,* 86(2): 103–24.

Answers

Activity 6.6

The social consequences of the listed behaviours could be:

- Hygiene problems due to not washing or bathing. This could have health implications due to infection which may exacerbate mental symptoms.
- Not eating may lead to weight loss and nutritional deficits that exacerbate mental symptoms.
- Suspension from work, leading to loss of earnings, leading to inability to pay bills, leading to electricity cut off so unable to cook or keep warm, so losing more weight, developing hypothermia (which exacerbates mental symptoms), not paying rent, leading to homelessness.

There is little chance at this point of getting back to former functioning without considerable help and support, due to increased inability to function effectively and increased distress due to other people's intolerance and ignorance.

Activity 6.9

In the nurse's desire to comfort and reassure Chris she stands very close to him and also touches him several times. While this may usually be reassuring and comforting, given Chris's feelings of suspicion and threat he may misinterpret the nurse's intentions as threatening, hostile or even aggressive. It is vital that the nurse establish whether Chris has taken an overdose, and if so, of what. In trying to find out, the nurse asks Chris lots of questions. Again, considering Chris' current emotional distress, he may become further unsettled by these questions. Some are answered by, and directed to, Chris' sister directly over Chris. This could also reinforce his feelings of suspicion.

Activity 6.10

Patient advice and liaison service (PALS). Information about:

- The hospital facilities
- The clinical team
- Meal times
- Visiting arrangements
- Financial assistance, for example, for car parking
- Welfare rights
- Telephone availability
- Food availablility
- Local facilities
- Mental Health Act information
- Mental Health Act commissioner visits
- Service user meetings

Activity 6.12

Some people drink alcohol as a way to manage their stress. However, this can, in fact, increase their experience of stress. Alcohol stimulates the secretion of adrenaline, which is associated with problems such as tension, irritability and insomnia. Excess alcohol increases fat deposits in the heart, decreases the effectiveness of the immune system and restricts the liver's capacity to remove toxins from the body. Excessive drinking is also associated with violent and aggressive behaviour.

Some people use non-prescribed soft or hard drugs to relieve stress levels. This may seem to provide some short-term relief from symptoms of stress, but in the long term hard drugs can cause serious medical harm. Becoming reliant on soft drugs avoids addressing the actual cause of stress. People who smoke may react to stressful situations by lighting a cigarette; however, being without a cigarette actually produces the symptoms of stress itself. There is actually no evidence that smoking helps stress in any way, and people tend to have their cigarette once they are away from the immediate source of their stress, when the body is starting to relax. Smoking is associated with several potentially fatal conditions including cardiovascular disease, cancer and chronic obstructive pulmonary disease.

Physical exercise can play a significant role in the prevention and treatment of a range of physiological and emotional conditions, including the relief of stress and has received increased attention in recent years, including the prescription of exercise by GPs. Although the potential benefits of exercise are acknowledged, there is an emerging focus within the literature on the concept of exercise addiction. The notion of exercise addiction suggests that the mood-enhancing and analgesic properties associated with exercise are influenced by chemicals in the brain which are akin to opiates. There is also an association between exercise addiction and eating disorders. Some individuals may even experience increased feelings of anxiety, depression, restlessness and guilt if they are unable to exercise.

Often, for physiological reasons following a period of increased stress, our body can crave foods that are rich in fat, sugar and salt, and as a result we may then eat inappropriate foods in excessive quantities. This is sometimes referred to as 'comfort eating', however, the overwhelming evidence suggests that eating unhealthy food is not good for stress and that in the long term a healthy diet is beneficial for dealing with stress.

Activity 6.13

This is a highly emotive issue which frequently results in strong negative reactions from some people. People with less training and experience in working with people who self-harm or who have attempted suicide tend to react more negatively than experienced individuals and tend to make more misjudged assumptions about the motives for the behaviour (Oliver *et al.* 1996; Huband and Tantam 2000). Untrained and inexperienced individuals are also more likely to unintentionally respond to self-harming behaviour in ways that might reinforce that behaviour, and therefore increase its frequency (Oliver *et al.* 1996). When individuals do not feel that they have a good understanding of self-harm or suicide, they often feel overwhelmed when faced with the challenges of working with this client group (Gough and Hawkins 2000; Jeffery and Warm 2002).

7

Self-care

Alison Brown

Chapter Contents

Learning objectives

The aim of this chapter is to explore the role of the nurse in relation to promoting self-care with patients. Throughout the chapter we will be referring to the accompanying Media Tool DVD. Please watch the video clips as directed as these will reinforce your learning and expand upon the information given in this book. After reading this chapter and working through the activities you should be able to:

- Define the term 'self-care'.
- Discuss your own views of health and what influences them.
- Discuss how you currently promote health with your patient/client group.
- Identify how you would assess a patient and their family in relation to self-care needs.
- Recognize your own and others' responsibilities in promoting self-care.
- Discuss how self-care fits with rehabilitation.
- Produce a list of agencies that support patients and families.

Introduction

Self-care has been defined as:

> *a broad term comprising all that people, patients and carers do to maintain health, prevent injury, seek and adhere to treatment, manage symptoms and side effects, accomplish recovery and rehabilitation and manage the impact of chronic illness and disability.*
>
> (Alliance for Self Care Research 2006: 2)

Recent research by the Department of Health (DoH 2005) indicated that over three-quarters of those surveyed believe that they are in good health, are satisfied and feel in control of their own lives. They believe they can manage their own minor ailments, can monitor their own illnesses when diagnosed and, where long-term conditions exist, 82 per cent believe they have an active role in caring for their condition themselves. In looking at these figures it is apparent that many individuals believe they are more than capable of managing their own care and health. If this is so, what is it that we, as nurses, can do to help them?

In this chapter, we will first look at self-care in relation to health and lifestyle, before going on to look at the knowledge and skills needed to manage self-care and how we can, through risk assessment of patients and carers, monitor their ability and condition, and diagnose any changes and actions to be facilitated.

We will then look at individual responsibilities in relation to self-care and how nurses can support the

Activity 7.1

Consider your definition of what a nurse is, and note it down before reading on.

If your definition includes doing things for people and acting on their behalf, you need to question whether this is appropriate when promoting self-care. You need to consider if this is fostering their dependence on you. You may feel that helping a patient to wash, or dress, when you know they are able to do these things themselves, albeit slowly and with some difficulty, is helpful. However, a wise patient will tell you that they won't have you at home to do these tasks, so by doing them for the patient we may actually not be doing them any favours. Instead, as nurses, we should be asking ourselves what steps we need to take to allow the patient to manage their own care, without absolving ourselves of all our responsibilities in ensuring that care is safe and appropriate.

patient and their family to take on this responsibility. As we explore responsibility, we will consider how this fits with the patient's journey home and their rehabilitation, together with the decisions they need to make. Finally we will consider discharge and look at the services that will be needed to support self-care activities during the transition from hospital to home. This will include looking at the environmental factors that need to be examined for a safe return to the community.

Self-care, health and lifestyle

As previously mentioned, in a recent survey by the Department of Health, three-quarters of the population identified that they are in good health and feel satisfied and in control of their life most of, or all of, the time. Interestingly, those who feel they are not in good health, or have less control over their lives, are most likely to be the elderly and less well off (DoH 2005). Currently in the UK we are facing a demographic time bomb with a falling birth rate and an increasingly elderly population living to more advanced ages (Scottish Executive 2005). The Scottish Executive, for example, has predicted that over the next 25 years 1 in 4 of the population will be aged 65 or over, with 1 in 12

over the age of 80. The elderly are not only more like to suffer from long-term illnesses but to have sever such illnesses which result in more admissions hospital and longer stays (Scottish Executive 200 DoH 2007). With this in mind it could be argued that the population is becoming more elderly, then there a potential for more people to feel less in control their lives and that the incidence of ill health ma increase. To address this, we need to consider ne ways of working within the healthcare service ensure that we can continue to provide an excelle health service. One suggestion as to how we can this is by becoming more focused on the issues health and prevention of illness and by facilitatir people to take care of their own health issues throug self-care (Scottish Executive 2005).

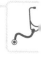

Activity 7.2

Note down what the terms 'health' and 'public health' mean to you.

First we need to consider what we mean by heal and public health. You may have already noticed th definitions of 'health' are many and varied and tend relate to ideas of 'wholeness'. They can be divided in two types: the *positive view* is that health is a sense well-being, while the *negative view* tends to focus the absence of illness, with health and illness seen opposite ends of a continuum (Naidoo and Wills 200 The WHO, in its definition of health, has move towards a more positive view, in that: 'Health is resource for everyday life, not the objective of livin rather it is a positive concept emphasising social an personal resources as well as physical capacitie (WHO 1984). This positive view of health is shared the population at large (Fryback 1993; DoH 200 Scottish Executive 2005), and most people, even thos with a chronic illness, see themselves as healthy, control of their own lives and able to self-care. nurses we need to think in this positive way abo those we meet, and focus on how we can help fost this approach in order to enable individuals to tak control of their own care needs.

'Public health', on the other hand is seen as bein about the health of populations or communities. On well-known definition is that of Sir Donald Acheso

(1988), who said it was 'the science and art of pre- venting disease, prolonging life, and promoting health through the organised effort of society'. If we consider this definition we again see the positivist viewpoint which suggests that by galvanizing the community, they can take control of their own health and it then becomes the norm to look after the health of yourself and others.

Yet it has been suggested that healthcare profes- sionals are often socialized by their profession to view health in a narrow way that relates more to absence of disease or illness (Naidoo and Wills 2000). By taking this narrow view we must ask ourselves if we com- municate that view to our patients and therefore cause them to question their own ability to monitor their own health and manage their own care.

Activity 7.3

Consider how you defined health and public health previously and review the four case study patients referred to in this book and on the Media Tool DVD – Chris, Tom, Margaret and Alex – focusing on their admission to hospital. Who do you view as healthy? Consider what has informed your thinking. How healthy do you think each of the case studies see themselves? What about their next of kin?

Having identified what your thoughts are on the health status of each of the case studies, can you identify whether you have taken a positive or negative view?

You will find that as you develop during your career in nursing, your views may change. It is easy at the start to see the individual as a diagnosis, such as stroke or diabetic, and think they are not healthy, whereas Tom has only broken his leg – therefore you might view him as healthy. People with chronic illnesses such as cancer or AIDS often view themselves as healthy; it is just that they happen to have a diagnosis (Fryback 1993). They feel that their view of health is widened by their illness and that in fact they are healthier after a diagnosis than before, as they re-evaluate their life. It is often not the diagnosis that makes them feel unhealthy; rather it is the inability to live their life as

they wish (Fryback 1993; Corner and Bailey 2001). If patients are encouraged to take a positive view and communicate this to their family, they may start to feel more in control of their life and their health. It could be argued that by fostering a positive approach with the patient we are assisting in empowering them to take control of their own care.

What is self-care?

Self-care is seen as part of daily living (DoH 2005) and has been the focus of several models of nursing over the years, such as Orem's Self-Care Deficit Model (2001). However, the most widely used model in the UK is that of Roper *et al.* (1983) and this model is under- pinned by the idea that care provided by the healthcare practitioner to address the activities of living is dependent on the patient's point on a dependence– independence continuum. That is to say, if the patient is independent when eating and drinking, as nurses, our care is directed at the monitoring of that activity rather than feeding them. However, if the patient can feed themselves but has difficulty in cutting up their food, then we should only cut up the food.

It could be argued therefore that as much of nursing over the past 60 years has been directed by models of nursing, that nursing is geared to facilitate self-care of patients and should therefore be based on the premise of patient health. Indeed, the focus of pre-registration nurse education since 1992, and with the advent of Project 2000, has been on a health-promoting curri- culum. Yet sitting in the first decade of the twenty-first century, we must ask ourselves: have we made a dif- ference to the nation's health and, if not, why not?

Scenario 7.1

Janey is a 15-year-old girl. She is overweight and has asthma, which she often uses as an excuse to avoid physical exercise. She has recently started seeing Steve, and feels under pressure to sleep with him. What do you see are Janey's needs in relation to promoting health and how would you support her in her choices to ensure she has responsibility for her own self-care? When you have considered this, check the sample answer at the end of the chapter.

It has been suggested (Scottish Executive 2005) that the health service is still focused on illness, with the bulk of funding still being spent on hospital care. To address this, the suggestion is that we make major changes to our health service, with a move away from large 'juggernaut' hospitals to a more community-focused healthcare service with patients undertaking more self-care activities, including responsibility for their own health. To take this first step in self-care, nurses need to consider how we promote health with our patients.

Managing self-care

Having first considered some steps we can take to prevent ill health, we then have to think about how we enable individuals to make choices about self-care. Research would suggest that one of the greatest ways to enable self-care is by providing individuals with the knowledge and understanding that will enable them to achieve this.

Box 7.1 The importance of knowledge and understanding

Ninety-five per cent of people say that they have the knowledge and understanding necessary to treat their own minor ailments, and 89 per cent of those who have long-term conditions feel confident that they have the knowledge and understanding to take care of their own health condition (DoH 2005). However, those who feel little confidence in their own knowledge and understanding of their own condition and health have less interest in self-care (DoH 2005).

Bandura (1997) writes about his theory of 'self-efficacy' in which he suggests that a person's ability to self-care is linked to their belief in their own ability to achieve results. This suggests that individuals need to be given information to help them understand their condition in order to support their belief in their ability to self-care. The first step to helping people to self-care is by doing a thorough assessment of their needs, physiologically, emotionally, psychologically, cognitively and socially (Frich 2003). By assessing the individual and listening to them and their loved ones we can ascertain what we need to put in place to help. For example, by assessing the patient we can find out if the reason they and their family are not self-caring is because no one has told them what they can do for themselves, or because they need some adaptations to their homes, or because they need to be advised of some support groups in their area.

Activity 7.4

Go to the Media Tool DVD, select **Case Studies** and read the introduction to each case study. It is anticipated that each of these patients will eventually be going home. What questions would you ask at the beginning of their journey to find out what they need to know to allow them to self-care? Check our suggested answers at the end of the chapter.

How you undertake the assessment will vary depending on the area you work in. Most areas base their assessment on a model of nursing. As mentioned previously, the best-known model related to self-care is that of Orem (2001), and even though your ward assessment may not be based on Orem's model, you can still apply her thoughts to your assessment. Orem's model is based on three theories. These are: theory of self-care; theory of self-care deficit; and theory of nursing systems. When considering assessing the patient we can think of the theory of self-care deficit, which identifies the areas where the individual can and cannot self-care. It is useful on admission to identify the areas where the patient has deficits in order to plan your promotion of their future self-care. This initial assessment records the baseline information you need to allow you, and the patient, to set goals for their care and eventual discharge. This baseline assessment occurs in the community as well as in hospital and will inform the patient's or client's healthcare record. You may wish to review Chapter 3 at this point to remind yourself of the important issues related to such records.

Once we have a baseline assessment, we then have an idea of what to work towards. Your admission records should then be reflected in your care plan for the patient. The care plan should detail what the patient can and cannot do for themselves and the

Scenario 7.2

Stan is a 70-year-old man. He developed an abdominal obstruction six weeks ago, and on investigation was diagnosed with cancer of the bowel. He had a colostomy formed. Since his surgery Stan has refused to self-care for his stoma, and instead identified early on that his wife Jean, 69, would care for it. The stoma nurse and the ward staff have spent time with Jean and she is competent to care for Stan's stoma. The day before Stan's planned discharge Jean comes to you in tears. She reveals that this is not an aspect of Stan's care that she can cope with on her own and that she has not been sleeping as she is so worried about the care of the stoma. She refuses to allow Stan to come home.

In this case, Stan was delayed from going home for a week until home care was established. Meanwhile he also made the decision that as he was so keen to go home, he would take on the care himself. The team worked with Stan to increase his confidence in his self-care management.

Here, perhaps the assessment initially focused too strongly on Stan's needs and desires. Perhaps Jean was pushed into acquiescence by feeling under pressure and out of a sense of duty for her husband's care. By undertaking an assessment of both the patient and the carer early on, it is easier to identify the risks that may face the patient and their loved one later on in their journey.

interventions that need to be undertaken for each of the patient's health needs.

For example, when admitting a patient, you note that they have difficulty in expressing themselves (as in the case study of Margaret) and you note that in relation to their food they cannot identify their likes and dislikes, so their partner sits with them and goes through the menu marking off the meal choices. This can still be considered as self-care, as the nurse is not taking over; rather they are allowing the couple to identify ways to maintain their ownership of care.

In Margaret's case it is important that we detail in her care plan the fact that her husband is closely involved, so that both parties are prepared for her discharge at a later date. However, you should always check with the carer that they *want* such involvement, as some do not. If this is identified early, the discharge plan can be prepared with it in mind. Consider how things can go wrong – as illustrated in Scenario 7.2.

If we now consider the case study of Chris, our assessment may indicate that the risk for him is that he continues to participate in risky behaviour. If we do not start to address his knowledge deficits early and we leave it to the last minute before discharge, the messages we give him may be ineffective, setting him and his family up to fail on discharge and risk readmission to hospital. This can cause increased pressure on healthcare resources and engender feelings of inadequacy in patients' ability to self-care (Bandura 1997).

One of the enablers of self-care is providing the patient or their carer with underpinning knowledge. Yet over half of the public have identified that they do not receive encouragement from healthcare professionals to engage in self-care and that their use and awareness of patient organizations related to long-term illnesses are low (DoH 2005). So the question has to be asked, how can we as healthcare professionals provide this education and support?

Once we have made our initial assessment of the patient in finding out what their current abilities are in relation to self-care, and have determined how much they can or cannot do for themselves, we then need to plan their care in order to inform their individual training for self-care.

The first step to planning individualized care is the setting of realistic goals which are meaningful to the patient. If we set unrealistic goals, then we are setting them up to fail and this will undermine their confidence in their own ability to self-care. By finding out how much time the next of kin has to support the patient in their activities while in hospital, we can assess their willingness to undertake the care of the patient at home and how able they are to take on some of that care.

However, as in Stan's case, we can still get it wrong. Perhaps if we had used a simple question and answer routine, as used when undertaking a risk assessment, when working with Stan and his wife, we would have discovered earlier her reluctance to participate and Stan's ability to self-care.

An example of assessing using simple questions and answers relates to mobility. You might ask, 'Can you stand up and walk by yourself?' If the patient says no, then ask, 'Can you move yourself forward in a chair? Can you wiggle your bottom forward? Can you place your feet one in front of the other?' By undertaking a step-by-step assessment of how much someone can do, we can identify more clearly the potential risks to the patient, ourselves and their carers. Once we have this basic knowledge the next step is to give the patient and their family permission to *do* things.

Activity 7.5

Go to the Media Tool DVD, select **Case Studies**, **Learning Disability (Alex)**. Watch the case study and then consider the information below.

Alex has been living at home with his mother and he is in for assessment of his ongoing care needs. He has been managing his diabetes with support. Therefore, by giving him permission to continue to do this with professional support, his independence is maintained. This also allows the nurse to see the areas where he needs further support and informs the type of information he is given, so that he can progress his self-care. It is easy to disempower patients when they come into hospital and take over responsibility for giving medicines, which in Alex's case he has taken for a period of time at home. Allowing Alex to maintain responsibility for taking his own medications encourages him to maintain his self-care ability.

By observing clients or patient in their daily tasks and activities we can identify where their motor or cognitive skills may need support. For example, Betty is an 83-year-old lady whose eyesight is failing. She takes medication for arthritis, hyperthyroidism and osteo-porosis and is now having problems reading labels on her medication. In order to allow Betty to maintain control of her own medicines she can be provided with a *Dosett box* which the nurse or carer can pre-load with her tablets, an eye test can be arranged to obtain glasses to allow her to read the labels, or identify whether she has any other problems with her sight that

need to be addressed. Remember, the problem may need only a simple solution. For example, Betty problem with her medicines may be due to her arthriti and *osteoporosis*, because she no longer has the moto ability to manage the child-proof bottles.

The hospital or other pharmacy can provide med cations in other forms, enabling patients like Betty t take their medication more easily. By allowing a patien to self-care in this way we not only identify thei knowledge deficits but their skills deficits, which w can address together with the multidisciplinary team However, it is also important to consider any risk fac tors and where ultimate responsibility for care lies.

Responsibility for self-care

Up to now, we have talked about how we can facilitat self-care by taking a positive approach with the patien and their family. Through a thorough assessment w can identify what they can and cannot do for them selves. However, self-care in hospital settings can b quite scary as we consider the question of who ha responsibility and what if something goes wrong where do we stand legally? Most patients coming int hospital will go home in due course. If we keep in th forefront of our minds that as we assess patients o admission we need to prepare them to go home agair we also need to consider our responsibilities, not onl while they are in hospital but when they go home, s that they are safe and do not need to be readmitted.

When you read Chapter 3 on record keeping, yo will have encountered a discussion on the legal aspect of this (see pages 45–50). In terms of the case studie in this book, how would you ensure that your record of care stand up to scrutiny in relation to self-care Remember that self-care is not about abdicating a responsibility as a healthcare professional to th patient and their family. It is *our responsibility* t ensure that the patient is safe to self-care.

Let us consider a patient who is self-medicating While in hospital, nurses need to work with the phar macists to ensure patient safety so that medication are only accessible by nursing and other qualified staf and in some cases by the relevant patient themselve (see below). Many ward areas now have locked cup boards at each patient's bedside. As you procee through your nurse education you may want to fin out how each area supports the patient in their sel care in relation to medicating. In some areas patients will have the key to their own locked box; in others the nurse maintains responsibility during the drug round for opening the locked cupboard for the patient to access. Both methods have their advantages and disadvantages.

If the patient has responsibility for their own medications, this maintains their ownership of their own care; however, it does not necessarily mean that they are taking their medicines safely and correctly. As nurses, we still have a responsibility for recording the patients' medications in the appropriate documentation and for ensuring that they are taken safely. We can do this by checking that the patient is taking the tablets (this could be done in conjunction with the pharmacist, counting the amount left each day), observing the patient taking their medication (checking that patients are not taking two doses at once, for example), recording the medications correctly and asking the patient how they take the medications. If we were to allow a patient to take the medication without checking, we would not know if the patient was ingesting inappropriately – for example, before food rather than after, with the result that the drug may not be working properly.

We also have a responsibility for noting the patient's ability to self-care in the care plan. The care plan will identify for other staff where the patient is having difficulty and will inform ongoing education and skills assessment and training for the patient throughout their time in hospital. This may seem to be time-consuming and some nurses may feel it is easier to take over the responsibility for giving the patient their medications when in hospital, especially if doses or medications are always being changed. However, if we take over responsibility for the drug administration when in hospital, while we will be assured that the drug is being taken correctly and at the correct time (according to the strict times used in hospital), we are not preparing the patient to take their medications when at home. If the patient is not given responsibility while in hospital, it may mean that when they go home they make errors in the timing of when they take the medication or with the drug itself because they are confused as to what to take when.

Many patients go home on several medications and if they do not know what to take and when, they can make errors. We may also impact on their own routine

at home where even meal and bed times may be affected because the patient thinks they have to rigidly stick to the times used in the hospital.

It is best then that we work with patients throughout their stay in hospital to establish a medication routine that fits with their own lifestyle, maintains their safety and prepares them for home as part of the rehabilitation process.

Activity 7.6

We have been discussing medication and self-care so far. Can you think of other activities in relation to the case studies where we can enable self-care in the hospital which prepares the patient for going home? Check your answers with those at the end of the chapter before reading any further.

Rehabilitation and decision-making

'Going home' is part of the process of rehabilitation. Rehabilitation is a process which starts on admission and progresses throughout the patient's stay in hospital with periodical reassessments as the patient's needs change over time. Rehabilitation has been defined by the WHO as 'helping patients to achieve and to maintain their maximum physical, emotional, spiritual, vocational and social potential, however limited this may be as a result of disease progression' (WHO 1987).

Dietz (1981), writing about rehabilitation in cancer patients, saw it as having four phases which could be applied equally to any patient with a chronic or acute condition. These phases are preventative, restorative, supportive and palliative rehabilitation. In Phase 1, the preventative phase, it is the engendering of hope and preventing deterioration in health that are important. In each of the case studies we could say that we engender hope in the patients by talking to them about going home, and by facilitating self-care we prevent dependence on the healthcare professional.

Phase 2, the restorative phase, is about 'putting right'. So following our assessment, and through helping the patient take over control of their care with our assistance or that of their next of kin, we start to 'restore'. In the case of Chris, for example, by giving him information on how his condition developed and his role in this, we could be seen to be restoring him to take responsibility and prevent further admissions.

Phase 3, the supportive phase, is where we are seen as sustaining life. For Margaret, we would begin in the supportive phase by trying to prevent deterioration in her health due to her stroke; however, as we progress through her time we will use the restorative phase to return her to self-care and the preventative phase to show her and her husband how to look after themselves to help prevent further strokes.

Phase 4, the palliative stage, is where we look at extending life and helping the patient to take care of themselves while providing more support to allow them to live with their condition. In this phase we could consider the case of Alex. We cannot take away his learning disability, however, we can provide support to allow him to live successfully with his condition and his diabetes, and to return him to some sort of independent living.

However, none of this can be done by nurses alone. As we look at the rehabilitation of these patients, we need to consider the input of the interdisciplinary team. When thinking about rehabilitation, the main objective of the interdisciplinary team is to coordinate the healthcare given by the individual team member (Frymark 1992). If we do not coordinate in this way, then the rehabilitation plan will break down and our attempts to promote self-care will fail.

As you consider the case studies and note all the work the interdisciplinary team undertakes to promote the rehabilitation of the patients and ultimately their return to self-care, it will become apparent that this does not just apply while they are in hospital. Rehabilitation and self-care, though starting on admission, will continue once the patients go home, with services in place to support self-care both in hospital and on discharge.

Services to support self-care

As we look to the discharge of a patient, we need to think about the ongoing support they will need to self-care in the community. One means of ensuring the patient is supported in their endeavours is by encouraging them to access schemes such as The Expert Patient Programme (DoH 2001). Through this, individuals can receive training and support from fellow patients and become part of the 'workforce' within the community of individuals who can support others to self-care and self-manage (Kennedy *et al.* 2005). This programme has been piloted in several sites and the results indicate that for those with long-term conditions, there is an increase in self-efficacy, energy, quality of life and well-being. The results also show better relationships with doctors (National Primary Care Research & Development Centre 2006). The major part of this programme is made up of a six-week self-care skills training course delivered by people who have personal experience of living with long-term conditions. There is funding to support individuals on this course and to continue training others.

Another way we can encourage patients is by advising them that when seeing healthcare professionals, they first write down a list of questions they need to ask. By supporting the patient to do this, the patient takes control of their condition and ensures that they receive the information they need to support them with their health issues.

Alternatively, patients could be put in touch with local and national support groups. One of the main complaints of patients is that they don't know where to go for help and advice on finance, aid and general support. To ask any nurse to be an expert on all support agencies would move us to the 'Super' status expected of Superman, however you can start small.

Scenario 7.3

Josephine is a 64-year-old lady of Caribbean origin who used to be a nurse. She has *multiple sclerosis* and though wheelchair-bound, is determined to live at home. She has three children who are all married with families of their own. She separated from her husband five years ago. She has two older sisters who live nearby and who help out with her shopping.

Draw up a list of services that may be consulted in order to facilitate Josephine's safe discharge home. Then consider the impact that discussing nursing homes might have on Josephine's self-worth. Compare it with the list at the end of the chapter.

As we look at services, we must also consider the environmental factors which impinge on self-care.

When in the ward setting, the environment is set up so that the patient is 'safe'. However, the ward environment may not reflect the patient's home circumstances. For example, there tends to be a lack of stairs in wards, or if access to baths is limited, there will be showers available. However, patients may not have a dedicated shower at home, and need to be able to get into a standard bath with an overhead shower. Even making tea and coffee may be restricted in hospital – patients normally have to wait until the ward maid provides this. All such environmental factors mean that often in the ward environment the patient's ability to self-care at home may not be reflected appropriately.

In order to address this discrepancy, patients may be taken to a home care setting by the occupational therapist and a physiotherapist to assess their ability to manage in a mocked-up environment. There is also often a home visit for patients where the social worker is involved in order to see the patient functioning in their own home, and to identify what aids and services need to be provided.

If we think about Josephine, when undertaking the home assessment, for example, it may be found that although she can manage perfectly well with support services in her home as it is all on one level, she may not be able to get in and out of the building as she is on the second floor with no lift. In situations such as this, the social worker in liaison with the local council and various health agencies may have to consider and discuss with Josephine finding her accommodation in a ground floor flat or a bungalow, or in a property where lifts are available.

When problems with the environment are identified, they can delay the patient's discharge. This is why it is so important that on admission to a ward we start to plan the patient's discharge. Can you imagine how Josephine would feel three days before going home if she found out that the health professionals were uncomfortable with her home setting and were starting to look at alternatives?

It is also important to consider the possibility that even where the appropriate resources are available to a patient, that patient may not choose to access them. It

Activity 7.7

In relation to the four case studies on the Media DVD and discussed in this book, can you identify any barriers to safe discharge? Before reading any further, draw up sample lists of services which could be accessed in your own area by each of the case study patients and their carers to ensure that they are able return to independent living.

may be that the patient or their family do not want other people 'interfering', or it may be a matter of not knowing that the services are available and what they offer. Other reasons may be that the health professionals have misunderstood what is available, how to access it and whom to contact to do so. You may also find that resources that are available in some parts of the community are not available in others. For example, the bereavement group CRUISE do not have counsellors in every town. It is useful when thinking about services and resources to discuss this with key people in the patient's locality to ensure that the services you are offering are actually available. The lack of consistency across the UK may appear to suggest that there are inequalities; however, it may be that the same services are offered by different groups, hence the need to liaise directly with the patient's own community staff.

Activity 7.8

Review the lists of services and resources you produced in the last activity. Pick a neighbouring county and identify which of the services and resources on your list would still be available there, and what options are available for a patient who comes from that county.

Summary and key points

As we have progressed through this chapter we have explored the ways in which we can promote self-care from admission to discharge. This process can be applied to any patient you may come across in your career. Self-care has been defined and its relevance to healthcare indicated. Self-care is an important element in how we view our own and the public's health. As nurses it is essential that, to ensure the health and safety of all whom we meet, we promote self-care, through our own work, the interdisciplinary team and with the help of support agencies.

It is important to remember that self-care is not about abdicating responsibilities to the patient and their relatives; it is about the ongoing facilitation of the patient and their family to take ownership of their care while ensuring that that ownership is safe.

Always remember the following key points:

- Self-care involves assessment of patients and their carers to identify their needs and to work to support them.
- Most people in the UK feel they have control over their life and that they are in good health.
- In order to achieve the vision of the NHS in the future – of a more community-focused healthcare service – those who feel they have less control over their health need to be assisted to regain this control.
- Responsible nurses allow their patients/clients to maintain and regain their independence as far as reasonably practical.

References

Acheson, D. (1988) *Public Health in England: The Report of the Committee of Inquiry into the Future Development of the Public Health Function.* London: HMSO. Cited by DoH (Department of Health) (2008) *What is Public Health?* para 3, available at www.dh.gov.uk/en/Aboutus/MinistersandDepartmentLeaders/ChiefMedicalOfficer/Features/FeaturesArchive/Browsable/DH_5017805, accessed 24 July 2008.

Bandura, A. (1997) *Self-efficacy: The Exercise of Control.* New York: Freeman.

Corner, J. and Bailey, C. (2001) *Cancer Nursing Care in Context.* Oxford: Blackwell Science.

Dietz, J. (1981) *Rehabilitation Oncology.* New York: Wiley.

DoH (Department of Health) (2005) *Public Attitudes to Self Care Baseline Survey.* London: DoH.

DoH (Department of Health) (2007) *Raising the Profile of Long-term Conditions Care: A Compendium of Information.* London: DoH.

Frich, L.M.H. (2003) Nursing interventions for patients with chronic conditions, *Journal of Advanced Nursing*, 44(2): 137–53.

Fryback, P.B. (1993) Health for people with a terminal diagnosis, *Nursing Science Quarterly*, 6(3): 147–59.

Frymark, S.L. (1992) Rehabilitation resources within the team and community, *Seminars in Oncology Nursing*, 8(3): 212–18.

Kennedy, A. Rogers, A. and Gately, C. (2005) From patients to providers: prospects for self-care skills trainers in the National Health Service, *Health and Social Care in the Community*, 13(95): 431–40.

Naidoo, J. and Wills, J. (2000) *Health Promotion Foundations for Practice*, 2nd edn. London: Baillière Tindall.

National Primary Care Research & Development Centre (2006) *The National Evaluation of the Pilot Phase of the Expert Patient Programme* (final report). Manchester: NPCRDC.

Orem, D. (2001) *Nursing: Concepts of Practice.* St Louis, MO: Mosby.

Roper N. Logan, W. and Tierney, A. (1983) *Using a Model for Nursing.* Edinburgh: Churchill Livingtone.

Scottish Executive (2005) *Building a Health Service Fit for the Future.* Edinburgh: Scottish Executive.

WHO (World Health Organization) (1984) *Health Promotion: A Discussion Document on the Concept and the Principles.* Copenhagen: WHO.

WHO (World Health Organization) (1987) *Palliative Cancer Care: Policy Statement.* Leeds: WHO.

Answers

Scenario 7.1

You may wish to consider how you can ensure that Janey is aware of what options are available to her, that she is fully informed as to what actions she needs to take and how you can ensure that information given to Janey is consistent among care staff and that there is ongoing monitoring of her health. The advice that you give Janey could be in relation to healthy eating – five portions of fruit and vegetables daily, reducing salt, avoiding of fatty foods, dietary advice related to medications, increased water intake – plus increased physical activity/exercise which raises the heart rate for 30 minutes a day, including walking, gentle exercise etc., and the monitoring of her own health, for instance, the correct and regular use of asthma inhalers. She may wish to seek self-screening for Chlamydia, and seek advice on contraception with family planning experts. You probably identified much more, but the important issue here is consistency and, for a young adult, that their choices are considered and respected.

Scenario 7.3

Your initial thoughts may have been to have a case conference with Josephine, her next of kin and members of the interdisciplinary team. Those involved would be the physiotherapist, occupational therapist, social worker, community liaison officer, nursing and medical staff. From there an initial discharge plan would be drawn up and relevant services involved. These would include community members of the interdisciplinary team, the MS Society, carers associations, etc. However, your list should be much more comprehensive than this.

Activity 7.4

As we don't know whether Chris's problems are drug induced or due to a diagnosis of schizophrenia, you might want to find out what support he has at home. At this early stage it is important not to make judgements about his behaviour or lifestyle, but rather find out what his interpretation of life is.

With Margaret, you will want to know how independent she has been to date, what her husband's abilities are and what they know about what is wrong with Margaret. If we have an idea of what she could do before her stroke, then we will have something to work towards during her recovery.

With Tom, it is important to find out how independent he was before his injury. At age 9 we would expect him to be independent in his mobilizing and toileting; however, with his leg in plaster this will be restricted. It is important to ask Tom and his mum how they will manage this and find out whether Tom's room at home is upstairs, and where the bathroom is.

Alex has been managing his diabetes successfully at home, so we need to find out if this can be facilitated successfully while in hospital by Alex himself, as we don't want to make him dependent.

Activity 7.6

You may have identified that Alex could monitor his own urine and blood glucose levels. All patients could choose their own meals or have their next of kin help them with this. All patients might wash themselves (or their own face, hands and upper bodies in the case of Margaret and Tom).

8

Personal and oral hygiene

Jane Ewen and Pamela Kirkpatrick

Chapter Contents

Learning objectives

The aim of this chapter is to explore the nurse's role in caring for patients' personal and oral hygiene needs. Throughout the chapter we will be referring to the accompanying Media Tool DVD. Please watch the video clips as directed as these will reinforce your learning and expand upon the information given in this book. After reading this chapter and interacting with the Media Tool DVD you will be able to:

- Assess, plan, implement and evaluate each aspect of care in relation to personal and oral hygiene.
- Recognize and respond to individual patient preferences while balancing an evidence-based approach to care delivery.
- Consider differing aspects of psychological, social, cultural and religious needs of different client groups in respect to personal and oral hygiene.
- Identify the relevant equipment required for undertaking specific clinical skills relating to personal and oral hygiene.
- Interpret and integrate local and national guidelines while undertaking procedures for all aspects of personal and oral hygiene.

Introduction

For most people, the ritual of personal and oral hygiene is a vital component in self-care and forms part of daily activities. Cleanliness is an individual standard and is normally carried out in a private setting, as it is a particularly intimate and personal element of self-care. When you support and provide personal and oral hygiene for a patient, it is one of the most fundamental elements of care and one that must be performed competently, respecting privacy and dignity to the highest level (see Chapter 5). As a nurse you are bound by a code of professional conduct (NMC 2008), ensuring that the highest standard of evidence-based individual care is provided to all patients in your care.

Washing the body is carried out for a number of reasons: it enhances the individual's self-esteem and is closely linked to sexuality, culture and religion, as well as having a comfort and cleanliness function to remove excess perspiration, dead skin cells and other body fluids (Pegram *et al.* 2007). From a nursing perspective, it is necessary to help patients wash at regular internals to keep the natural flora of micro-organisms under control and it is also a perfect opportunity to observe your patient's mood and mental health, monitor the skin for rashes or bruises and also check for infestations of the hair and skin (Lentz 2003). Before proceeding any further it is important to have a good understanding of the anatomy and physiology of the skin and the mouth. Access a suitable textbook and do some revision on this.

Cleaning the teeth and oral cavity is also a vital component of daily care. This activity helps to keep natural teeth clean, healthy and free from plaque and decay, and dentures clean. It also ensures that the mouth is clean and free from debris and infection, both of which can compromise communication and eating, chewing and swallowing.

A flexible approach to meeting patients' personal and oral hygiene needs is required in order to adapt to different settings where care delivery is carried out. For example, you may care for patients in hospitals, care homes, social care settings or in the patient's own home. When patients needs are being met in a community setting, daily routines and hygiene processes may differ slightly. Within these community settings personal and *social carers* normally attend to the personal hygiene needs of patients, having been planned in collaboration with the patient, family and healthcare professionals.

This chapter will begin by providing an overview of the general principles that must be considered by you, as a student nurse, in relation to meeting the personal and oral hygiene needs of patients and clients.

General principles

Communication

Communication during personal hygiene should be a two-way interaction between you and your patient and is an ideal opportunity to develop a rapport. At this time they will have your undivided attention and may talk in detail about themselves, their family and their condition, as well as how they are feeling – for example, whether they have pain. This requires you to have effective listening and observation skills (see Chapter 2) and this information can be invaluable when assessing, planning, undertaking or evaluating a patient's care.

Having an awareness of a patient's psychological needs and spending time with them allows you to pick up on any non-verbal cues. For example, you may be able to establish if the patient is in pain by their facial expression or ascertain their mood from their eye contact. It is also important to recognize that in some cases patients may not wish to speak during the procedure, due either to their physical or their psychological condition, and you should be sensitive to this and carry out their personal and oral hygiene in accordance with their individual preferences (Dougherty and Lister 2004).

Where two nurses are involved in assisting with personal hygiene needs, they must ensure that any conversation taking place includes the patient and does not occur above them or exclude them. The conversation should directly relate to the patient, their well-being and the processes involved in the care and not include the nurses' personal or other professional matters. In some cases, where the patient is acutely ill, it may be appropriate to keep communication to a minimum.

When attending to the hygiene needs of an unconscious patient, communication is of equal importance as hearing may still be present. Despite the patient's apparent lack of awareness of their surroundings and your presence, the use of non-verbal gestures including touch, as well as speech directed at them, is of paramount importance. This will give them a sense of understanding of their surroundings and make them feel included (Geraghty 2005).

However, communication issues may arise in the case of conscious patients as demonstrated in the Alex case study and it may be useful to review these communication issues at this stage.

Activity 8.1

Go to the Media Tool DVD, select **Case Studies**, then **Learning Disability (Alex)**. Watch both the video clips of the **nurses visiting Alex** and pay particular attention to the good and bad communication that takes place with and over Alex. Read the further information supplied in relation to these clips and note down your observations.

It may also be appropriate to involve a family member to assist personal and oral hygiene needs to ensure that individual preferences and needs continue to be met. This can be particularly helpful with children, or patients who have a learning disability, who may be less anxious around a familiar individual such as a carer or parent. Equally, it may be comforting for the relatives themselves, particularly in situations where their loved one is critically ill. Allowing the family to be included makes them feel involved, which can be comforting in difficult circumstances and may assist in the patient's care and can also contribute to their recovery and sense of well-being (Verhaeghe *et al.* 2005).

Patient-centred care

Prior to carrying out personal and oral hygiene it is important to assess the patient's ability to participate in washing or bathing as well as discussing the patient's likes and dislikes with them (Hooks and Roberts 2007). The type of care and level of support given to a patient's personal and oral hygiene needs can be dependent on a number of factors. For example, a child will require a different level of care to an adult patient and their needs may differ. In children, as they

grow physically and become more independent, their needs change and they may require less support (Trigg and Mohammed 2006). In addition, parents and siblings will want to be supportive in meeting these needs and may also be involved with their delivery when appropriate. In adult patients, an individual's physical and psychological condition or symptoms will dictate the approach to be taken to attend to their needs effectively and to their preferred standards, and you may wish to consider the fundamental questions listed in Box 8.1 when assessing a patient's preferences before helping with personal hygiene needs.

Box 8.1 Key questions to consider in the assessment of personal hygiene needs

- Does your patient prefer a bath or a shower?
- Does their condition necessitate that they should be bed bathed because mobility is challenged, or are they are too ill for alternatives?
- Does their culture or religion dictate where and how personal hygiene needs are attended to?

In some instances, the patient's mobility might be restricted, for example, with enforced bed rest following a lumbar puncture, during monitoring or following orthopaedic surgery for the fitting of external frames. Though immobility is enforced, a bed bath is still an effective option for many patients. In all cases, planned care is negotiated with patient and/or carers and is based on the assessment of their individual needs. The procedure should be clearly explained to your patient and you should gain cooperation and consent before proceeding.

Privacy

Most people prefer privacy while carrying out personal hygiene activities but this is not always easy to achieve. Although most hospital/care home/ward areas have bed screens or curtains that can be pulled around the bed area or a washbasin cubicle, these do not provide the same level of privacy as a self-contained bathroom. Curtains alone do not shield noise and conversation or ensure complete privacy. It is therefore important to endeavour to ensure that noise be kept to a minimum and any conversation between individuals is done quietly. This will help to reduce embarrassment for the patient, maintain privacy and protect patient confidentiality (Pegram *et al.* 2007). For more information refer to Chapter 5.

Cultural and religious preferences

The patient's cultural and religious beliefs also need to be taken into account as they may also have an impact on the level of care and the way in which it is delivered. Different cultures place differing values on cleanliness. For example, Muslims expect a high standard of personal hygiene both from a physical and spiritual perspective. This necessitates the more mobile patient having access to running water in which to carry out their personal hygiene needs (Arif 2005). Patients who may be restricted to bed, and where running water is less accessible, will also require assistance with their personal hygiene needs a number of times during the day (Peate 2005). This may mean that when a bedpan is provided, a container of clean water should also accompany it.

Cultural and religious practices also need to be taken into account when removing, or assisting a patient in the removal of their clothes for personal hygiene needs. Some cultures have strict guidelines on what clothing is worn and complete removal of items of clothing in some cultures and religions is not acceptable practice (Peate 2005). It is important that as a nurse you discuss cultural and religious needs and requirements in relation to personal hygiene with all patients and their families. Many hospitals have specific guidelines and information on different cultural and religious practices, which will help guide you in the care required, and you should endeavour to seek these out when in the clinical environment.

Consideration should also be given to the wearing of jewellery and other adornments, as these are often a display of sexuality and may also be worn by patients for religious and cultural reasons. Body piercing and the use of decorative jewellery in the ears, nose and mouth and around the eyes are common in society and attention must be given to cleanliness in this respect, ensuring that these sensitive areas are not damaged during personal hygiene practices. You can always

discuss with the patient how these may be best cared for and whether or not they can be removed for personal hygiene needs.

Activity 8.2

Identify and reflect on the key requirements in relation to the personal and oral hygiene needs of the most dominant religious and cultural groups that you are likely to nurse within your area of practice. Locate and compare your answers with local policies. The following website also offers further information: http://www.ethnicityonline.net/hygiene_good_prac.htm.

Assisting with personal and oral hygiene

In general, patients may require assistance with their personal hygiene in a number of circumstances including following a clinical procedure, surgical intervention or as part of their daily living activities in acute or ongoing care situations. In all cases, where possible, patients should be actively encouraged to participate in their care, with the promotion of self-care being advocated to promote independence (see Chapter 7). In certain circumstances – for example, in children or adults who have a learning disability – it may be entirely appropriate to involve a family member or carer in this aspect of care. Some patients who present with mental health conditions such as depression or schizophrenia, may refrain from attending to any of their personal or oral hygiene needs despite being physically able to do so. While respecting their individual preferences, these patients should be encouraged and motivated as much as possible to carry out these procedures with appropriate support. If a patient presents with severe depressive symptoms which prevent them from attending to their personal and oral hygiene needs due to complete lack of motivation, you should seek the patient's consent to assist them with this and respect their wishes if the response is negative.

Patients who may be restricted to bed or have restricted movement, and who are not necessarily in familiar surroundings can feel particularly anxious at the prospect of being less independent than they would normally be. Involving family or carers may help alleviate some of these anxieties. However, in your role you should ensure that caring for the patient's personal and oral hygiene needs is not rushed and also ensure that it is as relaxing and comforting as possible for them.

Standard infection control precautions

In carrying out personal and oral hygiene tasks you should ensure that standard infection control precautions are adhered to in order to minimize the risk of cross-contamination of micro-organisms between individuals. The wearing of disposable gloves and the appropriate plastic apron for all direct patient care where there is a chance of coming into contact with body fluids is advocated (Candlin and Stark 2005). This again will assist in reducing the transmission of micro-organisms and prevent risk of harm from contamination of body fluids (Trigg and Mohammed 2006). Careful and thorough hand washing is also fundamental before and after attending to the personal hygiene needs of a patient, together with the appropriate use of alcohol hand rubs. An example of an alcohol hand rub can be seen in Figure 8.1. Hand washing is an important skill that you should master before commencing clinical practice. You need to make sure that you understand when to use alcohol hand rubs and when you should wash your hands.

Activity 8.3

Go to the Media Tool DVD, select **Skill Sets**, **Infection Control and Hygiene**, and then **Hand washing**. Watch the video of hand washing and make a list of the step-by-step approach.

Practise the technique both at home and within your clinical area to gain competence and confidence in this important skill.

Bathing

Bed bathing is an important clinical skill for any nurse to carry out. It assists a patient with their personal hygiene when confined to bed for a period of time due to an acute or chronic condition. This can mean that during your career you will bed bath many patients from the elderly to the very young, in both conscious and unconscious states.

Care should be taken to ensure the patient's privacy and dignity are maintained throughout this process, particularly as the patient's nightclothes will require to be removed. This may make your patient feel very vulnerable as their skin will be exposed. In addition, due to the patient's reduced movement in bed together with the removal of clothes, the patient is at risk of cooling down very quickly. Therefore having two nurses to assist in carrying out the procedure allows one nurse to wash the patient while the other dries and ensures the bed bath is carried out in a timely manner, keeping the patient's skin exposed for as little time as possible. The patient may be restless, agitated or confused and having two nurses at the bedside will provide a safer environment for the patient at this time.

When preparing a patient for a bed bath, it is important that all the necessary equipment is prepared prior to commencing the procedure (see Box 8.2). Moving a patient during a bed bath should be kept to minimum and you should consider the patient's pain score before carrying out personal hygiene as

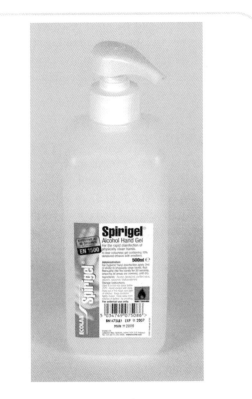

Figure 8.1 Alcohol hand rub

Scenario 8.1

John is a 56-year-old married man and a long-distance lorry driver who was admitted to a coronary care unit following an acute myocardial infarction. You may wish to revise the anatomy and physiology of the heart together with the care of a patient with this condition before answering the questions below. You could also talk to colleagues and your mentor in practice.

1 Outline how you would address John's personal and oral hygiene needs and how these may change during his hospital stay.

2 John voices concern and anxiety while you are bed bathing him. Taking consideration of his current condition, diagnosis, age and occupation, what anxieties may he discuss with you? Compare your response with the suggested answer at the end of the chapter.

Box 8.2 Equipment required for bed bathing

- Plastic apron and disposable gloves.
- Clean bed linen and linen bag (appropriate to local protocol and policy).
- Clinical waste bag.
- Disposable wipes/cloth.
- Basin (individual patient basin).
- Toiletries (patient's own where possible).
- Clean pyjamas/night dress.
- Two large towels.
- Brush/comb.
- Toothbrush, toothpaste and clean receiver/ bowl for patient to clean teeth; water or mouthwash.
- Denture pot if required.
- Razor and shaving foam if required.

movement during the procedure may exacerbate their pain. If the patient is experiencing discomfort, this should be addressed prior to carrying out the procedure in order to ensure the patient is more comfortable and relaxed. If the patient is pain-free and able to move with assistance, it may be appropriate for you or a

member of the multidisciplinary team such as a physiotherapist to undertake passive exercises of the limbs and assist with breathing exercises. This will help prevent complications of bed rest, for example, *deep vein thrombosis.*

At the outset the patient should be offered the opportunity to empty their bladder or bowel prior to commencing the bed bath. This will also aid their comfort during the procedure (see Chapter 10). Where possible, the patient's own toiletries should be used and you should be guided by them as well as local policy on the application of talcum powder, deodorant and make-up. If a patient has been admitted as an emergency they may have no toiletries or nightclothes with them. Although patients are expected to supply their own toiletries, there is usually a supply of individual soaps, disposable combs, toothbrushes and toothpaste in the clinical area for individual patient use.

When preparing the environment for bathing, you should ensure it is warm to promote patient comfort and prevent the patient from losing heat. The temperature of the room should ideally be between 22–25°C (Trigg and Mohammed 2006). A sheet, blanket or large bath towel should be used to cover the patient during the process to prevent unnecessary exposure and heat loss. In addition, a clean and clear surface or bed table is required along with the equipment listed in Box 8.2.

Bed bath procedure

Before carrying out any procedure, a full explanation should be given to your patient in order to gain cooperation and consent from them. Although you may be very used to carrying out bed baths, you should take into account that this may be your patient's first experience and they may feel quite anxious.

Frequently the procedure is undertaken in a ward environment at an appropriate time. The screens around the bed should be drawn, any doors closed and window curtains drawn. This will also help keep the area warm as well and assist in maintaining the patient's privacy and dignity (Dougherty and Lister 2004). Your hospital may also use privacy and dignity signs that may be attached to the curtains (see the Media Tool DVD).

Hand washing and application of a disposable apron

are crucial. The patient should be in a comfortable position in their bed, ideally semi-recumbent. However, the patient's condition and level of consciousness will dictate position, and a breathless patient is generally nursed sitting up. You should also ensure that the water in the basin is hand-hot and comfortably warm for the patient.

The patient's bed should be elevated to an appropriate height for both nurses. This will help prevent any unnecessary back strain and stretching while undertaking the procedure. The procedure should be carried out in accordance with local moving and handling policies to ensure the safety of both the nurses and the patient. Any excess linen should be removed and placed on the bed rail at the bottom of the bed. Assistance should be given to the patient to remove day/nightclothes where required.

A logical approach should be taken to carry out a full bed bath. Patients cool down quickly and you should therefore ensure that only the part of the body being washed is exposed. Box 8.3 suggests a logical order in which to carry out the procedure, however, local policy should always be considered. Each part of the patient's skin should be washed, rinsed and thoroughly dried as this will minimize the risk of loss of skin integrity. When washing the patient's limbs, the furthest limb should be washed first. This will allow the second nurse to dry the limb and also prevent water being splashed on already washed and dried skin (Pegram *et al.* 2007).

Box 8.3 Suggested washing order

- Face, including neck and ears.
- Arms.
- Chest and abdomen.
- Legs.
- Genital area.*
- Back.
- Buttocks.

*Water should be changed after genital area has been washed.

Individual preferences should be sought with regard to the use of soap, which can be harsh and drying on the skin (e.g. on the patient's face) and this may also be dependent on the patient's condition (Dougherty and Lister 2004). There are a number of alternatives to using soap for cleansing the face and body and these include lotions and emollient baths, which may be more soothing if the patient presents with an underlying skin condition or has a personal preference. Again, dignity should be maintained throughout. It may be appropriate to ask your patient if they would like to wash and dry their own face. If you are unsure of any aspect of care, you must seek advice and support from the nurse in charge.

When attending to the pubic and groin area, disposable wipes must always be used as this will prevent cross-infection. If patients are able to wash this area themselves, this should be encouraged to promote dignity and independence and reduce possible embarrassment. However, the patient may require assistance. In male patients, if the patient has not been circumcised, the foreskin should be retracted to expose the *glans penis*. This area should be washed, rinsed and dried thoroughly to prevent bacterial growth and the foreskin replaced to prevent any constriction of the penis. The scrotum should also be washed and dried. For female patients, each part of the labia should be cleaned from the area of minimal contamination (usually the pubic area) to that of the maximum (usually the rectal area) using one single wipe to avoid contamination. Again, this area must be rinsed and dried thoroughly. After perineal hygiene the water must be changed to reduce the risk of cross-infection from the normal skin flora. If a patient has a catheter, then catheter care should be carried out at this time (see Chapter 10).

To wash the patient's back they should be rolled onto their side. This will also allow the bottom sheet to be changed without the patient getting out of bed. Care should be taken to ensure that there are no creases in the bed linen with could lead to pressure ulcers (see Chapter 11).

The patient should be helped into clean night/day clothes and assistance should be given with brushing/combing their hair if they are unable to do this independently. When confined to bed, patients' hair can become tangled, therefore a thorough brush or comb is important. Care should be taken, however, not to apply too much pressure as sharp bristles on some brushes may scratch or tear a patient's scalp. It may be more appropriate to wash your patient's hair at this time and this will be discussed later in the chapter. Oral hygiene should be provided at this point and some patients may require minimal assistance while others may require this to be carried out for them; this will also be discussed in more detail later in the chapter.

For some patients it may be appropriate to carry out a facial shave or apply make-up. This can help promote their self-esteem at a time where they may be quite low in mood. Throughout the procedure the patient's skin should be observed for signs of redness, bruising, pain or rash as this may indicate areas of potential pressure sores.

Any significant findings regarding the condition of the patient, the condition of their skin, nails, eyes. etc. should be monitored and documented in the nursing records together with level of assistance required (see Chapter 3). Any changes should also be reported to the nurse in charge so that the individual patient care plan can be evaluated and updated accordingly. On completion of the bed bath, you are responsible for leaving the bed area clean and tidy. To prevent cross-infection, hand hygiene should take place prior to attending to the next patient.

Washing hair

There may be occasions where the more dependent patient who is restricted to bed requires their hair to be washed and some patients may find this procedure tiring, depending on their condition. Careful consideration should therefore be given to the time of day that hair washing is carried out and where possible the patient should be allowed time to rest following the procedure. There are a number of devices and receptacles available to undertake hair washing in bed and you should seek advice from your local procedure manual prior to carrying this out, but the information given here can act as a general guideline.

The bed head needs to be removed and stowed safely during the procedure and ideally two nurses should be present. The patient should be asked to lie on their back in a comfortable position with their head at the top of the bed and their shoulders and neck well supported with pillows, unless their physical condition dictates otherwise. Supporting the neck and shoulders will ensure patient comfort and will allow their hair, if long, to drape over the back of the bed giving greater access to the scalp for washing. Placing a large plastic

Scenario 8.2

Billy is a 44-year-old man who has been involved in a road traffic accident. He has sustained a fractured pelvis, ribs, tibia and fibula. He is on bed rest following surgery to his leg and has an internal fixator in place. He is a heavy smoker.

1. While attending to Billy's personal hygiene needs the nurse must be aware of the potential complications of bed rest. What complications do you think Billy could develop and why?

2. What actions could you take to help prevent these complications when attending to personal hygiene? Check the end of the chapter for a suggested answer.

sheet and towels over the pillows will protect the patient and absorb any water that is spilt. A jug of warm water will be required together with the patient's shampoo and conditioner, and a large empty basin which should be placed on a chair or small table for water collection.

Careful observation of the patient's scalp should be made prior to washing to identify any dry, flaky, red or broken areas which must be noted and reported. Clean warm water should be gently poured over the patient's hair ensuring that it is kept away from the eye and ear area. The patient may wish to hold a small cloth or wipe over their eyes and, where advocated, cotton wool to their ears to protect them from splashes of water or shampoo. Shampoo should be applied and thoroughly massaged in the scalp, which should then be rinsed with clean warm water. Care should be taken not to scratch the patient's scalp with fingernails. The process should be repeated with conditioner and the hair then gently combed or brushed.

The patient may wish their hair to be dried using a clean towel or hair dryer depending on individual preference. Once the procedure has been completed you should ensure that any damp or wet towels are removed, the bed head and pillows placed back onto the bed and the patient left in a comfortable position. The procedure should be recorded in the patient's notes and their care plan updated.

Assisted bathing

The principles discussed in the previous section also apply to patients who require assistance with a bath, shower or wash. The promotion of self-care is advocated (see Chapter 7) and in all cases the patient should be encouraged to do as much as they can for themselves. Some patients may have input from an occupational therapist who will work with them to assess their ability to wash and dress independently. Where assistance may be required, observations should be made of the skin, documenting and reporting any signs of redness, bruising or broken areas.

Safety in bathroom areas is crucial whether caring for an adult or a child. Comprehensive assessments of the risks are imperative for each patient in each situation. A child or baby should never be left unsupervised with water, or in a bath, as there is a risk of slipping, scalding or drowning. Similarly, when assisting someone with a mental health condition such as the case study patient, Chris, you should always check what supervision is required and give this as directed.

It is important to consider the temperature of the water for bathing and showering. The temperature needs to be between 32 and 42°C to be comfortable. However, you should bear in mind individual preferences and also consider whether the patient has compromised circulation or neurological sensation, which may mean that their judgement regarding the water temperature may not be accurate and they may be at risk of scalding.

When assisting a patient who is unsteady on their feet or immobile into and out of a bath or shower, it is

Activity 8.4

Go to the Media Tool DVD, select **Case Studies**, then **Mental Health (Chris)**. Review the case study of Chris who has mental health problems and consider what personal hygiene support he may require in order to maintain a safe environment for him and others before reading on.

It is important that a risk assessment is first carried out on Chris and that this is updated appropriately. He will also need careful observation and lots of encouragement. Self-care should always be promoted.

likely that the use of a mechanical bath hoist or a moveable shower chair will be required. Within different clinical areas the style of hoist may vary, some choosing one manufacturer over another. However, when operating any of these hoists you need to familiarize yourself with the manufacturer's instructions and use them only with the support and supervision of experienced staff. You are also required to have had adequate training in the use of hoists and it is important that you refer to local moving and handling protocols when using such equipment.

Activity 8.5

Identify the different hoists/chairs that you have seen used in the hospital or in the patient's home.

Maintaining a safe environment at all times is fundamental in the care of a patient. Care should also be taken to ensure any water and soap on the floor are mopped up immediately to prevent the possibility of the patient or staff member slipping or falling and causing injury to themselves.

Patients who are more independent and whose condition is stable may wish to be left alone in the bath or shower to relax and wash themselves. This decision should be made in conjunction with the patient's risk assessment and an experienced staff member. Be sure that a nurse call bell is in place in an accessible position in case the patient requires assistance at any time. It is deemed good practice to knock on the bathroom/shower room door periodically and check the patient is well.

If required, the patient may need assistance to wash and dry their hair, feet or back and when out of the bath or shower may require help to open or apply toiletries. Patients affected by a mental health disorder may require different levels of supervision, which will be agreed by the multidisciplinary team as part of their ongoing treatment and be influenced by local guidelines. Patients with mental health conditions must be informed of their 'observation status' prior to commencing any personal hygiene needs (see Chapter 6). This will prevent a situation escalating which could have an impact on the health and safety of others as well as yourself.

Bathing a baby or infant

When bathing a baby or child, the general principles discussed earlier should be adhered to. In general, it is not necessary for babies to have immersion baths daily as this can alter the natural pH balance of the skin (Trigg and Mohammed 2006). However, where babies are acutely unwell or have soiled nappies, bathing will be required more frequently.

In cases where a baby or infant is considered too ill or restless to be given an immersion bath, the use of the 'top and tail' approach is suitable. This procedure involves cleansing the face, hands and the nappy region and is a good alternative to an immersion bath.

Whatever approach is used, it is vital to stress to those supporting or delivering the care that a baby or infant will lose body heat quickly during the procedure due to their immature temperature regulation system. A suitably warm environment of 22–25ºC, free from draughts with windows closed will provide a comfortable setting and the use of warm towels will assist in maintaining the infant's body temperature. Box 8.4. provides a list of equipment required to carry out the top and tail procedure.

Whether bathing or 'top and tailing' a baby you should hold the baby securely as they can wriggle or slide away from you when the skin is wet. All skin creases should be washed and dried thoroughly to prevent any red or broken areas of skin developing. Advice should be sought regarding the use of talcum powder from trained members of staff and in line with local policy. Use may be contraindicated as it could increase the risk of irritation and, as with adults, may

irritate respiratory conditions (Trigg and Mohammed 2006).

Observations of the nails should also be made and, if long or sharp, these should be cut with blunt-ended scissors designed for this purpose. This will prevent the baby or infant from scratching their skin. The cleaning of orifices such as the ears and nostrils is not advocated as this may damage delicate organs. These orifices will in time naturally clean themselves (Trigg and Mohammed 2006). Local policy should be referred to for the cleansing of umbilical cords.

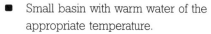

Activity 8.6

Go to the Media Tool DVD, select **Skill Sets**, **Infection Control and Hygiene**, then **Bathing a baby**. View the video clip for further information.

Shaving

Assisting your patient with shaving is an important element of caring for an individual's personal hygiene needs and can help lift the individual's mood and increase their self-esteem at a time when they may be feeling unwell and low. Shaving can be incorporated into the day-to-day personal hygiene routine, whether a bed bath or an assisted wash has been carried out. In all cases the assessment of the patient's capability dependent on their physical and psychological needs may determine the level of assistance required. It is also important to take into consideration the individual's culture and religious beliefs at this time as facial hair is significant in some cultures and any removal should not be carried out without consent. Individuals usually have a preference as to whether they have an electric or wet shave and this should be established through consultation with the patient or relatives together with the nursing care plan. The use of the patient's own toiletries is advocated together with the patient's own razor to prevent possible cross-infection.

Prior to carrying out this procedure you should ensure that standard infection control precautions have been carried out including hand washing and the wearing of disposable gloves and apron (Candlin and Stark 2005). When carrying out a wet shave, you will need the equipment listed in Box 8.5.

Box 8.4 Equipment needed for the top and tail procedure

- Small basin with warm water of the appropriate temperature.
- Soft, clean cloth or sponge.
- Disposable wipes.
- Disposable bag.
- Soap or soap alternative.
- Warm towels.
- Nappy if required.
- Hairbrush.
- Clean clothing.

Box 8.5 Equipment needed for facial hair removal

- Towel to place over the patient.
- Basin of warm water.
- Disposable wipe or patient's face cloth.
- Shaving foam/gel.
- Shaving brush.
- Razor (patient's own).
- Aftershave lotion or balm.

Where possible, the patient should be in a sitting position either in a chair or in bed, but if this is not feasible due to their condition, a suitably comfortable position should be adopted. Prior to carrying out an electric or wet shave the patient's skin should be inspected for any blemishes, moles or broken areas. When undertaking a wet shave the face should be warmed with water to open the hair follicles and shaving foam or gel then applied. The use of short straight strokes with the razor in the direction of facial hair growth should be performed while holding the skin taut in the opposite direction. Shaving in this direction it will promote patient comfort and ensure a cleaner shave for the individual, reducing the likelihood of skin abrasion. Throughout the procedure excess foam should be rinsed from the razor to prevent any clogging of the razor and to allow the free flow of the blades across the facial hair. This should be repeated until the entire face and neck are cleanly shaven. The patient's face should then be dried with a towel and, if preferred, aftershave or balm applied. Care must be taken throughout the procedure to ensure that the patient's skin is not nicked or cut with the razor, particularly if the patient has any underlying condition, for example, *haemophilia*, or if the patient is taking prescribed medication, such as *warfarin*, that may affect their blood-clotting mechanism.

It is not uncommon for female patients to require assistance with facial hair removal. This may be due to, for example, medication that they are prescribed, which has caused excess and undesired hair growth. Such cases should be treated sensitively, while maintaining the individual's privacy and dignity at all times.

Following a shave, you should ensure the safe disposal of the razor either into a sharps container (see Figure 8.2.) or into the patient's wash bag with the safety guard reattached. It is important to recognize that there may be particular patients (e.g. those with mental health conditions) for whom a bladed razor is inappropriate. In such cases the wet razor may be replaced by an electric razor. Always be guided by the patient's records as well as the nurse in charge.

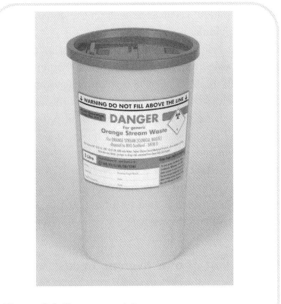

Figure 8.2 Sharps container

Patient education

Assisting a patient with personal hygiene provides an ideal opportunity to teach and educate them about many aspects of health and hygiene. For example, caring for the skin, mouth, feet, stoma, wound or catheter. You should use your judgement on the appropriateness and timing of education depending on the patient's condition. For instance, it may be more appropriate to involve the patient's family or carer in the education and use educational resources in

Activity 8.7

Go to the Media Tool DVD, select **Skill Sets**, **Infection Control and Hygiene**, then **Facial shaving**, and watch the video clip of a wet shave.

addition to an informational discussion. In all cases you should ensure sensitivity and tact and take an opportunistic approach when embarking on this role.

Oral hygiene

Nurses have a key role in promoting good oral health with patients and carers. The aim of good oral hygiene is to ensure that your patient has a clean, comfortable and healthy mouth, to promote patient comfort and to add to their well-being and quality of life.

A healthy mouth is clean, functional and comfortable, free from infection and essential for the maintenance of general health, effective communication, acceptable appearance and nutritional status (see Chapters 2 and 9). Poor oral heath can influence a patient's mood and dietary intake and can have an effect on patient comfort as well as the general health of the individual.

In your role you will nurse patients of all ages and cultures who require frequent oral hygiene for a number of reasons. Box 8.6 identifies some predisposing factors that contribute to poor oral health.

Oral hygiene must be provided to all patients who have these predisposing factors and include the dying patient, the elderly and the immobile. However, the level of assistance that you provide in this area may differ depending on how independent the patient is and whether they are able to attend to this aspect of personal hygiene themselves.

Assessment of oral hygiene needs

Before carrying out any oral hygiene, your patient's needs should be assessed and their consent and cooperation granted. Any problems with delivering oral hygiene should be noted and advice sought from the dental team or nurse specialist. All patients are assessed to identify the advice and care required to maintain and promote their individual oral hygiene and this will be met according to the patient's individual and clinical needs, which may change depending on their condition. The mouth, lips and teeth must be assessed to identify any sores, broken areas or infection in order that appropriate advice is given and care carried out.

This assessment should be made at the initial stage of care with ongoing reassessment when changes

Box 8.6 Poor oral health

- Inability to take adequate fluids/food orally.
- Poor nutritional status.
- Patients who are nauseated and vomiting.
- Insufficient saliva production leading to a dry mouth, collection of debris and possible infection.
- Major interventions altering oral status, i.e. surgery, radiotherapy or chemotherapy for malignant disease.
- Lack of knowledge or motivation for maintaining oral hygiene.
- Mouth-breathing in patients who have respiratory disease.
- Continuous oxygen therapy which leads to drying of the oral mucosa.
- Intermittent suctioning.

occur, or at frequent intervals. At this time nurses should take into account the patient's physical and mental ability to achieve self-care. When carrying out oral hygiene, there are a number of factors that need to be taken into account. These include whether your patient is in a conscious/unconscious state, whether they are dependent or independent and whether they have dentures or natural teeth, all of which can direct and dictate the way the care is carried out. For example, patients with limited manual dexterity (e.g. arthritic joints) or who have lost the function of one arm following a *cerebral vascular accident*, as in the case study of Margaret, may find it difficult to brush their teeth or dentures. Simply introducing a toothbrush with a modified handle or an electric toothbrush can be a useful aid to brushing and allows independence with this activity. There are a number of oral health assessment tools available and an example of one is shown in Figure 8.3 (NHS Grampian 2005). It is important to note that such tools should be used in conjunction with local policy and best practice statements where available.

Name: ....   DOB: ....   Unit no.: ....

Ward: ....   Date of admission: ....

		Yes/No	Action
1.	Does the client have natural teeth?	Yes	Brush teeth twice daily with toothpaste and toothbrush
		No	Rinse mouth with water after meals and before bed
2.	Does the client have dentures (full or partial)?	Yes	Clean daily with soap and water (do not use toothpaste), take dentures out at night
		No	No action required
3.	Are any dentures labelled?	Yes	No action required
		No	Label dentures with marking kit
4.	Does the client have their own toothbrush?	Yes	Check toothbrush is suitable
		No	Ensure client receives a suitable toothbrush
5.	Is the client able to clean their own teeth?	Yes	Ask if assistance is required
		No	Contact oral care resource nurse, OT hygienist or dentist for advice
6.	Is the client registered with a family dentist?	Yes	Note name and address of dentist below (see no.8)
		No	Contact community dental service
7.	Is the client having any dental problems?	Yes	Detail problem(s) below
		No	Review six-monthly if no abnormality or problem experienced
8.	Name and address of family dentist		
9	When did the client last have a dental check up?		
10a.	Does the client smoke?		
10b.	Has the client ever smoked?		
11.	Brief description of dental problems (see care plan overleaf for any actions):		
12.	Brief description of other oral care issues (see care plan overleaf for any actions):		

Name of Assessor: ....   Job Title: ....   Date: ....

If action is required, please refer to resource/pack on how to contact community dental service or contact the senior dental officer

Figure 8.3 Oral health assessment form

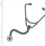
Activity 8.8

Access the local oral assessment tools used within your practice area and note your findings as appropriate.

Oral hygiene and dependent patients

The frequency with which oral hygiene is carried out is also determined by your patient's condition. If your patient has any of the previously indicated predisposing factors outlined in Box 8.6 or if they are extremely weak or unconscious, it may be appropriate to carry out oral hygiene every one to two hours. For example, in the case of Margaret, you will see her condition changing: she moves from an unconscious dependent state to a conscious dependent state. These changes will be documented in the patient's care plan and should guide your practice.

Before proceeding with oral hygiene, the mouth and lips should be assessed for sores, broken areas and infection. A small torch is helpful when doing this. Oral *Candida albicans* (thrush) is a common infection particularly with patients presenting with ill-fitting dentures, where there is evidence of poor oral hygiene or in patients who are *immuno-suppressed*. This fungal infection presents as small white spots that coat the tongue, the mucosa of the inner cheeks and sometimes the soft palate. Should this be detected, it must be reported to the nurse in charge and a doctor so that treatment can be prescribed and it should also be documented in the patient's care plan.

The use of a toothbrush and toothpaste is the most effective method for maintaining good oral hygiene (Geraghty 2005). Most patients are familiar with brushing their teeth so it would seem sensible for this practice to be encouraged. The use of other dental hygiene aids such as dental floss should be continued if they are part of the person's normal ritual. Even when providing oral hygiene to an unconscious patient's mouth, a toothbrush and toothpaste can be used and this is the most effective way of reducing the build-up of plaque and ensuring the enamel on all surfaces of the teeth is cleaned (Geraghty 2005). If a toothbrush and toothpaste are unsuitable, then sponge-tipped sticks, similar to the one shown in Figure 8.4, soaked in water, or gauze wrapped around a

gloved finger may be considered (NHS Quality Improvement Scotland 2005), but care must be taken to ensure the patient doesn't bite on the sponge-tipped stick.

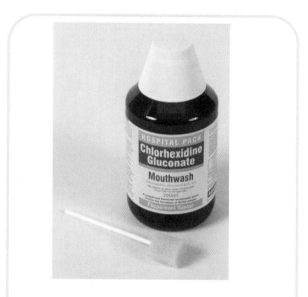

Figure 8.4 Sponge-tipped stick and mouthwash

There continues to be some debate concerning the use of sponge-tipped sticks for general oral hygiene. Such sticks are not effective in removing plaque from the surface of teeth but can be useful for refreshing the mouth (NHS Quality Improvement Scotland 2005). Patients who may be unconscious and receiving continuous oxygen therapy may benefit from the use of these sticks to ensure their mouth is moist and fresh. The action of rotating the sponge-tipped stick soaked in water gently over the mucosa will prevent trauma within the oral cavity. There are some contra-indications associated with the use of sponge-tipped sticks, which include an unpleasant feel in the mouth and the risk of the sponge being bitten off and swallowed. In light of this, it is essential that a risk assessment of your patient be carried out before using a sponge-tipped stick. Further details on the use of oral care tools and various solutions for cleaning and treatment can be found in Dougherty and Lister (2004).

Unconscious patients should have their dentures removed, as if they are ill-fitting they can potentially block the airway. Place dentures in water in a clearly marked denture pot. Yellow soft paraffin can also be applied to the lips of an unconscious patient if they are

Activity 8.9

Go to the Media Tool DVD, select **Skill Sets**, **Infection Control and Hygiene** and then **Oral care.** View the video clip **Oral care – Unconscious patient without toothbrush**. This provides a demonstration of how to carry out this procedure safely using sponge-tipped sticks.

dry. In this instance, the patient should be lying flat with their head turned to the side. Gentle suction with a suitable oral catheter may be required to remove any debris.

Denture care

Patients who wear dentures should remove and clean them after every meal and before they go to sleep. Leaving dentures out at night while sleeping allows the mouth to rest and recover, but many people can be embarrassed to do this. Some patients may undertake their denture care independently in the privacy of a toilet or washbasin cubicle, however, for patients who are confined to bed, the provision of a water-filled bowl, a cup of water for rinsing, toothbrush, toothpaste and a towel should be sufficient for them to care for their dentures.

Care should be taken when you are required to clean patients' dentures and this should be done over a bowl or sink of water so that if dropped they do not break. Disposable gloves and a plastic apron should be worn to perform this procedure, which is best carried out with a small soft brush, such as a toothbrush. The fitting surface as well as the teeth should be thoroughly cleaned and the patient should also be encouraged to brush their gums gently with a soft toothbrush before re-inserting the dentures. These should be rinsed after cleaning and left to soak overnight in hypochlorite denture-cleaning solution. This will help break down plaque, reducing calculus or tartar formation.

In hospital, patients should have a disposable denture bowl, clearly labelled with the patient's name and date of issue on it. The dentures themselves may be inscribed as appropriate to prevent any mix-up and/ or loss. This bowl should be changed weekly or as appropriate and the water emptied out when the dentures are removed. If dentures are not being worn,

the water they are stored in for soaking should be changed daily.

Tooth brushing

Patients who need help with toothbrushing should be in a comfortable position with a basin or bowl and mirror close by. An explanation of the procedure to the patient should be given and their co-operation and consent gained. The equipment required for this procedure is detailed in Box 8.7.

Box 8.7 Equipment needed for tooth brushing

- Patient's own toothbrush or denture brush.
- Toothpaste.
- Container with water.
- Gauze swabs.
- Gloves.
- Disposable bowl.
- Towel.
- Yellow soft paraffin if required.
- If nil by mouth, ensure suction is on standby.

Only a small amount of toothpaste (the size of a pea) should be applied to the toothbrush. You should protect the patient's clothes with a towel draped around their neck and shoulders and stand behind them, or slightly to one side, depending on what is comfortable. Take care not to use excessive pressure when brushing the teeth as this may lead to bleeding gums and patient discomfort.

If the patient has partial dentures, these should be removed before cleaning the natural teeth and the principles discussed earlier in the section on denture care adhered to. The patient's head should be supported gently and the lips drawn back with thumb or finger. A small-headed toothbrush should be used to brush one or two teeth and gums at a time with care being taken if there are any loose teeth. The patient, if able, should be asked to rinse their mouth with water. However, if unable to do this, to prevent the risk of aspiration, the use of gauze swabs wrapped around a gloved finger to mop up excess toothpaste and saliva is acceptable.

The above procedure can also be followed for

patients who have dentures using the same process to gently brush all tooth surfaces, the gums, the tongue, inside the cheeks and the palate. Yellow soft paraffin may be applied to the patient's lips at the end of the procedure to keep them moist and prevent any cracking. The patient, as always, should be left warm and comfortable.

Activity 8.9

Go to the Media Tool DVD, select **Case Studies**, **Adult Health (Margaret)**, **Margaret in bed** and watch the video clip. Then go to **Margaret and her husband choose from the menu** and watch the clip **Margaret objects to pureed food**. Discuss the oral hygiene requirements that will need to be carried out. What considerations are needed in relation to oral hygiene in both cases? Consider your answer before reading on. There is a suggested one at the end of the chapter.

Children

Oral hygiene in children is of great importance and should be undertaken from the point at which a child cuts its first tooth. It is important to involve both the child and family in oral hygiene. Children should be encouraged to brush their teeth after meals and before bedtime, using a soft toothbrush and toothpaste and small, gentle, circular motions to clean the teeth. However, it is generally agreed that most children under the age of 6 do not have the manual dexterity required to achieve effective plaque removal without assistance. Therefore, while it remains important with this group to encourage self-care, it should also be remembered that appropriate assistance and education should be given when required, from a parent, carer or healthcare professional (Mohebbi *et al.* 2008).

In children who are immuno-suppressed and who, for example, are undergoing chemotherapy for a malignant disease, specific problems may be experienced and assessment of the mouth should an essential part of their daily care. In addition to normal oral hygiene, these individuals may also require the use of a prescribed mouthwash to prevent any oral infection they are at risk of developing due to their

Activity 8.10

Go to the Media Tool DVD, select **Case Studies**, **Child Health (Tom)**, **Tom brushes his teeth** and watch the video clip. Observe the joint approach to this aspect of care. Describe the advantages of taking this approach with children before reading on.

You will probably have noted the consistency of care, promotion of independence and reduction of anxiety shown in this clip.

physical condition. Within family-centred care there is opportunity for health promotion on the subject of dental care and this should also be encouraged where appropriate.

The discussion so far has focused on the main elements of personal and oral hygiene. Consideration will now be given to the delicate structures of the eyes, ears and nose. Further detail on these elements of personal hygiene can be found in Dougherty and Lister (2004).

Eye care

The eye has its own effective cleansing system that maintains the correct moisture balance and normally requires little specific care. Eye care may be required during the daily routine of personal hygiene, however, to remove a build-up of discharge and/or crusty matter, prevent drying of the cornea, assess for and treat infection and administer medication. Great care is required to carry out this delicate procedure effectively. It is also vital to ensure infection is not introduced into the eye, therefore hand hygiene and the use of an aseptic technique are of paramount importance.

Eye care, or eye swabbing as it is sometimes called, may be required once daily or more frequently depending on an individual's needs and circumstances. As with other aspects of patient care, before commencing, the procedure must be explained fully and discussed with the patient, and informed consent obtained. The procedure is described in Box 8.9.

There is some debate as to which material is optimal for swabbing the eyes. In some clinical areas the use of non-woven swabs may be advocated to prevent the cotton fibres scratching the cornea.

Box 8.8 Equipment needed for eye swabbing

- A clean tray to hold all the equipment.
- A sterile eye-care pack containing a sterile towel, gallipot and cotton balls or non-woven swabs.
- Sterile water or 0.9 per cent Sodium Chloride (normal saline) solution.
- A disposal bag for clinical waste.
- Plastic apron.
- Sterile gloves if appropriate.
- Medication if required.

With an unconscious patient, the lid closure (blink) is inhibited and tear production reduced, which easily leads to drying of the eyes (Geraghty 2005). The use of a gel eye pad is sometimes advocated in this case, which remains placed on top of the closed eye. This helps to prevent corneal drying and trauma in the unconscious patient. The use of artificial tears may be required if dryness is problematic. Contact lenses should always be removed carefully and with guidance from an appropriately experienced member of staff.

Consideration should also be given to the appropriate care and cleaning of vision aids such as spectacles and contact lenses by following the patient's instructions or manufacturer's guidelines. This is also appropriate for patients who have an artificial eye. A holistic approach to caring for the eyes and vision will help prevent potentially serious conditions and maximize the visual function, ensuring patient comfort and safety.

Activity 8.11

Go to the Media Tool DVD, select **Skill Sets**, **Infection control and hygiene**, then **eye care**, and watch the clip showing eye swabbing on an adult.

Ear care

Ear care is another element of the daily routine of personal hygiene. The ear is a sensitive organ that can be easily damaged. Prior to washing the ears they must be carefully inspected in order to check the skin

Box 8.9 Procedure for eye swabbing

- Prepare the patient and help them settle into the correct position (either sitting up with head tilted back or lying down flat on their back). An additional light source may be useful depending on the situation
- Arrange the equipment and open out the pack onto a suitable work surface.
- Put gloves on.
- Protect the patient's clothing by draping a sterile towel around their neck.
- Fill the gallipot with cleansing solution.
- Moisten cotton wool or gauze with cleansing solution.
- With the patient's eyes closed, gently swab the upper lid from inside (nose) to the outer aspect in a single sweep, using each swab once only. This action should be repeated until all traces of matter have been removed.
- Repeat these steps on the lower lid.
- Dry both lids in the same way as above using each swab once only.
- If required, administer medication as prescribed. The patient should be left in a comfortable position.
- Tidy, remove and dispose of all equipment safely in accordance with local policy and wash and dry hands.
- Document the procedure in the patient's notes, noting any changes or abnormal findings. These findings should also be reported to the senior nurse.

If either eye has infection present, this should be swabbed last. If infection is present in both eyes, this procedure should be undertaken separately using new equipment.

integrity and also for the presence of a build-up of wax that may affect hearing. Observations should be made for signs of inflammation or infection such as pain, redness and swelling. The external auditory meatus should be inspected for signs of discharge or wax and, if present, these should be referred to a nurse who is trained in aural care for further assessment and examination.

Ears are very prone to the effects of pressure. This is equally applicable for the elderly and the young, including premature infants. If the ear has been resting on a surface for a period of time it should be carefully inspected to ensure the tissues are fully perfused and not showing signs of pressure-related damage. Pressure damage in and around the ear may also be the result of a badly fitting hearing device or from the use of oxygen therapy where the tubing or mask fastening can traumatize the delicate tissues. Care must be taken in all these respects to prevent harm.

Activity 8.12

Go to the Media Tool DVD, select **Skill Sets**, **Administration of Medicines**, then **Oxygen administration with dialogue** and view the clip. What nursing interventions do you think are appropriate to prevent pressure damage from occurring with this patient? Make a note of your answers before reading on, and compare them to the sample answer at the end of the chapter.

The pinna and the lobe (front and back) should be cleansed with a soft cloth using warm water with minimal soap or wash cream. If the patient is free from dermatitis, then soap is an acceptable cleansing solution. Drying the ear needs special attention and gentle patting on and around the lobe is required to ensure it is dried fully. If necessary, cotton-tipped buds can be used in the folds of the pinna to ensure all traces of soap and moisture are removed completely. Never insert an object into the ear canal as the drum as the cillial membrane can be very easily damaged. Hairgrips and cotton buds have been noted to cause trauma to the inner ear.

Once you are appropriately skilled and experienced, the use of a *tympanic thermometer* for temperature

recording and an *auroscope* for examining the ear canal is appropriate. Any concerns regarding the ear and its function should be referred to a nurse trained in aural care or medical staff for further examination (NHS Quality Improvement Scotland 2006).

Nasal care

The nasal cavity, like the ear, is delicate and very easily damaged. If a nasal cannula or naso-gastric tube is being used, careful inspection is needed as damage from pressure can occur. Moist cotton-tipped buds or swabs are useful in cleansing the nasal passages and removing dried mucus in the lower cavity. As with the aural cavity, care must be taken to ensure the cotton bud is not pushed too far or too hard into the nasal passages, causing discomfort or trauma. Use a small amount of yellow soft paraffin, or an alternative, to keep the mucosa moisturized and reduce dryness. This will enhance patient comfort, particularly if oxygen therapy or enteral feeding is being administered. If tape or another fixture is used for securing a naso-gastric tube on or around the nose, this must be replaced regularly and the area under the fixation should be checked frequently.

Hand and foot care

The hands and feet are often neglected aspects of personal hygiene, however, their care and maintenance are important for individual cleanliness standards as well as for safety and infection prevention reasons. Long fingernails and toenails not only harbour dirt and microorganisms, but if ragged, can cause superficial damage to skin tissues.

Hand washing is best done as part of the showering or immersion bathing process, but if this is not possible, a small bowl of warm water can be used. Thorough washing between the fingers with a small cloth helps to remove dirt and dead skill cells. The areas between the digits require careful drying to ensure moisture is fully removed, thus minimizing the moist environment in which fungal infections thrive.

Nails should be kept as short as the patient requests by cutting straight across with nail clippers or small scissors, ideally to the level of the finger. The nail can then be smoothed with a nail file to remove sharp edges. Hand cream or lotion can be applied as desired or if hands show signs of dryness.

You may clean and cut toenails as outlined above. It is important not to file into the corners to prevent ingrowing toenails. The use of powders or creams may already be part of the patient's treatment plan for skin, odour control or fungal conditions. These should be applied according to the prescription and individual care plan. In general, care should be taken not to over-use products such as talcum powder or aerosols as a build-up of these may lead to a breakdown in skin integrity and irritate some patients with respiratory conditions.

Because toenails are much tougher than fingernails, it may be necessary to refer the patient for specialist advice from a chiropodist for support and care. Patients with certain conditions causing poor periph-

> **Activity 8.13**
>
> Go to the Media Tool DVD, select **Skill Sets**, **Infection Control and Hygiene**, then **Hand and nail care**. View the video clips there.

eral circulation and neurological impairment, such as diabetes, for example, should always be referred for specialist foot assessment and maintenance of nail care. This should be done in accordance with local guidelines ensuring appropriate expert care and monitoring is obtained and that inadvertent, superficial damage by the nurse or carer does not occur.

Summary and key points

This chapter has considered an essential element of caring for any patient in your practice. The general principles including the importance of communication, self-care and family inclusion have been explored, together with consideration of an individual's religious and cultural background, all of which impact on the type and level of personal care and oral hygiene being performed. A number of procedures have been outlined to aid your practice, however, it is stressed that these cannot be used in isolation and local policies and procedures should be adhered to. Remember the following key points:

- Assisting a patient with their personal hygiene needs can provide an ideal opportunity to develop a rapport and gain important information to inform the assessment, planning and evaluation of their care.
- The family plays an important role in personal hygiene, particularly in children or patients with a learning disability.
- Personal hygiene must be patient-centred.
- Privacy and dignity must be maintained during personal hygiene activities.

References

Arif, Z. (2005) Shower scene, *Nursing Standard,* 19(26): 20.

Candlin, J. and Stark, S. (2005) Plastic apron wear during direct patient care, *Nursing Standard,* 20(2): 41–6.

Dougherty, L. and Lister, S. (2004) *The Royal Marsden Hospital Manual of Clinical Nursing Procedures,* 6th edn.Oxford: Blackwell Science.

Geraghty, M. (2005) Nursing the unconscious patient, *Nursing Standard,* 20(1): 54–64.

Hooks, R. and Roberts, J. (2007) Older people's personal care needs, an analysis of care provision: care provision and the roles of key healthcare personnel, *International Journal of Older People Nursing,* 2(4): 263–9.

Lentz, J. (2003) Daily baths: torment or comfort at end of life? *Journal of Hospice and Palliative Nursing,* 5(1): 34–9.

Mohebbi, S. Virtanen, J. Murtomaa, H., Vahid-Golpayegani, M. and Vehkalahti, M. (2008) Mothers as facilitators of oral hygiene in early childhood, *International Journal of Paediatric Dentistry,* 18(1): 48–55.

NHS Grampian (2005) *Oral Assessment Tool.* Aberdeen: NHS Grampian.

NHS Quality Improvement Scotland (2005) Working with dependent older people to achieve good oral health, www.nhshealthquality.org/nhsqis/files/21412%20NHSQIS%20Oral%20BPS.pdf, accessed 30 November 2007.

NHS Quality Improvement Scotland (2006) Ear care, www.nhshealthquality.org/nhsqis/files/22241%20NHSQIS%20Ear%20Care%20BPS.pdf, accessed 30 November 2007.

NMC (Nursing and Midwifery Council) (2008) *The Code, Standards of Conduct, Performance and Ethics for Nurses and Midwives.* London: Nursing and Midwifery Council.

Peate, I. (ed.) (2005) *Compendium of Clinical Skills for Student Nurses.* London: Whurr.

Pegram, A. Bloomfield, J. and Jones, A. (2007) Clinical skills: bed bathing and personal hygiene needs of patients, *British Journal of Nursing,* 16(6): 356–8.

Trigg, E. and Mohammed, T.A. (eds) (2006) *Practices in Children's Nursing: Guidelines for Hospital and Community,* 2nd edn. Edinburgh: Churchill Livingstone.

Verhaeghe, S. Defloor, T. Van Zuuren, F. Duijnstee, M. and Grypdonck, M. (2005) The needs and experiences of family members of adult patients in an intensive care unit: a review of the literature, *Journal of Clinical Nursing,* 14(4): 501–9.

Answers

Scenario 8.1

You will probably have noted that John will require a bed bath initially to reduce any strain on the cardiac muscle. John will also be extremely tired. As each day passes he may gradually become more independent, from requiring assistance with washing and oral hygiene at his bedside while sitting in a chair to becoming fully independent and bathing or showering himself.

John may have fear of a further attack or may voice fear of death. He is currently employed although the condition may affect his occupation. This may have an impact in terms of supporting his family financially. You should report his concerns so that the appropriate help and support can be offered.

Scenario 8.2

Because of his restricted movement and fear of potential pain Billy may be afraid of moving very much and you will probably have noted the complications of deep venous thrombosis, pulmonary embolism, chest infection and pressure ulcers. He is also a heavy smoker so this may cause him to be agitated as well.

When attending to personal hygiene you should encourage passive exercises on the lower limbs as Billy is at risk of developing deep vein thrombosis due to his lack of mobility and because he is a heavy smoker. Encourage deep breathing using exercises provided by the physiotherapist, as Billy is at risk of developing a chest infection as a result of his fractured ribs and smoking. Encourage active and passive movement where appropriate, in conjunction with pressure-relieving equipment as Billy is at risk of developing pressure ulcers in a number of areas, again due to his lack of mobility.

Activity 8.9

An assessment of Margaret's mouth should be made (using a torch if need be) and the nurse should communicate with her during this procedure. It may be appropriate to consider sponge-tipped sticks here or, if Margaret has her own teeth, to use toothpaste.

When Margaret's food arrives there should be promotion of self-care, and perhaps some input from an occupational therapist if the use of an adapted toothbrush is required. A mirror should be provided and the nurse should check that food has not gathered in the mouth. If food is left in the mouth it could cause a mouth infection and potential inhalation problems, a common complication in patients who have suffered from a stroke.

Activity 8.12

In this case it is appropriate to perform regular turning according to local policy, observation of the skin and observation and assessment of the positioning and fitment of the oxygen administration device.

9

Food and nutrition

Karen Staniland and Frances Gascoigne

Chapter Contents

Learning objectives

The aim of this chapter is to explore your role in relation to the principles of nutritional assessment and in the planning, managing and evaluation of patient care. The accompanying Media Tool DVD will also help you to participate in the appropriate nursing interventions when helping a patient to eat and drink. Please watch the video clips as directed as these will reinforce your learning and expand upon the information given in this book.

After reading this chapter and interacting with the Media Tool DVD you will be able to:

- Identify the principles of screening and assessment.
- Categorize, plan, implement and evaluate the care for patients requiring nutritional assessment.
- Recognize the factors that contribute to creating a conducive environment for eating and drinking.
- Identify how and when patients need assistance with eating and drinking.
- Monitor, record and act appropriately in relation to patients' nutritional needs.
- Provide and promote information for heath in relation to eating and drinking.

Introduction

The importance of food to patients is well recognized and research has shown that recovery time can be shortened if the nutritional status of a patient can be improved (Rollins 1997). Later in the chapter you will be introduced to the components of a *balanced diet* so that you can offer appropriate healthy and nourishing food (especially if a patient requires a modified diet), and check that food and drink are served in the correct proportion and at the correct temperature for patient preference and safety. You will be able to offer help and assistance to a patient in order for them to make their own choices and enjoy the food presented. You may need to take cultural and religious dietary observations into account and note any difficulties with chewing and swallowing. However, remember that a speech and language therapist or appropriately trained nurse should assess anyone exhibiting swallowing difficulties, to ensure the correct textures of foods and liquids are provided, and you should report any concerns that you might have, however irrelevant they may appear.

The Nutrition Action Plan was launched by the

Box 9.1 Web links – nutrition

The Nutrition Action Plan is available at www.dh.gov.uk/en/Publicationsandstatistics/Publications/PublicationsPolicyAndGuidance/DH_079931. The Department of Health free online training in nutritional care for all nurses working in the NHS and other healthcare professionals working in the social care sector is available at www.corelearningunit.com/index.php?id=1.2.

Further support for nurses is provided in the form of a toolkit from the NPSA which aims to help staff implement the Council of Europe Alliance UK's ten key characteristics of good nutritional care in hospital. The document acts as a checklist for readers to refer to and the NPSA is supporting it from a patient safety perspective to ensure that malnutrition does not become a risk.

The NPSA fact sheets are available at:
www.npsa.nhs.uk/patientsafety/alerts-and-directives/cleaning-and-nutrition/nutrition/.
See also Traffic Light food labelling: http://www.fphm.org.uk/resourses/AtoZ/ps_food_labelling.pdf

Department of Health in October 2007 (DoH 2007) and sub-groups were convened to drive forward each of the priorities identified within it, including free online training for healthcare professionals as identified in Box 9.1.

It is important to remember that there are many influences on diet including cultural, social and economic factors. Eating well is an essential part in the treatment and care of patients, but it is not unusual for a patient to lose their appetite when they are unwell. This may be because of the illness itself, the treatment, or through fear and anxiety. You may also come across patients being treated for illnesses associated with *obesity* and *anorexia*. Obesity is a government-wide priority and one of the major public health issues in the developed world. Although obesity and anorexia are not covered specifically in this chapter, it is useful to have some knowledge of their effects and Box 9.2 can help here.

Box 9.2 Web links – obesity and anorexia

Further information about obesity and anorexia is located on the following websites: www.dh.gov.uk/en/Policyandguidance/Healthandsocialcaretopics/Obesity/index.htm; www.nhsdirect.nhs.uk/articles/article.aspx?articleId=27.

Screening and assessment

To begin this section, we offer you a definition of food and nutrition in Box 9.3.

Box 9.3 Food and nutrition definitions

Food: substances that provide carbohydrates, lipids and proteins as an energy source to organisms.

Nutrition: the taking in and *metabolism* of nutrients (food and other nourishing material) by an organism so that life is maintained and growth can take place.

An adequate food and liquid intake provides energy for necessary activities, maintains healthy body tissues and regulates bodily functions such as temperature, blood pressure and pulse with adequate tissue perfusion as measured by capillary refill and the temperature of the extremities.

Qualified dieticians are the resource for expert knowledge in nutrition, but it is you, the nurse, who is in a key location to assess and offer general advice to patients as well as ensuring that they have a good nutritional diet. If a patient requires a special diet as part of their treatment, a dietician will ensure that their individual dietary needs are provided for, but you are in a position to observe if the patient is actually eating the food provided.

To begin, it is fundamental that routine nutritional

Activity 9.1

Before you go any further in this chapter, it may be useful to go to the Media Tool DVD, select **Skill Sets**, then **Nutritional Intake**, and read the **Key points** lecture **Nutrition Across the Lifespan**. This introduces you to the importance of nutrition, some of the complications of not eating properly and the nutritional needs across the human lifespan. It will provide background information for this chapter.

screening is carried out on every patient on admission to hospital including whether any assistance will be needed at mealtimes. This should be recorded and referred to by all the relevant staff. It is also important that if and when there is a requirement, a daily record of food and fluid intake is kept.

The purpose of nutritional screening and assessment is to identify those patients who are 'at risk' of not receiving appropriate nutrition to meet their physical and emotional needs. The process is ongoing and, if necessary, the screening and assessment will be repeated at appropriate intervals to determine the progress of the patient and evaluate the interventions. Any further assessment will depend on the patient and it is extremely useful to consult with any patient carers involved in order to gain information for record keeping. You may also wish to refer to Chapter 3 in this book. It is also important for the screening and assessment to be documented, as will be explained later in the chapter.

'At risk' is a term used to identify factors that may contribute towards a negative outcome. There are too many possible negative outcomes to list here so we provide just two examples that you may see in practice:

(1) Wound healing may be impaired or delayed with a poor nutritional intake as tissues require certain basic dietary elements such as amino acids, which come from proteins, to promote wound healing.

(2) A lack of calcium, which is an essential element in the diet, may contribute to the poor building of bone tissue.

Unqualified staff, students and carers can screen patients if they have received the necessary education and training and have been assessed as competent to undertake the assessment. The qualified nurse must

have a level of knowledge that enables adequate teaching and we stress that it is important for the qualified nurse to be aware that accountability remains with them. It is also the responsibility of the qualified nurse to liaise with the multidisciplinary care team if necessary, which may include dieticians and doctors, to ensure complete assessment and screening.

Activity 9.2

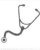

What do you think the purpose of nutritional screening and assessment is? Try to answer this before reading any further. The answer is given at the end of the chapter.

The screening and assessment of a patient's nutritional status require you to use background knowledge of the current best evidence regarding nutrition, and there are screening tools available to help you do this. The use of screening and assessment tools should be applied to practice in a way which is appropriate for each individual patient, both in the community and hospital care settings. Initially it is important for you to assess the physical appearance of the patient to identify any potential risks associated with inadequate or inappropriate nutrition, and then mutually agree with the multidisciplinary team (which includes everybody involved in the care of the patient) the interventions that are considered necessary to promote or maintain the well-being of the patient.

A screening or assessment tool is one that uses a questionnaire-type format, contains more than one risk factor for malnutrition and gives an assessment of risk (Green and Watson 2005).

Box 9.4 Web link – the Malnutrition Universal Screening Tool (MUST)

The MUST is available at the British Association for Parenteral and Enteral Nutrition website, along with advice on how it is used: www.bapen.org.uk/must_tool.html.

Those at a high level of risk require a referral for a further comprehensive nutritional assessment. It is your responsibility when admitting a patient to try to recognize and report any concerns that you feel might put the patient at risk from inadequate or inappropriate nutrition. Such patients may need to be referred to the appropriate professionals, such as the nutritionist, or the dietician. For example, a patient with diabetes may require intervention from the dietician and the specialist diabetic nurse.

Activity 9.3

Go to the Media Tool DVD, select **Case Studies, Learning Disability (Alex)**, then **Introduction to Alex**. Watch the clip which introduces Alex, who has recently been diagnosed with diabetes. Then watch **The nurses visiting Alex demonstrate good practice** and compare it with **The nurses visiting Alex demonstrate poor practice**. Think about the differences in approach.

Before reading any further, it is important that you revise your knowledge of the anatomy and physiology of the alimentary tract (also called the gastrointestinal tract and the digestive tract) which is associated with eating and drinking.

The alimentary tract is necessary for breaking down the food we eat, followed by the absorption and finally excretion of the waste products of digestion. The alimentary tract is a continuous tube that runs from the mouth to the anus and has the physiological responsibility of providing the body cells with all their nutritional requirements. The digestive system carries out these functions by motility (peristalsis), secretion, digestion and absorption, then excreting the byproducts in the form of *stools* and flatulence. The physiological process of digestion is broken down into mechanical and chemical digestion. *Mechanical digestion* involves the controlled movement of food through the digestive tract and the preparation of that food for the *chemical* process of digestion – the activity of breaking down the food into smaller particles by digestive enzymes. Physical and chemical digestion depends on exocrine and endocrine secretions.

The alimentary tract needs to be intact structurally and able to move the food from the mouth down to the anus. Along the way the food is broken down into

smaller particles so that they can be absorbed into the bloodstream and finally be used by the cells in the body. When there is a structural or chemical malfunction, the process of breaking down the food into smaller particles will be impaired.

For example, if a patient has lost their teeth or their mouth is painful due to ulceration, they are not going to be able to bite and then chew their food satisfactorily. This inability to chew will inhibit the mixing of the food into a moist bolus which is easier to swallow. As chewing is the first physiological function of nutrition, this may be a simple reason why a patient is malnourished.

Activity 9.4

Go to the Media Tool DVD, select **Skill Sets, Nutritional Intake**, then play the **Keypoints lecture – Digestive system** on the overview of the digestive system. This will give you more background information on the alimentary tract.

The risk factors which should be considered during screening and assessment vary with different age groups. If an older age group is under consideration, Activity 9.5 gives some examples of what you should try to establish when completing an assessment. However, remember that the information provided here is to increase your own background knowledge and you should not be expected to undertake an assessment on your own.

Having outlined some of the risk factors which might be identified by assessment and screening, we can now think about the social, clinical and physical assessment of a patient in more detail. The clinical and physical assessment will involve taking a history from the patient (and carers if appropriate), with particular reference to social features and their diet.

The NICE clinical guidelines on nutrition support in adults cover the care of patients with malnutrition or at risk of malnutrition, whether they are in hospital or at home, although the guidelines do not cover malnutrition or its treatments in detail (see Box 9.5).

The body's nutritional status influences the effectiveness of metabolic processes. Numerous

Activity 9.5

The following areas are important to consider when undertaking an admission assessment on an elderly patient. Can you identify why? Think about this when you go through the list. Some points to think about in relation to each are located at the end of the chapter.

1. The structural condition of the patient's alimentary tract, for example, teeth and gums.

2. The patient's ability to swallow.

3. Any associated discomfort or pain.

4. Desired or undesired weight gain or loss. Has this change has been rapid or slow? What is the total weight loss or gain?

5. Social situation: does the patient have adequate income for food purchases?

6. Does the patient live alone and/or feel isolated (related to psychosocial factors which include separation from family and lack of social interaction at mealtimes)?

7. Does the patient have transport to obtain food?

8. Does the patient have adequate facilities such as a fridge to keep the food fresh?

9. Is the patient interested in food and/or meal preparation?

10. Does the patient have adequate time to eat?

11. Is the patient able to concentrate to eat?

12. What are the patient's eating habits and patterns – for example, number of daily meals and snacks? Look for food group avoidance (e.g. eggs may make someone with liver disease feel nauseous).

13. What are the patient's energy levels and exercise tolerance? Do they take regular exercise?

14. Is there any evidence of diarrhoea, constipation, vomiting, excessive thirst or frequent urination?

15. Does the patient have any preoccupation with their body weight/shape?

16. Does the patient have any cravings and habits such as smoking or alcohol intake?

17. Is there evidence of chronic illnesses, for example, diabetes, renal disease, cancer, heart disease?

18. What is the family history and past medical history?

19. Is there evidence of acute illness such as fever or trauma?

20. Is there evidence of external losses (e.g. fistulas, wounds, abscesses, chronic blood loss, chronic dialysis)?

21. What medication is the patient is taking, if any?

Remember to look at the answers at the end of the chapter.

Scenario 9.1

Mary Jones is an 87-year-old lady living alone who has some difficulty in mobility due to arthritis and breathlessness. She has been admitted for a general assessment as her GP believes she is not coping at home.

Try and think about any significant social, clinical and physical features that you might generally look for with Mary while undertaking a nutritional assessment.

Box 9.5 Web links – nutrition guidelines

The NICE clinical guidelines on nutrition can be found at www.nice.org.uk/guidance/CG32#summary.

The British Association for Parenteral and Enteral Nutrition website offers information on malnutrition at www.bapen.org.uk.

See The Royal College of Nursing Nutrition Now campaign for better patient nutrition http://www.rcn.org.uk

Activity 9.6

Before you progress any further with this chapter, we would advise you to go to the Media Tool DVD, select **Chapter Resources**, then **Nutrition** and **Activity 9.6** and answer the questions there in relation to **Screening and assessment** and **Planning, implementation and evaluation** to reinforce your understanding of the information given here.

vitamins, minerals and other co-factors, along with water, contribute to the environment for cellular metabolism to function effectively and efficiently. The activity level is the primary factor determining the daily energy requirement, assuming a stable body weight. A

person's energy requirements are based on their physical activity, their body weight and height, and their body mass index (BMI).

The management of care

Screening and assessment are ongoing and it is often the responsibility of a nurse to coordinate these. The role of the coordinator is to ensure that all the mem-

Activity 9.7

BMI is a height versus weight calculation of body fat. Many websites will help you work out your own BMI: look up BMI using an internet search engine and calculate your own.

bers of the multidisciplinary team involved in the nutritional care of the patient work together to plan the care. This care plan must be accessible. Regular review meetings at appropriate time intervals may be arranged, and suitable channels for contact should be clearly evident, especially if the patient is in the community, so that the carers are supported and know who to contact when they want advice or assistance. This communication should be evident in a documented care plan which is the focus of this section. You should also refer to Chapter 3.

Comprehensive screening and assessment which lead to the implementation of an appropriate care plan for nutrition will go a long way to providing the best available care and promote the well-being of individual patients. In addition, this will help to avoid complications such as prolonged wound healing which may result in further disability.

The outcome of the assessment will depend on the nutritional factors and the general health of the patient (Kondrup et al. 2002). Part of the screening and assessment described in the last section is to establish how the interventions influence the outcome; therefore, the outcome must be influenced by the care implemented. This results in the formulation of a care plan. You will not be expected to write a care plan for nutrition on your own, but may be involved as a member of the ward team in the planning of one.

Box 9.6 Web links – nutrition care plan

An example of a care plan for nutrition can be found at:
www.mcht.nhs.uk/documents/Standards/
Essence%20of%20Care/Food%20and%20
Nutrition%20-%20Action%20Plan.pdf.

A balanced diet

Before you can advise or help a patient to eat and drink, it is useful to review what the components of a balanced diet are. A balanced diet is said to provide a range of nutrients that include vitamins, dietary fibre, minerals, carbohydrates, fat and protein in order to maintain a healthy body weight and health.

Food nourishes the body by supplying necessary nutrients and calories to function in one or all of three ways:

1. To provide *energy* for necessary activities.
2. To provide for the *building* and *maintenance* of body tissues.
3. To *regulate* body processes such as temperature (homeostasis).

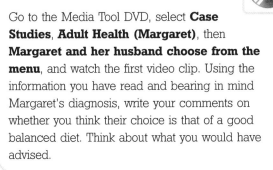

Activity 9.8

Go to the Media Tool DVD, select **Case Studies**, **Adult Health (Margaret)**, then **Margaret and her husband choose from the menu**, and watch the first video clip. Using the information you have read and bearing in mind Margaret's diagnosis, write your comments on whether you think their choice is that of a good balanced diet. Think about what you would have advised.

The nutrients necessary to the body are classified as *macro* nutrients, *micro* nutrients, and *water*. Energy requirements are based on the balance of energy expenditure associated with an individual's body size and composition, and the level of physical activity. An appropriate balance contributes to long-term health and allows for the maintenance of desirable physical activity.

Activity 9.9

Go to the Media Tool DVD, select **Case Studies**, **Child Health (Tom)**, then **Tom painting and getting ready for lunch** and watch the first video clip on this page. Using the information here write your comments on whether you think the choice is a good balanced diet. Would you have done anything differently?

There are some excellent resources available on nutrition and a few are detailed in Box 9.7.

Box 9.7 Web links

Useful websites which offer further information about nutrition and related areas can be found via the following links.

Nutrition
www.bbc.co.uk/health/healthy_living/nutrition/

Healthy living
www.jr2.ox.ac.uk/Bandolier/booth/booths/
hliving.html

Food Standards Agency
www.food.gov.uk/healthiereating/

Water and elderly people
www.caredirections.co.uk/

Special diets

Often you will come across patients who have a need for a special diet. This might be through illness, or a request due to cultural, religious or personal preferences, such as snacks, kosher meals or vegetarian meals. It is imperative, however, not to make assumptions about patients' preferences on the basis of their cultural background. They should always be asked what their actual preferences are. Qualified dieticians in hospital aim to ensure that all patients receive a nutritionally adequate diet and will liaise with other health professionals to enable optimal nutritional care. However, when a patient requires a special diet and the qualified dietician becomes involved, the nurse is still responsible for ensuring that the correct patient receives the correct diet.

Diets might include diabetic, gluten free, renal, low or high fibre, low fat, low sodium or low protein. Modified in consistency diets may also include clear liquid, full liquid, puréed, mechanical soft (such as a ground meat with gravy, soft cooked vegetables and canned fruit), selected soft (meat, fruit and vegetables cut into bite-size portions), or just soft (textured foods, omitting fresh fruit and vegetables).

It is very important that this type of food still appears appetizing and, where food needs to be puréed, it is helpful to use moulds to keep foods separate and indicate what they are – for instance, a fish-shaped mould for fish.

Box 9.8 Web link – religion and diet

Religious needs also need to be considered and information is available in the form of useful guides such as McCabe (2005). See http://diversiton.com/downloads/checkUp.pdf.

Sometimes it is necessary for patients to remain on special diets when they go home. In this case dieticians prepare written information and follow-up appointments can be arranged at either the hospital or at a community clinic.

It is important to remember that illness may affect a patient's ability to taste and eat. For the sense of taste, for example, chemicals are detected and transduced by chemo-receptors located in the taste buds. When people have had a stroke, their taste may become altered. Tastes are mixtures of four elementary taste qualities: salty, sweet, sour and bitter. Sweet taste is detected best at the tip of the tongue, with salty and sour detected along the sides and bitter sensed best at the base.

Disorders associated with the sense of taste are not life-threatening, but they can impair the quality of life, impair nutritional status and increase the possibility of accidental poisoning. Taste disorders can include an absence of taste, decreased or increased taste sensitivity and a distortion of taste. The senses of gustation

Activity 9.10

Having worked further through the chapter, you may wish to visit the Media Tool DVD, select **Case Studies, Learning Disability (Alex)**, then **The nurses visiting Alex demonstrate good practice** and watch the video clip on this page again to check if you identified all the relevant points earlier. The following link will also provide further information on diabetes: www.nhsdirect.nhs.uk/articles/article.aspx?articleId=128

As Alex has special needs, this link might also be useful:

www.nursing-standard.co.uk/archives/ldp_pdfs/ldpvol2-1/ldpv2n1p2935.pdf.

(taste) and olfaction (smell) depend on chemical stimuli that are present either in food and drink or in the air, and they contribute considerably to quality of life and are important stimulants of digestion. For example, giving a patient a drink in a plastic cup may alter both the texture and taste of the drink. Plastic consistency is altered when exposed to heat repeatedly and cups are often washed in dishwashers in hospitals, so the nurse must make sure the plastic is in good condition by looking at its colour and testing its 'stiffness'.

The chemoreceptor cells located in taste buds are continuously replaced, and may become altered or less effective in their sensing ability when there is cerebral damage; patients may find their food preferences have altered because of this.

Activity 9.11

Go to the Media Tool DVD, select **Case studies, Adult Health (Margaret)**, then **Margaret and her husband choose from the menu**. Scroll down to watch the video clip **'Margaret objects to pureed food'**. Think about what might be done differently in this situation.

Helping patients to eat and drink

Eating is an essential activity which should be made as enjoyable as possible by the nurse for the patient. The patient should be assisted to sit in the most comfortable position, either in a bed or a chair, so that they are able to reach their food easily, and the food should be placed within easy reach of the arm and hand that the patient normally uses to eat with. However, staff on a busy ward sometimes forget these basic principles and you may encounter bad practice which, after completing this section, you should easily recognize and be able to avoid. It is necessary to demonstrate many practical points in this section and you will often be referred to the accompanying Media Tool DVD for demonstration purposes.

Any food given to a patient should be at a safe temperature and served with appropriate utensils. The patient may find gripping things difficult and require adapted cutlery and crockery. They may need encouragement from you to eat and you could make sure that there is someone to provide social interaction if the patient desires it. As it is necessary to make sure the patient understands the importance of having a drink

---

Activity 9.12

Go to the Media Tool DVD, select **Skill Sets – Nutritional Intake** then **Assisting patients to eat – good practice** and watch the following clips:

- **Jayne brings Lyn her dinner nicely!**
- **Example of how to assist a patient who has perceptual or cognitive difficulties**
- **Lyn eating lying down, good practice**
- **Assisting a patient to have a drink**

Now answer the following questions.

(**1**) What *good* practice points can you identify from the clip concerned with eating lying flat?

(**2**) List six elements of good practice shown in the clip relating to helping a patient have a hot drink.

(**3**) What other feeding utensils could have been offered to the patient instead of a beaker?

Check your answers with those given at the end of the chapter.

Activity 9.13

Go to the Media Tool DVD, select **Skill Sets – Nutritional Intake** then **Assisting patients to eat – poor practice** and watch the following clips:

- **How not to leave a patient with food**
- **How not to feed a patient!**
- **How not to give a patient who is lying down a drink**

Now answer the following questions.

(**1**) From the clip **How not to leave a patient with food** list five elements of bad practice.

(**2**) List at least five elements of bad practice in **How not to feed a patient!**

(**3**) List the points that might concern you in the clip **How not to give a patient who is lying down a drink**.

Check your answers with those given at the end of the chapter.

during a meal, the container must be assessed as appropriate. A straw, for example, can be difficult to use if the muscles in the face are not agile enough, as with partial paralysis. It may be dangerous to provide a drink in a spouted beaker if the patient is unable to control the container and tip it appropriately, as too much fluid entering the oro-pharynx at any one time causes choking. Everybody therefore must constantly be on the alert for any difficulty patients may experience physiologically when obtaining food.

Patients' perceptions of care are very important and there is now much more emphasis on these within the NHS. It is useful at this stage to find out how patients feel when care is inappropriate.

Activity 9.14

Go to the Media Tool DVD, select **Skill Sets**, then **Nutritional Intake** and then **Assisting patients to eat – poor practice** and watch the following clips to gain a patient perspective.

- **Lyn's reactions to being fed by Jayne**
- **Another nurse comments on the poor feeding technique**
- **Lyn's reactions to Helen trying to give her a drink lying down**

Of course, helping an adult to eat is a bit different from helping a child or a baby. Further information on helping a child and feeding a baby is available on the Media Tool DVD (see **Case Study**, **Tom paints and gets ready for lunch** and **Feeding a baby** in the **Skill Sets** section).

The accurate recording of a patient's food and fluid intake is important and you will need to familiarize yourself with the various charts available for food and drink monitoring in use on your own ward.

Activity 9.15

Go to the Media Tool DVD, select **Skill Sets**, then **Nutritional intake** and **Fluid balance** and work through the activities outlined there.

If a patient is deemed to be at risk following an appropriate nutritional assessment, a subsequent nutritional care plan should be written. In these cases, monitoring of a patient's food and fluid intake may be commenced and undertaken over a period of time. Height and weight recording is a primary part of this assessment. Healthcare professionals recording dietary and fluid intake should be skilled and knowledgeable. Identified staff should be responsible for ensuring that the food and drink offered to a vulnerable patient will meet their specific needs in the type, amount and appropriate supplement. It is particularly important for the person removing plates from the bedside to be well informed about the need for the recording, reporting and monitoring of a patient's nutritional intake.

Marson *et al.* (2003) evaluated the extent of food wastage on a renal ward in a large NHS Trust hospital, which demonstrated the extent of the problem. Nurses should be extremely observant in terms of what their vulnerable patients are (or are not) eating.

Swallowing

Care must be taken to make sure the patient is able to chew and swallow. A patient with poor coordination may, for example, be unable to transfer the food from the plate towards their mouth. It is also very hard to move your mouth around to chew if your cheek is pushed into a pillow and it may be necessary to support the patient's head in such a case. However, there may be other causes of difficulty in swallowing and

---

Box 9.9 Web links

There are many useful and comprehensive resources in respect of highlighting best practice for patients with dysphagia. These include risk assessments, guides to levels of risk and eating, drinking and swallowing care plans. Some of these are located on the Media Tool DVD under **Chapter Resources**, **Chapter 6 Weblinks and activities**, **Box 9.9**.

You may also like to access the following web links for more information: www.npsa.nhs.uk/patientsafety/resources/dysphagia/ and www.nice.org.uk/guidance/CG32.

---

there are many useful resources in respect of high-lighting good practice for dysphagia. Dysphagia refers to difficulty in eating, drinking or swallowing and can lead to *malnutrition, dehydration*, reduced quality of life and even choking.

Enteral feeding

If a patient's swallowing assessment has shown that they are not able to swallow, an alternative source of feeding is required. You may come across some patients who receive 'enteral' tube feeding and 'par-enteral' nutrition both in hospital and at home.

In adults the commonest reason for starting tube feeding is swallowing difficulties. These are commonly experienced by patients with neurological disorders, such as motor neurone disease, multiple sclerosis and *Parkinson's disease*, but the commonest single cause is cerebrovascular disease. It is therefore necessary to intermittently assess the swallowing capabilities of patients in order to avoid unnecessary tube feeding. The patients and/or carers should have adequate training, contacts with appropriate health professions and a reliable delivery service for feeds and ancillary equipment. They should also be clear about how to manage simple problems associated with the feeding tube, which is usually a gastrostomy tube rather than a *naso-gastric tube*. The nasogastric tube is generally used as a short-term measure until a more permanent tube is inserted.

Enteral nutrition means using the gastrointestinal tract for the delivery of food (carbohydrates, proteins and fats) along with vitamins, minerals, liquids and medication. The routes of enteral feeding are:

1. Nasogastric tubes.
2. Percutaneous endoscopic gastrostomy tubes.
3. Naso-jejunal and jejunostomy (used if it is inappropriate to feed into or via the stomach).

Intravenous routes

An intravenous (into a vein) route of fluid administration is used to provide volume replacement when patients are not able to absorb adequate nutritional requirements via the alimentary tract. This may be due to dehydration, being nil by mouth before or after an

Activity 9.16

You may see and care for a patient with a nasogastric tube inserted. If you haven't had the opportunity to see or do this yet, go to the accompanying Media Tool DVD, select **Skill Sets**, **Nutrition**, **nasogastric tube insertion** then **Explaining nasogastric intubation to a patient** and answer the questions.

Then please go to **Skill Sets**, **Nutritional Intake**, **Passing a nasogastric tube** and answer the accompanying questions.

The next clip involves explaining and giving a patient a feed when a nasogastric tube is in place. There is also a tutorial here that you may find helpful.

Activity 9.17

You may now wish to consolidate this section by answering the questions on the Media Tool DVD under **Adult Health (Margaret)**, **Nurse explains the nasogastric tube**, where the nurse explains the nasogastric tube to Margaret.

operation, a structural defect such as a tumour, or *inflammatory bowel disease*. An intravenous route may also be used as a route for drug administration.

'Parenteral' nutrition is a method of delivering nutrition or other substances directly into a vein. It is not covered in great detail here, but various procedures are available to watch on the Media Tool DVD (see Activity 9.18).

Box 9.10 Web link – parenteral nutrition

For more information go to: http://cancerweb.ncl.ac.uk/cgi-bin/omd?parenteral+nutrition.

Activity 9.18

For detailed demonstrations of the factors and care involved in parental nutrition, go the Media Tool DVD and select **Skill Sets: Nutritional intake**

- **IV cannulation and care of a patient having IV therapy**
- **Explaining IV therapy to a patient; assessing the veins**
- **Demonstration of the procedure of cannulation on a model arm**
- **Priming the giving set**
- **Attaching the giving set to the cannula and setting the drip rate**
- **What to do as a student when the IV infusion pump alarms**

Try to answer the accompanying questions.

Promoting healthy eating

It has long been recognized that there has been a continuing need to improve nutrition, especially in hospitals, and in this respect Patient Environment Action Teams (PEATs) were established in 2000 to assess NHS hospitals. Under the PEAT programme every inpatient healthcare facility in England with more than ten beds is assessed annually and given a rating of excellent, good, acceptable, poor or unacceptable. The PEAT data for 2006 showed a continued improvement in the standard of hospital food (and cleaning), which is a clear indication that nutrition in hospitals is improving and that the nutritional needs of patients are being met.

Box 9.11 Web link – PEAT

More information on the PEAT 2006 data may be located at www.npsa.nhs.uk/patientsafety/alerts-and-directives/cleaning-and-nutrition/nutrition/.

In order to help you understand the current situation, this section will provide you with some background information in respect of the work that has been carried out on the provision of hospital food services. In 2001, the government looked at how hospital food services could be improved. This became known as the Better Hospital Food Programme. The aim was to improve the quality, availability of, and access to food in hospitals.

Box 9.12 Web links – Better Hospital Food Programme

A good resource for more information is the Better Hospital Food website which contains best practice guidance, resources, background information and research study results to support the delivery of food in NHS healthcare facilities. Go to http://195.92.246.148/nhsestates/ better_hospital_food/bhf_content/introduction/ home.asp.

The designated website for the Better Hospital Food Programme states that it was designed to make effective changes to hospital food services countrywide in order to:

- produce a comprehensive range of tasty, nutritious and interesting recipes that every NHS hospital could use;
- redesign hospital printed menus to make them more accessible and easier to understand;
- introduce 24-hour catering services to ensure food is available night and day;
- ensure hot food is available in hospitals at both midday and early evening mealtimes – research showed that a few changes could make a huge difference to patients' mealtime experience.

The programme set out key elements to providing a better food service to patients so that food is available and accessible between mealtimes:

- 'flexi menu': providing patients with a greater choice of meals;
- protected mealtimes: guaranteeing patients' undisturbed meals;
- 24-hour catering: providing food any time of the day or night;
- sustainability: reducing the environmental impact of food production;
- nutrition: a key issue for caterers and dieticians.

Box 9.13 Web link – Faculty of Public Health

A useful website is that of the Faculty of Public Health. This has an interesting section on food and health and can be found at www.fph.org.uk/resources.

Activity 9.19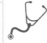

Find out which of the key elements your own Trust has in the provision of a better food service so that you are in a position to advise patients about what is available.

The government disbanded the Better Hospital Food Programme in 2006, after spending £40 million on investment in catering facilities. However, despite the good intentions of the Programme, it is useful for any healthcare professional to balance all the evidence in respect of whether or not it has been successful. A Food Watch campaign by Patient and Public Involvement (PPI) Forums in 2006, following a national survey of over 97 health Trusts and 2200 patients, which looked at the cost, quality and availability of food and drink for inpatients, their visitors and outpatients, showed that the Programme may not have improved anything at all despite the huge investment.

The survey indicated that there is still widespread dissatisfaction with hospital food and that NHS hospitals are slowing patients' recovery by serving meals that are tepid, unappetizing or downright inedible. It found that 40 per cent of patients were having their meals supplemented by food brought in by relatives and friends and that more than a third of patients (37 per cent) reported leaving a meal uneaten because it looked, smelled or tasted disgusting. Other findings were also worrying in that more than a fifth of patients said hospital meals were either too hot or too cold. A quarter of infirm patients, who needed help with eating, did not get it. There was frequent criticism of lack of choice on the menu. Four-fifths of patients were not given the opportunity to choose meals in advance, and 18 per cent said the dish of the day they liked sometimes ran out before the trolley reached their bedside. Among long-term patients, 37 per cent said menus were changed on a daily basis and 22 per cent said they were changed weekly, but 13 per cent said they were changed less often.

Box 9.14 Web link – Food Watch

The PPI forum's findings contrasted with evidence in the annual report of the health inspectorate, suggesting 96 per cent of Trusts met national standards on food. See www.cppih.org/documents/FoodWatchNationalSummary.doc.

This information would indicate that some Trusts can get it right when it comes to serving patients food that is appetizing and an aid to recovery. However, many Trusts are still failing patients by not providing meals that are meeting their needs and this is the point where nurses can try to make a difference.

This background information is important as it provides the necessary tools for healthcare professionals to consider patients' needs. This becomes more complicated when some patients are restricted in what they are able to eat and may have to be prescribed a special diet. It is also important that staff receive the appropriate training to equip them with the skills to communicate with patients who have dementia and communication difficulties. Visual aids (such as graphic menus) and non-verbal communication skills may help people to make choices. Relatives may also help you to identify food preferences.

The eating environment

We will now consider some factors concerning the environment when a patient is eating. The environment ought to be free of chemicals (such as cleaning liquids) during mealtimes and free of loud noise and other distractions. Some patients may find it difficult to concentrate and may forget they are eating if disturbed by cleaners, doctors' rounds and excessive numbers of visitors. Medicine rounds must be coordinated to suit the individual patient. Some patients may take their medicines with their meals as a regular routine, while others may find this reduces their appetite.

Food safety

Hospital wards are provided with basic kitchens which are subject to the Food Safety Act 1990, The Food Safety (General Food Hygiene) Regulations 1995 and the Food Safety (Temperature Control) Regulations 1995. The ward sister, charge nurse or senior nurse on duty is responsible for maintaining day-to-day standards of hygiene and food safety at ward level, and a formal inspection of food handling areas applies to ward kitchens.

To reduce the risk of cross-infection, many hospitals have policies in place where healthcare professionals and domestic staff wear different colour-coded aprons and gloves when serving meals and cleaning/washing up in the kitchen, and for other general activities. It is important to establish which coloured apron and gloves are worn for which task.

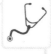

Activity 9.20

Identify what policy your own hospital has in respect of different colour-coded aprons and gloves for the serving of food and cleaning/washing up. Next time you are on the ward, observe whether or not the policy is implemented correctly.

Mealtimes

Nurses are in an ideal position to control the surrounding environment when patients are eating. In the past, patients' meals were frequently interrupted by clinical staff (e.g. doctors' ward rounds, phlebotomists taking blood samples, high noise levels, cleaning, maintenance and bed-making) but there have been many changes to enable the promotion of a suitable environment for patients when eating. This has become known as 'protected mealtimes'.

In 1859, Florence Nightingale stated 'Nothing shall be done in the ward while the patients are having their meal', but it is interesting that nearly 150 years later the introduction of protected mealtimes required a culture change for staff, patients and visitors. Protected mealtimes are periods on a hospital ward when all non-urgent clinical activity stops. Patients are able to eat without being interrupted and these protected periods give nurses time to offer and give assistance to

patients who need help. Many wards operate protected mealtimes and research indicates that patients who are not interrupted and receive appropriate service and support during mealtimes are happier, more relaxed and eat more. Remember, the better nutrition a patient receives, the higher the chances are of their recovering. You will see indications on the wards where protected mealtimes are implemented in a variety of formats such as notices and fact sheets for patients and relatives.

Protected mealtimes are generally liked by patients, who have commented on how they provide a feeling of dignity and respect. Protected mealtimes give patients time to eat when they are not rushed. You may find that on some wards a protected mealtime is followed by a quiet rest period for patients.

Activity 9.21

Go to the Media Tool DVD, select **Chapter Resources**, **Nutritional intake**, Activity 9.21 and read the information on protected mealtimes.

Information on protected mealtimes may also be obtained from http://195.92.246.148/nhsestates/better_hospital_food/bhf_content/protected_mealtimes/overview.asp.

Identify what tips the NPSA gives in respect of making protected mealtimes work. Your answer should include the following:

- Identify a 'champion' to lead and promote protected mealtimes.
- Use the Food and Nutrition benchmark in your Trust and communicate the results.
- Engage with all healthcare professionals.
- Promote protected mealtimes prior to launch.

NHS menus conventionally change daily over a one- to three-week cycle; therefore patients have a wider choice of dishes over a week but a fairly limited choice for each day. There are various trials running that you may experience when working on the wards which were initiated by the Better Hospital Food Programme. For instance, you may come across the 'flexi menu' trials, designed to test the viability of offering the same fixed menu for both lunch and evening meals. This allows patients to select foods they enjoy and to have the same dish more than once.

Another initiative is that of 24-hour catering. Hot food has not always been available to hospital patients who are admitted late in the day or who miss meal-times due to treatment or investigation, but with the introduction of 24-hour catering, patients should be able to ask a nurse or a ward housekeeper for hot food, snacks and drinks at any time of the day or night. Under this initiative patients may ask for light bite hot meals, ward kitchen service (light refreshments) or snack boxes (cold snacks such as sandwiches and a drink). Even if such an initiative is not in place, the hospital kitchen will usually help to meet any ward requests.

It is evident that there has been a lot of effort made to improve food choice and quality for patients, which in turn helps to promote eating healthily and con-tributes to patient recovery times. It is still the responsibility of the nurse, however, to ensure that patients in their care are receiving adequate nutrition on the ward.

Mealtimes are generally a social activity so, if appropriate, this should be encouraged. You may see the provision of dining areas and tables on various wards, with tablecloths to improve the dining envir-onment. This is quite popular on later-life wards. It is equally imperative, however, to remember that, while socializing during mealtimes should be encouraged, patients are different, and privacy should be offered to patients especially if they have difficulties with eating, to avoid embarrassment or any loss of dignity. Where necessary, assistance should be given discreetly and if the patient wishes it.

Fundamental practices before food is offered should include appropriate positioning and the use of napkins (not bibs) to protect clothing. 'Finger' food might be offered to patients who have difficulty using cutlery, but provision of adapted crockery and cutlery may enable such patients to feed themselves perfectly well. There should be enough staff on duty at mealtimes to provide assistance to those patients who need it. Some wards engage volunteer staff at this time. Drinking is also important and fresh water should be available throughout the day.

It is important that food served to patients should be made to look as appetizing as possible. A lot of plated food delivered to wards has a protective cover over it and this should be removed before the patient receives the food. Food should be served at an appropriate temperature and left within easy reach, with the patient being asked if there is anything else they require at that time.

Activity 9.22

Go to the Media Tool DVD, select **Chapter Resources**, **Nutritional intake**, Activity 9.22. Review the good practice in this area.

When you are next on the ward, try to identify as many good practices as you can in relation to the presentation of food.

Many hospitals have adopted various systems to identify the needs and maintain the dignity of patients at mealtimes. These include the use of different coloured trays, various symbols placed above a patient's bed (such as a knife and fork), and awareness projects including posters, information leaflets and best practice guidelines. The Social Care Institute for Excellence website (see Box 9.15) offers information concerning mealtimes and nutritional care and some practical advice that is useful for all healthcare pro-fessionals when presenting patients with food.

Box 9.15 Web link – Social Care Institute for Excellence

The institute's website can be found at www.scie.org.uk/publications/practiceguides/practiceguide09/mealtimes/index.asp.

Health promotion

Health promotion is the process of enabling people to increase control over, and improve, their health. The full definition of health promotion as provided in the Ottawa Charter (see Box 9.16) is widely accepted (WHO 1986).

So, health promotion is about keeping healthy, liv-ing a healthy lifestyle, preventing illness, and pre-venting any existing illness from becoming worse. Hospitals have a central role in treating diet-related

Box 9.16 Definition of health promotion

Health promotion is the process of enabling people to increase control over, and to improve, their health. To reach a state of complete physical, mental and social wellbeing, an individual or group must be able to identify and to realize aspirations, to satisfy needs, and to change or cope with the environment. Health is, therefore, seen as a resource for everyday life, not the objective of living. Health is a positive concept emphasizing social and personal resources, as well as physical capacities. Therefore, health promotion is not just the responsibility of the health sector, but goes beyond healthy lifestyles to wellbeing.

(WHO 1986)

The full Ottawa Charter can be viewed at www.phac-aspc.gc.ca/ph-sp/phdd/pdf/charter.pdf.

illness and encouraging physical activity. It would be logical then that they should be at the forefront of promoting and providing healthier food. However, a Soil Association report (2007), sponsored by Organix and entitled *Not What the Doctor Ordered*, identified inconsistencies between the government's policy on healthy eating and the dominance of junk food on sale in many hospitals.

Box 9.17 Web link – *Not What the Doctor Ordered*

The Soil Association report can be located at www.soilassociation.org/vending.

The main finding when the Soil Association visited five NHS hospitals and 17 sports and leisure centres across England and Wales was that much of the food on sale was of appalling nutritional quality, dominated by fatty snacks, fizzy drinks and confectionery. It would appear that while the hospitals had healthy eating policies, many did not adhere to them. This situation therefore makes it more difficult for nurses to promote healthy eating for patients.

Activity 9.23

- Find out if your hospital has a healthy eating policy.
- Locate and count the number of hospital vending machines and analyse the contents in terms of providing a healthy diet or junk food.
- Identify what you might be able to do about this.

Many useful websites provide information about health promotion and these can be viewed for up-to-date information. For example,

www.equip.nhs.uk/topics/promotion/promotion.html.

The health promotion departments in Primary Health Care Trusts provide leaflets, information and training days on many key health promotion issues. It is useful to always have plentiful supplies of these leaflets and posters (if applicable) on the wards for patients and visitors.

Summary and key points

The aim of this chapter has been to explore your role in relation to the principles of nutritional assessment and in the planning, managing and evaluation of patient care. It is evident from the literature that not all hospitals have consistent guidelines, protocols and practice regarding the nutritional well-being of patients in their care. Many hospitals do not yet have protected meal times, but there appears to be movement towards them. It is important to remember the following key points:

- Before being able to screen or assess the nutritional status of a patient the trained nurse should have a background level of information that will provide the necessary knowledge to use the screening and assessment tools available, recognize patients who are at risk and educate those individuals (e.g. the student nurse) who are providing care to the patient.
- The provision of a 24-hour food has yet to be realized and the choice and availability of food need to improve.
- The role of the nurse is clear. It is to make the environment and provision of food as pleasant as possible and to assess, assist and document the care given to any patient who requires help with eating and drinking. Finally, reporting any concern to a qualified member of staff should always be a priority.

References

DoH (Department of Health) (2007) *The Nutrition Action Plan*, www.dh.gov.uk/en/Publicationsandstatistics/Publications/PublicationsPolicyAndGuidance/DH_079931, accessed 3 May 2008.

Green, S. and Watson, R. (2005) Nutritional screening and assessment tools for use by nurses: literature review, *Journal of Advanced Nursing*, 50(1): 69–83.

Kondrup, J., Allison, Y., Elia, M., Vellas, Z. and Plauth, Y. (2002) *ESPEN Guidelines for Nutrition Screening*, Elsevier, www.espen.org/Education/documents/Screening.pdf, accessed 22 February 2008.

McCabe, D. (2005) *Check Up: A Guide to the Special Healthcare Needs of Ethno-religious Minority Communities*. New Activity Publications, http://diversiton.com/downloads/checkUp.pdf, accessed 22 February 2008 .

Nightingale, F. (1859) *Notes on Nursing, What it is and What it is Not*. London: Harrison.

Rollins, H. (1997) Nutrition and wound healing, *Nursing Standard*, 11(51): 49–52.

Soil Association (2007) *Not What the Doctor Ordered*, *www.soilassociation.org/web/sa/saweb.nsf/Living/vending_machines.html, accessed 28 July 2008.*

WHO (World Health Organization) (1986) *Ottawa Charter for Health Promotion* Geneva: WHO.

Answers

Activity 9.2

The purpose of nutritional screening and assessment is to identify those patients who are at risk of not receiving appropriate nutrition to meet their physical and emotional needs. Screening is also appropriate for those individuals who are unfit and/or unwell and who may be eating inappropriately – for example a patient with angina who may be eating a lot of food with a high fat content.

Activity 9.5

1   We need teeth to chew and sore gums make chewing difficult. The alimentary tract acts as a passageway for the food.
2   We need to be able to pass the food from the mouth into the oesophagus.
3   Discomfort or pain may indicate damage, blockage or regurgitation.
4   Desired or undesired weight gain or loss is an indicator of inadequate intake or absorption.
5   There may be financial problems.
6   There may be loneliness or depression problems.
7   There may be travel and carrying problems.
8   If the patient does not have adequate facilities such as a fridge, extra help may be needed from social services.
9   Disinterest in food and meal preparation may be an indication of physical or mental ill health.
10 A patient's lifestyle may not allow time to eat properly
11 Concentration may be impaired by an illness such as Alzheimer's disease.
12 Look for food group avoidance.
13 Energy levels, exercise tolerance, regular exercise and activities are markers of nutrition.
14 Diarrhoea, constipation, vomiting, excessive thirst and frequent urination are markers of organic disease.
15 Preoccupation with body weight/shape may indicate an eating disorder.
16 Cravings and habits such as smoking and alcohol intake may require intervention.to stop/modify.
17 Chronic illnesses such as diabetes, renal disease, cancer and heart disease all require further investigation.
18 Family history and past medical history are markers for genetic trends.
19 Acute illness such as fever and trauma may mean the patient is too ill to eat.
20 External losses may indicate the patient is dehydrated.
21 Medication may affect nutritional intake, absorption, metabolism and excretion, and increase/alter nutritional needs.

Activity 9.12

1

- A clear explanation was given to the patient.
- The patient was given a choice.
- The patient was offered a drink.
- The food was nicely presented.
- The nurse cut up and left the food within reach.
- The patient was given a napkin.
- The drink container was changed.
- The patient was assisted as required.
- The procedure was not hurried.
- The patient was left comfortable.

2

- The drink is at the right temperature.
- The patient was protected from potential spillage with a napkin.
- The patient was positioned correctly.
- The nurse explained what was happening and why a beaker was being used.
- The nurse assisted the patient to take the right-sized sips and to drink the whole cup.
- The nurse stayed and reassured the patient throughout.

3

- A cup, perhaps with a straw.

Activity 9.13

1

- The bed table was too far away from the patient.
- The patient was offered no assistance, despite having limited dexterity.
- The patient was only given a spoon to use to eat.
- The patient was only left a beaker which again was too far away. The patient knocked the beaker over so was unable to take a drink, compromising fluid intake.
- The patient became frustrated and pushed the food away, thus compromising nutritional intake.

2

- The food provided by the service did not meet the needs of this patient because the patient was not asked if she liked or disliked any of the food being offered.
- The environment was not conducive to enable the patient to eat because the plate of food was too close to the patient's face. She was not able to see or smell it clearly in order to choose what to eat.
- The nurse did not protect the patient's pyjamas, risking food spillage, and this compromised the patient's dignity.

- The patient did not receive the assistance she required with eating and drinking in several respects: the spoonfuls offered were too large which created difficulty in chewing and some food spilled out of the patient's mouth which was distressing and undignified; the food was offered too quickly, which did not allow the patient enough time to chew before swallowing and could have led to the risk of pocketing of food in the cheek and consequent mouth infections; mouth care was not offered following the meal.
- The nurse was rough and impatient with the patient.
- The nurse failed to give the patient the entire meal, thus compromising nutritional requirements and leaving the patient hungry.
- The nurse used both a spoon and her own hand to wipe the patient's mouth so did not maintain the dignity of the patient.
- No drink was offered.
- The nurse left the patient still chewing.
- The nurse did not record the amount of food eaten.

3

- The nurse did not explain to the relative that because of the awkward head position it was important to give the drink in small sips to prevent too much fluid entering the oro-pharynx at any one time – this could cause the patient to choke.
- The nurse did not warn the relative that the drink was hot.
- The nurse did not explain to the patient why the beaker was being used.
- The nurse did not explain the flavour of the tea would be affected by the beaker.
- The nurse did not explain to the patient and the relative the importance of drinking fluids in order to remain hydrated.
- No record was made of any drink taken.
- The relative was given no instruction from the nurse who should have stayed to check that all was well.
- The relative called repeatedly for assistance but nobody came.

Scenario 9.1

Your answer might have included some of the following:

Psychosocial

- Depression, loneliness, social situation, living alone, contact with friends. Her ability to shop, prepare food and store food, preparation equipment (e.g. refrigerator or oven).
- Income.
- Medication – some drugs may alter appetite.

Clinical and physical

- Her physical appearance, for example, sunken eyes, pallor, dentures, missing teeth, gum disease or mouth infections.
- Her appetite, usual calorie intake, type of diet (e.g. vegetarian).
- Her normal and current height and weight and interest in food.

Continence, bowel and bladder care

Susan H. Walker

10

Chapter Contents

Learning objectives

The aim of this chapter is to explore how skilled nursing care can improve the quality of life for an individual with bladder, bowel and/or continence compromise. Throughout the chapter we will be referring to the accompanying Media Tool DVD. Please watch the video clips as directed as these will reinforce your learning. After reading this chapter and interacting with the Media Tool DVD you will be able to:

- Relate the anatomy and physiology of the bladder and bowel to nursing decisions and interventions which promote continence.
- Assess the bladder and bowel activity and continence status of an individual patient.
- Plan, implement and evaluate care based on an assessment of an individual's bladder and bowel activity and their continence status.
- Provide education for individuals and their carers and the wider community to promote continence and health of the bladder and bowel.
- Promote independence with the physical activities of urination, defecation and management of continence.

Introduction

Assisting a person with the physical activity of elimination of *urine* and *faeces* is often referred to as *basic care*. This term is used because the activity of elimination is essential and fundamental to life. However, the amount of assistance a person may require is determined following a skilled nursing assessment and the interventions used to assist a person require the care-giver to be sensitive to issues such as privacy, dignity and the therapeutic and appropriate use of touch. So, rather than 'basic care', this is *essential care* which requires the input of a skilled and knowledgeable care-giver.

To give skilled care, you will be required to apply knowledge and provide a rationale and evidence base for your decision (under guidance) in relation to supporting a person with the activity of *elimination* and the promotion of *continence.* This knowledge begins with an understanding of the structure and function of the lower urinary tract and the lower gastrointestinal tract.

Activity 10.1

Go to the Media Tool DVD, select **Skill Sets**, then **Meeting elimination needs** and watch the Keypoints Lecture of the urinary system. You may also wish to revise the anatomy and physiology of the urinary tract (the kidneys, ureters, bladder and the urethra) by using an appropriate anatomy and physiology book.

The functions of the kidneys, ureters, bladder and urethra in relation to elimination include production of urine by filtration of blood contents, reabsorption of useful substances and secretion of waste products, regulation and maintenance of electrolyte and water balance required for health, and the storage and passage of urine to the external environment.

Steggall (2007) refers to the process of *micturition* as an extremely complex one. Involuntary or *autonomic urination* occurs as a reflex action in the infant and young child, as they have not yet gained voluntary control of the bladder. Once the bladder contains enough urine to initiate the stretch response of the *detrusor muscle*, the muscle will contract, aided by excitatory impulses and micturition will occur.

When urinary continence has been gained (usually by the age of 2), this reflex can be overridden as the nerve supply from the bladder to the spinal cord becomes complete and the external sphincter contracts and relaxes through voluntary control.

When the bladder is full and the bladder wall stretched, the stretch receptors send impulses via the *parasympathetic sensory nerves* to the sacral centre. Nerve impulses are then relayed upwards to the sensory cortex and the individual becomes aware of the need to pass urine. Micturition is withheld until a convenient time and a socially acceptable place to void urine is reached. The elimination of urine is aided by contraction of the abdominal muscles to increase abdominal pressure.

As with *urination*, involuntary or autonomic reflex controls the normal process of *defecation* (passing faeces) in the infant and young child, until voluntary control of the external sphincter is gained. A developing child usually gains this control in the second or third year of life. The defecation reflex is initiated when the stretch receptors in the rectal walls respond to pressure of faeces entering the rectum. The defecation reflex is a spinal cord-mediated reflex that causes the walls of the sigmoid colon and the rectum to contract and the internal anal sphincter to relax, allowing faeces to pass into the anal canal. The contractions bring with them a feeling of fullness. Once voluntary control of the external sphincter through the *pudendal nerve* is gained, it is possible to delay defecation until an appropriate place to defecate is reached (Waugh and Grant 2006). If defecation is delayed for long, the feeling of fullness will fade as the rectal walls relax, until the next defecation reflex is initiated.

The process of defecation is aided by the *Valsalva manoeuvre*, which includes a period of breath holding and contraction of the diaphragm and abdominal walls in an effort to increase abdominal pressure and force faeces downwards (Marieb 2006). This is similar to the contraction of the abdominal muscles and the pelvic floor muscles that occurs to aid the voiding of urine.

Activity 10.2

You may want to revise the anatomy and physiology of the digestive tract by consulting an appropriate anatomy and physiology book before completing this activity.

Go to the Media Tool DVD, select **Skill Sets**, **Meeting elimination needs** and watch the Keypoints Lecture of digestion and defecation. Chapter 9 is also a helpful resource.

Continence

Continence can be defined as being able to maintain voluntary control over the reflex action to empty one's bladder and bowel until an appropriate time and place are reached. For continence to be achieved, it is essential that both the lower urinary and gastrointestinal tract are intact and all organs of these tracts receive a good blood and nerve supply. The detrusor muscle in the bladder and the muscle of the colon are required to respond to the stretch stimulus of urine filling the bladder, and any faecal mass within the colon. The diaphragm and the intra-abdominal muscles of the pelvic floor need the ability to contract to assist the process of elimination of urine and faeces.

It is also important that there is an absence of any psychological and environmental factors that may inhibit the elimination process, such as a fear of small spaces or a lack of privacy.

Scenario 10.1

Amy is aged 18 months and is responding well to potty training. What physical, psychological and social interventions do you think can encourage a child to develop continence effectively?

For potty/toilet training to be successful, it is necessary for voluntary control over the external sphincters in the bladder and bowel to be gained. This is usually achieved by the second or third year of life. A child is required to recognize the need to eliminate and be able to convey this need to a parent or carer so an appropriate facility can be provided. The child needs to recognize the discomfort of being wet and soiled and must have developed the motor skills required to sit for a period of time on a potty or toilet. Using the potty or toilet successfully will lead to an association with the feeling of being clean and dry. Positive responses by means of praise and hugs from parents and carers need to be associated with successful use of the potty or toilet to reinforce the activity.

It is imperative to remember to always respond immediately when a child conveys the need to eliminate and to give praise to the child when they reach the toilet and eliminate successfully. It is also important to give praise when they have conveyed the need, even if the toilet is not reached in time, for example, 'Never mind, you did well to tell mummy you needed the toilet, we will try and be a little quicker next time.' It is important to remember to teach hand washing following elimination so that this becomes a normal part of a child's routine.

Incontinence

Faecal incontinence tends to be under-reported. Exact figures regarding faecal incontinence are difficult to specify as it is a taboo subject and people are reluctant to discuss their problems or seek help, due to embarrassment, anxiety and fear. However, it is known that faecal incontinence is more common in older people, particularly women. The *Good Practice in Continence Services* Report (DoH 2000) estimates that faecal incontinence is experienced by 1 per cent of the healthy adult population living at home, with an estimated 17 per cent of the very elderly reporting symptoms. This number increases to 25 per cent for those in institutional care (Irwin 2001).

Causes

There are several causes of faecal incontinence in adults, as follows:

- Impaction with overflow diarrhoea in the frail elderly, or those with dementia or physical disability.
- Diarrhoea/intestinal hurry due to *Crohn's disease*, *ulcerative colitis*, and medications such as antibiotics.
- Neurological disease which may include spinal cord injury, spina bifida, stroke and diseases such as multiple sclerosis and Parkinson's.
- Anal sphincter damage due to direct trauma, trauma caused during childbirth or surgery.

The main causes of *urinary incontinence* in adults are:

- Childbirth.
- Obesity.
- Chronic constipation.
- Weak pelvic floor muscles.
- Urinary infection.
- Prostate disease in men which leads to obstruction of urine flow and post-micturition dribbling.
- Menopause in women as a result of hormonal changes and a reduction in oestrogen levels.

There are different types of urinary incontinence and these are described in Box 10.1.

Box 10.1 Types of urinary incontinence

- *Stress incontinence* – an increase in intra-abdominal pressure which leads to involuntary leakage of urine when laughing, sneezing and coughing, or on effort and exertion (Scottish Intercollegiate Guidelines Network 2004). Stress incontinence is often experienced by women who have had multiple births and have a weakened pelvic floor.
- *Urge incontinence* – an urge to frequently rush to pass urine, often leaking some urine before a suitable place to pass is reached. Again common in women who have weakened pelvic floor muscles.
- *Overactive bladder syndrome* – when there is urgency with or without urge incontinence of urine, but usually with frequency and occurring often in the night.
- *Detrusor over-activity/instability* – incontinence due to involuntary detrusor muscle activity.
- *Overflow incontinence* – the bladder is full and over-distended leading to involuntary leakage. Overflow incontinence is often experienced in men with an enlarged prostate gland.
- *Reflex incontinence* – incontinence of urine occurs without warning.
- *Immobility incontinence* – a person has to pass urine in an inappropriate place due to their inability to access acceptable toilet facilities and their dependency on others to assist them.

Box 10.2 Treatment for stress and urge incontinence

- *Conservative pelvic floor muscle training* – an exercise plan is introduced to the patient which if followed regularly will strengthen the pelvic floor muscles.
- *Bladder training* – a timed toileting plan is introduced which helps the patient avoid episodes of incontinence and to become familiar with the need to empty their bladder.
- *Drug therapy* – oxybutanin if bladder training has been ineffective. This drug reduces the instability and spasmodic contraction of the bladder muscle and so can often reduce episodes of incontinence.
- *Surgical sacral nerve stimulation* – recommended for overactive detrusor muscle and if conservative treatment has failed.
- *Retro pubic mid-urethral tape procedures.*
- *Non-therapeutic intermittent self-catheterization* – the patient is taught how to pass a small urinary catheter themselves, at regular times, to empty their bladder. This gives the patient control over the emptying of their bladder and so reduces episodes of incontinence.
- *Indwelling urinary catheterization* – the patient is catheterized with a urinary catheter placed via the urethra, which remains in the bladder and constantly drains away urine.
- *Supra pubic indwelling catheterization* – the patient undergoes a short surgical procedure to have the catheter sited through the abdominal wall, into the bladder. The catheter remains in the bladder to drain away urine.
- *Adapted lifestyle to the use of absorbent products* – should only be long term when all other treatment options have been explored (NICE 2006).

It is important to know what the symptoms of urinary incontinence in adults are because it will aid your recognition of continence difficulties when assessing and caring for patients. Adults who have developed urinary incontinence often complain of the need to pass urine frequently. Their sleep is often disturbed by the need to use the toilet during the night and sometimes they may be incontinent during their sleep.

When awake, they may complain of feeling a sense

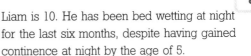

of urgency to pass urine, which results in leakage of urine if a toilet cannot be accessed quickly. Some adults experience leakage of urine when coughing, sneezing or laughing. All of these symptoms cause embarrassment and impact on an individual's ability to function normally. An outline of the treatment for stress and urge incontinence is given in Box 10.2. Box 10.3 provides more information on treating incontinence with drugs.

Box 10.3 Drug therapy

Drug therapy used to treat incontinence is usually considered when conservative treatment has been unsuccessful as a first line approach. However, bladder re-education can be undertaken with drug therapy and is reported by the Royal College of Physicians (1995) to be more effective when used in combination. Drugs such as Oxybutanin and Tolterodine are anti-cholinergic drugs with antispasmodic properties which are used in the management of detrusor instability. These drugs decrease the amplitude of detrusor contractions and also increase bladder capacity. Good improvements in symptoms have been reported, but side-effects include blurred vision, dry mouth and constipation (National Prescribing Centre 2006).

Enuresis

Enuresis is the term used when a child is unable to control their bladder during the day or night. A child may wet in the day time due to a delay in accessing the toilet or lack of a suitable facility. Most children remain dry at night by the age of 5. Parents and carers usually view an occasional wet bed at night time as part of continence training, however, if bed wetting continues beyond this age without physical cause this is referred to as nocturnal enuresis. According to the DOH (2000), there are 500,000 children in the UK with nocturnal enuresis, with prevalence decreasing with age. Secondary enuresis is the term used when a child who has achieved continence begins to bed wet. This may be due to psychological distress and insecurity such as the birth of a sibling, bullying or a move to a new house or school.

It is useful to reflect on the impact of incontinence on a child. Read the following scenario and try to answer the questions.

Scenario 10.2

Liam is 10. He has been bed wetting at night for the last six months, despite having gained continence at night by the age of 5.

He has been referred to a child psychologist by his paediatric consultant. While in the waiting room Liam becomes fidgety and his mother informs the staff that he has wet himself. Consider the possible causes and the impact of incontinence on the activities of living for a boy of Liam's age, before reading further. There is a sample answer at the end of the chapter.

Encopresis

Children can experience faecal incontinence which can have an equal impact on their self-esteem and toilet habits as urinary incontinence. *Encopresis* is the term used for faecal incontinence and soiling in children. Heins and Ritchie (1985) state that the cause of most cases of encopresis is prolonged constipation and impaction due to the constant stretching of the rectal walls, when the normal signals and muscle contraction of the rectum which would initiate the need to defecate are prohibited. Heins and Ritchie refer to the diagnosis of encopresis as difficult, stating that some children may faecally soil clothing and smear faeces as a result of psychological distress or as a symptom of an emotional disorder. This behaviour is distressing, but it is different to encopresis in that the child does have control over, or the ability to control, the defecation process.

Assessing risk

It is always important for any patient to undergo a full assessment of bladder, bowel and continence function on admission to hospital.

It is recommended by the NHS Modernization Agency (2003) that you use a trigger question to initiate conversation about this personal activity that most individuals find difficult to discuss. This allows a patient or client to respond and provide information about their bladder, bowel or continence status. For example, one question might be, 'Do you experience any difficulties in passing urine or moving your bowels, or controlling your bladder or bowel?'

The fact that you have prompted the discussion gives the patient an opportunity to discuss this personal and private bodily function without having to initiate the topic themselves. This demonstrates that the nurse sees this as an important activity of daily living, which can impact greatly on an individual's health status and quality of life. If a patient responds positively to an initial trigger question, then a more in-depth assessment can follow.

Patients who present themselves with a continence problem should automatically be afforded an in-depth and thorough assessment (DoH 2003). When assessing and taking a history of an individual's bladder, bowel habit and continence status, it is helpful if you (under supervision) gain information about normal bladder and bowel habits and any changes that may have occurred. It is important to note when any changes first occurred and for how long they have been present. Often the presence of unexplained changes will indicate infection and possible diseases such as cancer. It is often fear of an invasive examination and a cancer diagnosis that prevents people seeking help early.

Box 10.4 Web link – bowel cancer

Early diagnosis and commencement of treatment greatly improve prognosis and the chances of a full recovery, particularly for bowel cancer. For more information on the support available, go to www.cancerbackup.org.uk/Home.

An individual holistic assessment must also take into account how (or if) a person's culture, beliefs and religious practices influence their elimination habits. Acknowledging this individuality will ensure that the patient's needs are met (Holland *et al.* 2003). As with any patient assessment and history taking, a suitable environment should be sought where the patient is able to answer questions and provide information in confidence, knowing their privacy is secure (refer to Chapter 5 for more information). The nurse needs to

ensure a professional manner at all times, avoiding the use of jargon which can often lead to confusion for patients who are not familiar with medical terminology. Age-appropriate language is also important. A child or person with learning difficulties may have special names for urine and faeces such as 'wee wee' and 'poo', or 'number 1' and 'number 2'. It is important to ensure that the patient is aware of the necessity for the assessment and the importance of the information they offer, as this will be utilized to formulate their plan of care.

Some people will resist the urge to eliminate if this means using a lavatory other than their own. An individual bladder and bowel assessment must incorporate any psychological and environmental factors that may affect elimination habit.

Activity 10.3

Go to the Media Tool DVD, select **Case Studies**, **Adult Health (Margaret)**, then **Margaret arrives in hospital** and watch the video clip. How would you begin to plan care for Margaret, taking into account the fact that Margaret is unable to offer information about her normal elimination pattern at this time? The answer can be found at the end of the chapter.

There are specific questions that you may find useful when assessing bladder habit:

- How often does the patient pass urine, what time of day and how frequently?
- Does the patient wake in the night to pass urine?
- Is there any associated pain?
- Has the patient noticed a distinct smell or colour to their urine?
- Do they still feel the need to empty the bladder and feel uncomfortable after passing urine?
- How much fluid do they consume in a day?
- Do they experience urgency to void urine or can they hold urine for any length of time?
- Does the patient experience dribbling or urinary incontinence?
- Have they had any past investigations or interventions for bladder abnormalities and, if so, what were the results and outcomes?

Does the patient have an indwelling catheter or urostomy?

There are also specific questions that you may find useful to remember when assessing bowel habit:

- How frequently does the patient have a bowel movement; at what time of day; is the bowel movement stimulated by eating a meal or taking a hot drink?
- Does the patient respond straightaway to the need to defecate?
- What is the normal shape, colour and consistency of their faecal stool?
- Have they noticed any distinct odour or colour to their faecal stool?
- Have they experienced pain, need for excessive straining and increased flatus?
- Have they noticed blood in their stool?
- What type of foods and dietary preferences do they have?
- Do they take fibre regularly in their diet?
- How frequently do they eat and when is the main meal taken?
- Have they experienced any faecal soiling or incontinence?

- Have they had any past investigations or interventions for bowel abnormalities and, if so, what were the results and outcomes?
- Does the patient have a stoma, what is its anatomical position and the frequency and consistency of faecal matter?

Box 10.5 identifies more general information that a nurse should seek to find out from a patient during the assessment of bladder and bowel activity.

Factors affecting elimination

There can be a number of factors that can affect the process of elimination. These are identified below.

Physical

- Age (consider stages of development).
- Ignoring the urge to urinate or defecate (possibly due to embarrassment about the need for assistance or lack of assistance when required).
- Diet and fluid intake.
- Hormones (constipation is common in pregnancy).
- Immobility or reduced manual dexterity.
- Effect of medication such as opiods, antibiotics, diuretics, laxatives and iron.

Box 10.5 General information in the assessment of bladder and bowel activity

- Assessment of an individual's usual level of mobility, manual dexterity and exercise pattern.
- Does the patient use the lavatory, commode, bedpan or potty?
- Is the patient's lavatory modified (e.g. handrails or raised seat)?
- Is the person independent with bladder and bowel care or do they need assistance?
- Are they on any medication (over-the-counter and prescribed) or do they use an illegal drug?
- Do they have a history of previous medical conditions that might affect urination/defecation – for example, irritable bowel syndrome, haemorrhoids, spinal injury, enlarged prostate or related surgery?
- Use of any continence aids/devises such as penile sheaths, incontinence pads or intermittent self-catheterization.
- Oral health status that may affect ability to chew and swallow.
- Changes in behaviour – for example, a child who develops faecal incontinence after the birth of a sibling; an individual who begins to behave strangely; increasing confusion or aggression in an older adult with dementia.
- Change of environment and routine in both eating and bladder/bowel habit.
- Anxiety about using a public facility or requiring assistance.
- Recent changes in their overall health status.

Environmental/social/economic

- Lack of facilities or poor facilities which may be cold, dark and dirty.
- Lack of privacy which is often a problem for those in a multiple-bedded bay and needing to use a bedpan or commode.
- Change in familiar environment due to admission to hospital or a care setting.
- Having to use a bedpan or commode.
- Cost of aids and adaptations to facilities for elimination.

Psychological

- Anxiety and stress.
- Life events such as bereavement, bullying, new school, birth of a sibling.

Pre-existing conditions

- Congenital deformity, bladder or bowel disease.
- Inflammatory bowel disease or cancer.
- Neurological conditions such as multiple sclerosis, motor neurone disease or stroke.
- Systemic conditions (e.g. thyroid disease or infection) can all affect the elimination process.

According to Nakayama *et al.* (1997), incontinence of urine and faeces is a common complication immediately after stroke, caused by damage to the nervous system. In some cases the nervous system will recover and with good nursing and rehabilitation, continence can be regained.

A suitable environment

The NHS Modernization Agency (2003) recognizes the need for bladder and bowel care to be given in an environment that is conducive to the patient's individual needs. It is necessary that in any care setting patients know where lavatory facilities are if they are mobile and able to meet their own elimination needs. If a patient is immobile or requires assistance with elimination, then access to a nurse call bell, or directions to verbally call, is essential so that patients can summon help. Nurses should respond immediately to a patient's need to eliminate.

The lavatory area needs to be fit for purpose. This requires the environment and the lavatory itself to be

Activity 10.4

Go to the Media Tool DVD, select **Case Studies**, **Adult Health (Margaret)**, then **Margaret arrives in hospital** and watch the video clip. Margaret is semi-conscious in the A&E department but is aware of the fact that she has become incontinent of urine and faeces. This has caused her to become distressed. Incontinence is often associated with regression and loss of independence (Van Dongen 2001). You are required to provide a safe environment for Margaret, promote her physical comfort and protect her privacy and dignity (see Chapter 5). Why is it important that you deal with Margaret's personal hygiene needs at this point? Make a note of your answer and compare to the sample one at the end of the chapter.

private, clean and comfortable, warm and well lit. There should be a constant supply of toilet tissue and appropriate hand washing and hand drying facilities.

In identifying the particular needs of patients it will be necessary to take cultural differences into consideration. Patients should be assessed to determine cultural preferences and the amount of assistance required. For instance, Muslims prefer to wash their genitalia under running water after using the lavatory and by simply providing access to a jug in the privacy of the lavatory this need may be met. Some individuals will need assistance with access to the lavatory while others may need assistance to manipulate clothing due to a lack of dexterity or immobility. There is a legal requirement for lavatories to be available for a disabled person who may require assistance, with enough space to transfer from a wheelchair and with handles fixed to the walls to aid transfer onto the lavatory. Where hoists are used to assist patients onto the lavatory or a bedpan, the hoist slings should be allocated to individual patients and washed or changed if soiled as per the manufacturer's instructions.

Often odour eliminators or air fresheners may be used discreetly by individual patients (but not by or around those patients who may have allergies or breathing difficulties). This can help reduce embarrassment if bowel movements are malodorous, such as diarrhoea. Be aware of your own response to a patient's need to eliminate. A negative or delayed response from a nurse may result in continence difficulties and can delay recovery of continence status.

Activity 10.5

Consider your own thoughts and feelings in relation to the activity of elimination. What do you consider to be a suitable environment? Think about the times you have been required to use a public toilet, perhaps when travelling. What has made you feel comfortable when using such a facility? What has deterred you from using such a facility?

Common conditions

Let us now consider some common conditions associated with the process of elimination.

Diarrhoea

Diarrhoea may be acute or chronic, a symptom associated with infection, or a symptom of a disease such as ulcerative colitis. Severe or prolonged bouts of diarrhoea may lead to dehydration with infants and small children being particularly susceptible.

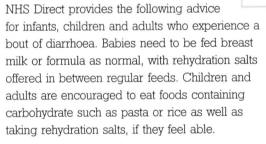

Box 10.6 Web link – NHS Direct

NHS Direct provides the following advice for infants, children and adults who experience a bout of diarrhoea. Babies need to be fed breast milk or formula as normal, with rehydration salts offered in between regular feeds. Children and adults are encouraged to eat foods containing carbohydrate such as pasta or rice as well as taking rehydration salts, if they feel able.

See www.nhsdirect.nhs.uk for more information.

When caring for a person with diarrhoea, the following aspects of care should be offered:

- Close access to a toilet cubicle or immediate response to a request for a bedpan or commode.
- Unlimited provision of toilet tissue and wipes.

- Ventilation and discreet use of air fresheners to reduce embarrassment.
- Access to washing facilities and assistance with personal cleansing as required.
- Good hand hygiene. Nurses need to consider implementation of cross-infection control measures.

It is also important to observe for signs of dehydration such as dry skin, dry mouth, sunken eyes, tiredness and confusion. Infants and young children may be disinterested in favourite toys and irritable. Adequate fluid replacement is essential. You may wish to refer to Chapter 9 for further information on this. Individuals should be assessed by a doctor if their symptoms persist or their condition deteriorates.

Activity 10.6

Hindus and Muslims require that nurses of the same sex meet their intimate hygiene and elimination needs (Holland *et al.* 2003). What strategies could your area of practice develop to ensure this need is always met? Refer to the answer at the end of the chapter.

You may come across various situations in practice such as the one highlighted in Scenario 10.3.

Urinary tract infection

Sudden onset of frequency in the need to pass urine with associated discomfort may indicate the presence of a urinary tract infection. The amount of urine passed may also be reduced, dark in colour and strong in smell.

Urinary infection in the bladder is known as cystitis, while infection present within the kidney is known as pylonephritis. Infection of the urinary tract is more common in females than males, due to the closeness of the vagina and the urethral opening, allowing organisms to pass from the bowel and perineum into the urinary tract. The short length of the female urethra allows quick passage of organisms to the bladder. Infection will usually be accompanied by pyrexia, nausea and vomiting and if in the kidney acute loin pain. Soloman (2003) names the organisms most likely

Scenario 10.3

Joan is 72 and was admitted to a medical ward having been found by her daughter in a distressed and confused state, after falling at home. Joan was taken to A&E by ambulance. Following a medical and nursing assessment and investigations it is established that Joan has no physical injuries and she is admitted to the ward. The ward is a 'Nightingale'-style ward, with bathing and toilet facilities at either end. You and your nursing colleagues note that whenever you respond to a patient's need to eliminate, Joan also calls for a bedpan or commode. When you reach Joan she has either been incontinent of urine while in bed or sitting in her chair, or is unable to use the commode when it is provided. Joan is mobile but unsteady on her feet and appears agitated or mildly confused most of the time. Prior to admission Joan was fully continent and her daughter reports that her mother has never previously displayed any signs of confusion.

1 What nursing actions and management issues should you consider in relation to Joan's incontinence?

2 What factors could be causing Joan's agitation and what could you do about it?

Check your answers with those at the end of the chapter before you move on to the next section.

---

to be involved as Escherichia coli, Streptococcus faecalis and Staphylococcus albus.

To eliminate or confirm the diagnosis of a urinary tract infection you may be asked to obtain a midstream specimen of urine (MSU) to send for a culture and sensitivity testing. Once the bacterial organism has been identified, an appropriate antibiotic can be prescribed.

Activity 10.7

Go to the Media Tool DVD, select **Case Studies**, **Adult Health (Margaret)**, then **Margaret in bed** and answer the associated questions.

Margaret has become unconscious. During this time the nurses will need to ensure that all her physical needs are met. Her husband has been informed of necessary interventions that will be required to maintain Margaret's homeostatic state. Margaret is obviously unable to take fluids or food while unconscious and will begin to receive fluids intravenously. You may wish to refer to Chapter 9 at this point. Now go to **Skill Sets, Nutritional Intake, IV cannulation** to watch care of a patient having IV therapy and answer the accompanying questions.

Catheterization

A urinary catheter is a hollow tube inserted along the urethra into the bladder to drain urine or to introduce medication. Urinary catheters may also be sited suprapublicly, through the abdominal and bladder wall.

Catheters can be intermittently inserted to empty the bladder or be left in situ for a period of time depending on the individual patient's circumstances and condition.

Activity 10.8

Go to the Media Tool DVD, select **Skill Sets**, **Meeting elimination needs**, then **Urinary catheterization and catheter care**. Watch the demonstration of catheterization and answer the accompanying questions.

If you remember, Margaret is receiving fluids intravenously. The nurses are required to monitor and record the amount of fluid she receives and also to monitor and record the amount of urine she passes to accurately maintain a positive fluid balance. It is imperative that a good fluid balance is maintained and recorded to prevent dehydration and organ failure. It is also important to keep a record of Margaret's input and output (see Chapter 3).

It is necessary to seek informed consent from any patient requiring an indwelling urinary catheter. The patient should understand why the catheter is

Activity 10.9

Go to the Media Tool DVD, select **Skill Sets**, **Meeting elimination needs**, then **Fluid balance**. Work through the keypoints lecture and extra resources.

Apart from the need to accurately measure urine output in an unconscious, traumatized and/or very ill person, what other circumstances may indicate the need for an indwelling urinary catheter? The answer is at the end of the chapter.

required and should also receive information regarding the procedure. Making an informed decision can only happen when this information has been provided. If the patient is unconscious, then the hospital staff will perform the procedure out of a duty of care, applying the rule of beneficence (Beauchamp and Childress 2001). In Margaret's case, the nursing and medical staff must ensure that her next of kin is informed of the clinical reasoning for catheterization.

Activity 10.10

Go to the Media Tool DVD, select **Skill Sets**, **Meeting elimination needs**, then **Urinary catheterization and catheter care** and observe the video clip of explaining catheterisation to an adult for the procedure of urinary catheterization.

When caring for a patient with an indwelling catheter, it is important to try and prevent associated catheter complications such as the risk of developing a urinary tract infection. A closed drainage system will reduce the risk of catheter-associated infection and should always be used whenever a patient has an indwelling urinary catheter. A closed drainage system is one which has a non-returnable/one-way valve to prevent the tracking of infection up the catheter tube. This system allows for drainage of the urine from the catheter bag without the bag having to be disconnected from the catheter itself.

Laurent (1998) estimated that 50 per cent of patients in hospital with an indwelling catheter will develop problems due to infection. Care must therefore focus on the prevention of infection. However, as infection for most patients with a long-term indwelling urinary catheter seems almost inevitable, catheterization is best avoided as an intervention if at all possible (NICE 2003).

According to Steggall (2007), to reduce the risk of infection, catheter hygiene should be performed twice daily, in the morning as part of a patient's personal hygiene activity and at night, before going to sleep. This involves the patient (or the nurse if required) thoroughly cleansing their genital area with warm soapy water. In male patients, if uncircumcised, the foreskin should be retracted to allow the urinary meatus to be thoroughly cleansed.

When removing a catheter, a clean, rather than aseptic, technique is used. It is essential to maintain hand hygiene by using an antibacterial solution and to wear an apron and disposable gloves. Gauze swabs, a disposal bag and a sterile syringe are also required. An indwelling urinary catheter is secured by a self-retaining balloon which when inflated sits at the neck of the bladder to hold the catheter in position. The balloon is inflated as part of the insertion procedure and the amount of water used to inflate the balloon along with the catheter size and date of insertion should be documented in the patient's records. The amount of water required to inflate the balloon is also on the hub of the catheter itself. This specified amount (usually 10mls) is removed by using a sterile syringe to withdraw it and so deflate the balloon prior to removal of the catheter. A catheter specimen of urine may be required prior to removal of the catheter to detect any possible presence of infection.

Bladder training

You may come across patients undergoing various forms of bladder retraining while on the wards. Bladder training programmes will involve regularly visiting the toilet with assistance from a nurse with mobilization, manipulation of clothing and post-elimination cleansing. For a stroke patient with bladder dysfunction, for example, bladder training will focus on increasing urine storage and promoting bladder emptying. Habit training and timed voiding, prompted voiding and pelvic floor exercises should be introduced into a plan of care for a patient as required. These are known as behavioural techniques.

Box 10.7 Best practice when taking a patient to the toilet

- Respond immediately to the patient's request.
- Put on a plastic apron and non-sterile gloves if help is needed with personal hygiene.
- Ascertain whether a stool or urine specimen is required.
- Assist the patient from the bed or chair as required.
- Ensure the patient is wearing slippers and dressing gown to promote a safe environment and promote dignity.
- Collect any personal items such as toiletries, sanitary towels and fresh underwear.
- Guide the patient to the lavatory cubicle or take them in a wheelchair.
- Offer assistance with clothing if required.
- Remain in the immediate vicinity if necessary and maintain privacy.
- Once the patient has eliminated, offer assistance with personal hygiene, ensuring the perianal area is clean and dry and helping with clothing. Consider cultural preferences, for example, running water for hygiene purposes. When assisting females with personal hygiene, wipe from front to back to avoid bacterial contamination of the urethra.
- Offer hand-washing facilities to the patient.
- Remove gloves if you have assisted with personal hygiene and wash your hands.
- Escort the patient back to bed or chair, making sure that they are comfortable and have everything they need within reach.
- Document the amount of urine or bowel movement as appropriate on fluid balance charts and in patient records.

Assisting patients

We have already determined that assisting patients with elimination needs requires skill, tact and diplomacy. Box 10.7 gives an example of best practice. You may wish to read this and compare it to your current practice and identify ways in which you could improve.

If a patient (like Margaret in the case study) is initially unable to walk to the toilet, then you may provide a bedpan or commode. The commode should not be used by the bedside unless total privacy can be assured. Alternatively the patient may be transferred from the bed to a wheelchair, taken to the lavatory and there transferred to the commode, which may then be moved over the lavatory. The advantage of using the commode rather than a bedpan is that it allows the patient to assume a position which aids elimination – the Valsalva manoeuvre is easier to achieve when the hips and knee are flexed. A risk assessment should be undertaken and safe moving and handling procedures adhered to when assisting patients with mobility difficulties. The commode chair should never be used as a mode of transport between the bed and the lavatory, due to the risk of cross-infection. Elimination is often inhibited when a bedpan is offered, due to fear of accidents on the bedclothes, difficult positioning and lack of privacy.

Very often you will look after patients whose conditions will affect their ability to get to the toilet in time

Activity 10.11

Go to the Media Tool DVD, select **Case Studies**, then **Learning Disability (Alex)**. Alex has developed non-insulin-dependent diabetes and is receiving help and advice on how to manage his condition. He has had some urgency to visit the toilet to pass urine as a response to his increased fluid intake, as excessive thirst is a side-effect of his illness. Sometimes Alex does not respond quickly enough to the need to pass urine and as a result he is occasionally incontinent. Alex finds this very distressing so he has decided to drink very little. What can you do to help Alex maintain and improve his continence status? A sample answer can be found at the end of the chapter.

Box 10.8 Providing a bedpan or commode

Providing a bedpan or commode is an essential nursing skill. The following is an example of best practice. You may wish to read this and compare it to your current practice and identify ways in which you could improve.

- Respond immediately to request.
- Put on a plastic apron and non-sterile gloves.
- Collect either the clean bedpan and a bedpan cover, or the commode from the sluice. Check that the brakes are in working order and the commode seat, handles and foot rests are clean.
- Take the bedpan or commode to the bedside. Position the commode and apply the brakes.
- Draw curtains around the bed to promote privacy and dignity for the patient.
- Ensure wipes and tissues are readily available.
- Assist the patient onto the bedpan/commode so they are well supported in an upright position.
- Offer further assistance if needed to remove/move clothing. Placing a disposable incontinence sheet under the bedpan will aid personal cleansing following defecation.
- If a commode is used, ensure slippers are worn by the patient to prevent slipping. Assist the patient from the bed to the commode, offering further assistance if needed to remove or move clothing. Once the patient is safely seated on the commode, cover their knees with a sheet or blanket to promote dignity and keep them warm.
- Once the patient is safely seated on the bedpan or commode, ensure support with balance is offered as required.
- Instruct the patient not to remove themselves from the bedpan unaided as this may lead to injury or spillage of contents.
- Stay inside the curtains if the patient wishes or requires constant supervision.
- If waiting outside the curtains, ensure that the patient can reach the call bell to indicate when they have finished.
- Remove the commode or bedpan and ensure that the protective sheet is in place.
- Offer assistance with perianal washing and wiping as required and remove the incontinence sheet from beneath the patient. When assisting girls and women with personal hygiene, wipe from front to back to avoid bacterial contamination of the urethra.
- Take the commode or covered bedpan with protective sheet to the sluice.
- Observe the colour, amount or urine and the consistency of the stool passed.
- Take any required samples, before disposing of urine or stool.
- Wash, sterilize or dispose of the bedpan and clean the commode according to local policy.
- Remove and dispose of apron and gloves and wash hands. Return to the patient to offer hand-washing equipment, wet and dry wipes, or a bowl, jug of water and hand towels.
- Ensure that the patient is comfortable and has everything they need within reach.
- Make sure the immediate environment is tidy, use air-freshener as necessary and open the curtains .
- Document bowel action or urine output in patient records and report any abnormalities.

and this might cause some distress. Activity 10.11 examines this issue further.

Now let us consider another age group from the case studies, 9-year-old Tom.

Activity 10.12

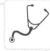

Tom has a fractured femur which has been immobilized in a Thomas splint. He is being nursed on traction. He is able to use a monkey pole to lift himself onto a bedpan when he needs to eliminate. Answer the following questions and then refer to the answers at the end of the chapter.

1 What terminology might a 9-year-old use to indicate this need?

2 How might you deal with this to ensure Tom is clean and dry?

3 Due to his immobility and possible fear of discomfort when using a bedpan, Tom is at risk of developing constipation. What can the nurse do to prevent this?

Constipation

All the patients referred to in the case studies are at risk of developing constipation. It is important to be able to recognize contributing factors and symptoms in order to promote prevention through practice and patient education, and to treat appropriately if constipation has already developed.

Constipation is the infrequent and uncomfortable passage of hard stools, with associated straining and a sensation of incomplete evacuation. Bowel movements are reduced in number from an individual's normal habit to three or fewer per week (Thompson *et al.* 1999). Constipation can affect anyone at any time during their life, but it mostly affects the very young and the very old. People worry more about their bowels as they age, but Norton (1996) concludes that ageing itself does not slow down stool movement in the colon. Constipation is not a disease, but often a symptom of disease or lifestyle.

Constipation can reduce comfort and quality of life and lead to the development of unpleasant symptoms which include flatulence, abdominal bloating, lethargy and irritability, fretfulness in children, halitosis, nausea and abdominal colic. Increased confusion may occur in those with dementia, and behavioural changes may occur in young children or those with a learning disability. The sudden development, or further worsening, of urinary incontinence can be due to hard faeces

pressing on the bladder or urethra. It is also possible for hard faeces to occlude the urethra completely, leading to retention of urine and great patient discomfort.

According to Kyle (2006), those who are ill in hospital or institutionalized are particularly at risk of developing constipation which can become a chronic problem.

Once a thorough history and assessment of a patient's bowel habit have been undertaken, it should be possible to identify contributing factors to the development of constipation. A physical examination will include abdominal palpation to feel for any faecal mass and a digital rectal examination to assess the tone of the anal sphincter and rectal contents.

Activity 10.13

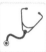

A digital rectal examination and abdominal palpation can only be performed by a doctor or a nurse who has received specific training. Explicit consent must be obtained from the patient or carer and documented in both medical and nursing records. Go to www.rcn.org.uk/__data/assets/ pdf_file/0009/78588/002062.pdf for guidance on obtaining consent for a digital rectal examination and by whom and how such an examination should be performed.

For a patient who is diagnosed with *faecal impaction*, faecal incontinence (overflow diarrhoea) usually develops if the impaction is untreated. For most people increasing the fibre content of their diet, taking more exercise and increasing their fluid intake can rectify the symptoms of constipation. Laxatives can help in the short term to relieve constipation and although they can be bought over the counter at a chemist, any person with prolonged symptoms should be seen by a doctor to ensure there is no underlying cause such as an intestinal obstruction.

It can be helpful for patients or parents to keep a diary of bowel actions to establish a pattern. This is particularly useful when bowel training programmes are in progress. Nurses should record bowel actions in the nursing notes and on the appropriate charts – for example, a stool record chart and episodes of diarrhoea are measured and recorded on the fluid intake and output chart.

Bristol Stool Chart

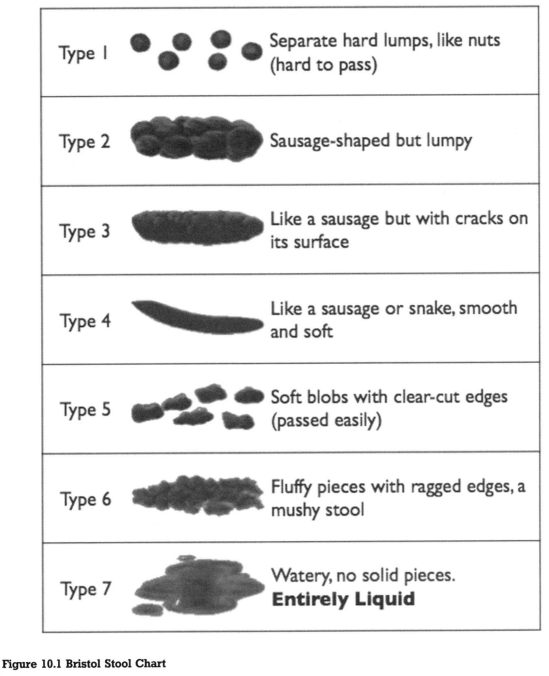

Type 1		Separate hard lumps, like nuts (hard to pass)
Type 2		Sausage-shaped but lumpy
Type 3		Like a sausage but with cracks on its surface
Type 4		Like a sausage or snake, smooth and soft
Type 5		Soft blobs with clear-cut edges (passed easily)
Type 6		Fluffy pieces with ragged edges, a mushy stool
Type 7		Watery, no solid pieces. **Entirely Liquid**

Figure 10.1 Bristol Stool Chart

There are some useful resources available for measuring and recording such as the Bristol stool chart shown in Figure 10.1.

Many people will self-diagnose and treat their own constipation with medications known as *laxatives*. Laxatives are often prescribed for patients in hospitals and care homes, but they should be administered with caution. Over-use of laxatives can lead to urea and electrolyte imbalances and impaired elimination patterns.

Laxatives can be given orally, rectally as suppositories, or in the form of an enema for severe constipation. Laxatives can be classified as bulking agents such as bran and methylcellulose (also a faecal softener). They work by increasing fibre content of the stool and water retention making the stool bulkier and softer to pass. Faecal softeners such as an Arachis oil retention enema will also soften the stool. Retention enemas are retained within the bowel for as long as possible to produce the desired effect. These are only useful if the patient is able to hold on to the enema solution through good muscle tone and therefore they are not usually suitable for the frail or elderly.

Senna and sodium picosulfate taken orally or glycerol suppositories (a semi-solid pellet given rectally) are known as stimulants. Glycerol suppositories also soften the stool. They work by stimulating the nerves in the colon to increase intestinal motility. Osmotic agents include the use of oral lactulose which draws water into the colon by osmosis, causing distension of the colon and peristalsis to aid faecal movement. Phosphate and sodium citrate enemas are also osmotic agents. Known as an evacuant enema, the phosphate and sodium citrate solution is only required to be retained in the bowel by the patient for a short time and is expelled from the bowel with any faecal matter.

An enema may be given as a method of emptying the bowels to relieve constipation, or sometimes as part of pre-operative preparation for patients undergoing bowel investigations and surgery.

Box 10.9 gives examples of best practice which you may wish to follow if required to support a patient through this procedure, or if participating in the administration of a prescribed enema.

Continence beyond hospital

It is important that patients have access to 'need specific' supplies that assist in the management of their continence (DoH 2003). When in hospital patients must be able to access continence aids. They will require time to consider advice from nurses and continence specialists to discover product preferences and what is most suitable for their individual needs. Once discharged to a residential care setting or back to their own home in the community, being able to access supplies is of paramount importance. Limited or unavailable supplies will increase patient anxiety and decrease their ability and/or their carers' ability to manage their continence.

Continence aids such as absorbent pads, adapted pants and anal plugs can be used to contain urine and faecal matter. They may also carry and/or collect urine and faecal matter. Other aids include urinary sheaths, pubic pressure urinals, urinary catheters for intermittent self-catheterization and long-term indwelling urinary catheters and drainage devices. Should a patient be discharged with a urostomy or colostomy, then a continual supply of skin wafers, stoma bags and other associated equipment is imperative. The stoma care nurse will advise about obtaining supplies following discharge. The stoma nurse specialist and the continence nurse are both a source of support for a patient with a stoma.

Activity 10.14

Go to the Media Tool DVD, select **Case Studies**, then **Mental Health (Chris)**. Chris is at risk of developing constipation as he is taking recreational drugs, many of which can cause this condition. As well as assisting with Chris's psychological needs, it is important that the nurses provide some health education for him in relation to the prevention of some of the side-effects of his recreational drug use.

1 Can you identify three types of drugs that may affect Chris's bowel habit? You may find the following link useful: www.bnf.org/bnf/bnf/current/104945.htm.

2 Should Chris require suppositories to relieve the effects of constipation, how should these be administered? Consider how the nurse would work to reduce patient anxiety and embarrassment in relation to this procedure.

Check your answers with those at the end of the chapter.

Activity 10.15

Look back at your answer to question 2 in Activity 10.14 and compare it to the following best practice guide to administration of a suppository. Can you identify areas for improvement in your own practice?

Equipment required:

- Incontinence pads to protect bed.
- Disposable gloves and apron to prevent contamination from bodily fluids.
- Disposable wipes and tissues.
- Suppositories as required/prescribed.
- Topical swab.
- Lubricating jelly.

Procedure:

- Explain the procedure to the patient to gain informed consent.
- Ensure privacy by using a treatment room or pull curtains around the bed. Ask staff to avoid interruptions.
- Assist the patient into the left lateral position, with knees flexed. Buttocks should be towards the edge of the bed to aid exit from the bed and to reduce bed soiling.
- Place an incontinence pad under the patient's hips and buttocks to help promote patient comfort and relieve distress and embarrassment of soiled linen.
- Ensure lower body is covered by a blanket to maintain dignity.
- Put on a protective apron, wash your hands using a bactericidal soap and put on disposable gloves to minimize the risk of cross-infection.
- Place lubricating jelly on a topical swab and lubricate the blunt end of the suppository to reduce anal trauma on insertion.
- Separate the patient's buttocks and insert the suppository blunt end first. Using your index finger, advance the suppository 4–5cms to aid retention. According to Abd-El-Mahmoud *et al.* (1991), cited in Mallet and Doherty (2004), suppositories are more readily retained if inserted blunt end first,
- Repeat for a second suppository.
- Ensure the patient's perianal/perineal area is clean and dry to promote comfort.
- Ask the patient to retain the suppositories for as long as possible, up to 20 minutes, to allow them to dissolve and have a softening effect on the faeces, making it easier to pass.
- Ensure patient access to a nurse call bell, a bedpan, a commode or a lavatory.
- When called, give any assistance required using safe moving and handling techniques.
- Observe the amount, colour, consistency and content of any expelled faeces (consider use of the Bristol stool chart).
- Take any faecal specimen required for examination.
- Dispose of and/or clean equipment for future use, remove apron and disposable gloves and wash hands using a bactericidal soap to reduce risk of cross-infection.
- Record the result from the suppositories and any specimens taken in the patient's nursing and medical records.
- Ensure the patient is comfortable following the procedure.
- Continue to monitor bowel function, along with reassessment and evaluation of the patient's presenting symptoms.

Box 10.9 Enema administration for adults

Equipment required:

- Incontinence pads to protect bed.
- Disposable gloves and apron.
- Disposable wipes and tissues.
- Prescribed enema/prescription chart.
- Jug of water at required temperature.
- Bath thermometer.
- Lubricating gel.
- Commode or bedpan and tissue, or access to a lavatory

Preparation:

- Explain the procedure to gain informed consent.
- Check that patient does not have a peanut/groundnut allergy before giving an Arachis oil enema.
- Ensure privacy by using a treatment room or pull curtains around the bed. Ask other staff to avoid interruptions.
- Warm the enema in a jug of warm water, until the required temperature is reached. Follow the manufacturer's recommendations for single, pre-prepared products. Mallet and Doherty (2004) recommend that the enema be warmed to body temperature, or just above. Oil retention enemas are warmed to 37.8°C.
- Assist the patient into the left lateral position, with knees flexed. This allows the nozzle or tubing of the enema to follow the natural anatomy of the colon and gravity will also help flow and/or retention of any solution used (Mallet and Doherty 2004).
- Place an incontinence pad under the patient's hips and buttocks to protect the bedding and relieve potential distress if fluid is expelled from the anus.
- Cover the lower body with a blanket to maintain dignity.
- Put on a protective apron, wash hands and put on non-sterile gloves.

Procedure:

- Lubricate the enema nozzle to minimize anal/rectal trauma.
- Separate the patient's buttocks and observe for soreness or other abnormalities.
- Introduce the nozzle into the anal canal, which is approximately 3.8cm in length in adults and then advance to approximately 10cm to ensure the tip reaches the rectum. This is normally the full length of the nozzle for pre-prepared enemas.
- To administer an evacuant enema, roll the packaging slowly from bottom to top to prevent backflow of the solution into the packet.
- Remove the nozzle slowly while still keeping the bag rolled and encourage the patient to hold on to the solution for as long as prescribed; the effect can be rapid and the patient should not be left without easy access to a nurse call bell.
- Wipe the patient's perianal/perineal area and leave them clean and dry. Cover the patient.
- Ensure access to a nurse call bell, a bedpan, a commode or lavatory. When called, give any assistance required.
- Take the commode or covered bedpan with protective sheet to the sluice.
- Observe the colour, amount and consistency of the stool passed.
- Collect faecal specimen if required.
- Wash/sterilize/dispose of the bedpan, or clean the commode according to local policy.
- Remove and dispose of apron and gloves, and wash hands.
- Return to the patient to offer facilities for personal hygiene and hand washing.

- Ensure that the patient is comfortable and has everything they need within reach.
- Make sure the immediate environment is tidy, use air-freshener as necessary and open the curtains.
- Document the type of enema given, the resultant bowel action and any specimens collected in patient records and report any abnormalities.
- Continue to monitor bowel function, along with reassessment and evaluation of the patient's presenting symptoms.

Box 10.10 Web links

Most of continence aids are provided by the health authority on prescription from a GP. A Continence Products Directory is now available online, providing independent, unbiased information on over 3000 continence products and appliances available in the UK, whether through the NHS, retail or mail order. The following websites provide more information.

www.continence-foundation.org.uk/

tenadirect.co.uk/

www.handyhealthcare.co.uk/

Good Practice in Continence Services (DoH 2000) provides a framework of practice for health services. People with continence problems and their carers can also access professional organizations and specialized charities to ensure their needs and rights are met. Most hospitals provide the support of a specialist team including specialist continence nurses and continence physiotherapists who work between the hospital and community to provide a seamless service. The continence service can supply continence aids and provide education for patients, carers and professionals. Specialist continence nurses can liaise with community services to arrange the loan of commodes and bedpans and recommend further assessment and adaptation to a patient's home that may aid continence.

Health education and promotion

The nurse as a giver of skilled, essential aspects of care has an excellent opportunity to promote continence and a healthy bladder and bowel with patients both in hospital and the wider community (DoH 2003). Nurses are well placed in primary, secondary and tertiary settings to promote continence and a healthy bladder and bowel, and to support those who have adapted their lifestyle to manage an altered continence status.

For a healthy bladder, individuals should be encouraged to:

- Learn pelvic floor exercises and do them daily. If pregnant or post-delivery, then pelvic floor exercises should be carried out regularly both during and after the pregnancy to maintain the strength of the pelvic floor muscles. Men can also be taught how to do pelvic floor exercises
- Drink six to eight glasses of water daily.
- Respond immediately to the feeling of a full bladder.
- Maintain a healthy body weight in relation to height and age. Weight puts extra strain on your pelvic floor muscles.
- Avoid constipation as this can affect the passage of urine due to pressure on the ureters from an extended bowel.
- Should pain be present when passing urine, or dribbling or incontinence occur, seek advice as soon as possible.

For a healthy bowel, individuals should be encouraged to:

- Drink six to eight glasses of water daily to help keep faeces soft and aid its passage.
- Eat a healthy, well-balanced diet which includes five portions of fruit or vegetables a day. Add fibre to maintain and improve motility within the gut.
- Take as much regular exercise as possible to stimulate gut motility.
- Respond immediately to the need to defecate.
- If pain, blood or mucus is present when passing faeces, seek advice as soon as possible.

Box 10.11 Bowel cancer

For individuals who have a family history of bowel cancer, a blood test in now available to people over the age of 55 years in the UK. Faecal specimens are tested to check for any hidden blood in the stool. Most people receive a normal result. An unclear result means that people will be offered further investigation to find a cause, surveillance, or treatment if necessary. An unclear result does not always indicate cancer and can often be attributed to haemorrhoids or stomach ulcers, but early detection and treatment of bowel cancer can result in a 90 per cent chance of survival.

tinence more difficult. Incontinence is a primary cause for many people admitted to nursing homes as family and carers feel unable to cope (Edwards and Jones 2001).

Information that patients will require includes dietary advice as described above. They also need to know how to access continence aids and products and how to correctly dispose of these. Advice about disposal of aids and products can be sought from the local authority as well as the continence service. Individuals and carers will need to know how to care for the skin and use barrier creams to prevent excoriation and breakdown in anyone with reduced mobility.

Washing soiled linen and clothes puts extra strain on finances and local authorities will sometimes provide a continence laundry service. Advice on prevention of cross-infection is imperative. Good hand washing, the use of disposable gloves and disinfectants need to be ensured. The storage and cleansing of bedpans and commodes used at home need to be explained to reduce the risk of spreading infection.

Advice and support are necessary for anyone living with an altered continence status and also for their family and carers. Any physical or cognitive disability present can make the issue of dealing with incon-

Summary and key points

This chapter has discussed elimination as a normal bodily function. When the process of elimination or continence status is impaired, it will impact on an individual's ability to cope and can greatly lower their self-esteem, regardless of age. It is necessary for the nurse to understand the normal process of elimination of both urine and faeces to be able to detect when this process is impaired.

An individual's lifestyle, attitudes, beliefs and culture influence their elimination habits and do not change when they go into hospital or a care setting. Care needs to be delivered that is sensitive to such beliefs and culture.

It is important to remember the following key points:

- Nurses require knowledge of factors and conditions that can affect a person's bowel, bladder and continence status. When care is needed, the nurse is required to assess, plan, implement and evaluate individualized care, which promotes independence whenever possible, ensuring sensitivity and personal dignity in all aspects of this process.
- Bowel, bladder and continence care is never basic. Knowledge and skill are required for the recognition of elimination impairment, through assessment.
- All individuals experiencing bowel, bladder or continence problems should have ease of access to continence services which offer the best advice, and equity in the quality of service provision provided.
- Nurses are best placed to play a role in the promotion of continence through health education. It is vital that nurses view continence care and continence promotion as a skilled intervention and recognize the value of this as part of the patient experience.

References

Abd-El-Mahmoud et al. (1991) Rectal suppository commonsense mode of insertion, *The Lancet* 338: 798–800.

Beauchamp, T.L. and Childress, J.F. (2001) *Principles of Biomedical Ethics*, 5th edn. London: Oxford University Press.

DoH (Department of Health) (2000) *Good Practice in Continence Services*. London: DoH.

DoH (Department of Health) (2003) *The Essence of Care: Patient-focused Benchmarking for Health Care Practitioners*. London: The Stationery Office.

Edwards, N.I. and Jones, D. (2001) The prevalence of faecal incontinence in older people living at home, *Age and Ageing*, 30: 503–7.

Ersser, J.S. Getliffe, K. Voegeli, D. and Regan, S. (2005) A critical review of the inter-relationship between skin vulnerability and urinary incontinence and related nursing intervention, *International Journal of Nursing Studies*, 42(7): 823–35.

Heins, T. and Ritchie, K. (1985) *Beating Sneaky Poo*. Canberra: Canberra Publishing and Printing Co.

Holland, K. Jenkins, J. Soloman, J. and Whittam, S. (2003) *Applying the Roper Logan Tierney Model in Practice*. Edinburgh: Churchill Livingstone.

Irwin, K. (2001) Managing adult faecal incontinence, *Journal of Community Nursing*, 15(2).

Kyle, G. (2006) Assessment and treatment of older people with constipation, *Nursing Standard*, 21(8): 41–6.

Laurent, C. (1998) Preventing infection from indwelling catheters, *Nursing Times*, 94(25): 60–6.

Mallett, J. and Dougherty, L. (2004) *The Royal Marsden Hospital Manual of Clinical Nursing Procedures*, 6th edn. Oxford: Blackwell Science.

Marieb, E. (2006) *Human Anatomy and Physiology*, 7th edn. California: Addison Wesley.

Nakayama, H. Jorgenson, H.S. Pederson, P.M. Raaschou, H.O. and Olsen, T.S. (1997) Prevalence and risk factors of incontinence after stroke: the Copenhagen Study, *Stroke*, 28: 58–62.

National Prescribing Centre (2006) MeRec Bulletin Number 3: Drug treatment of urinary incontinence in adults, 11(3), www.medicinescomplete.com/mc/, accessed 24 February 2008.

NHS Modernization Agency (2003) *Essence of Care Guidance – Patient Focused Benchmarks for Clinical Governance*, www.dh.gov.uk/Publications.

NICE (National Institute for Health and Clinical Excellence) (2003) *Infection Control: Prevention of Healthcare-associated Infection in Primary and Community Care*, www.nice.org.uk.

NICE (National Institute for Health and Clinical Excellence) (2006) *Urinary Incontinence: The Management of Urinary Incontinence in Women*, clinical guideline 40. London: NICE.

Norton, C. (1996) The causes and nursing management of constipation, *British Journal of Nursing*, 5(20): 1252–8.

Royal College of Physicians (1995) Incontinence: causes, management and provision of services, *Journal of the Royal College of Physicians*, 29(4): 272–4.

Soloman, J. (2003) Eliminating, in K. Holland, J. Jenkins, J. Soloman and S. Whittam (2003) *Applying the Roper Logan Tierney Model in Practice*. Edinburgh: Churchill Livingstone.

Steggall, M. (2007) Elimination – urine, in C. Brooker and A. Waugh (eds) *Foundations of Nursing Practice: Fundamentals of Holistic Care*. Edinburgh. Mosby.

Thompson, W.G. Longstreath, G.F. Drossman, D.A. Heaton, K.W. Irvine, E.J. and Muller-Lissner, S.A. (1999) Functional bowel disorders and functional abdominal pain, *Gut*, 45, Suppl. 2: 1143–7.

Van Dongen, E. (2001) It isn't something to yodel about, but it exists! Faeces, nurses, social relations and status within a mental hospital, *Ageing and Mental Health*, 5(3): 205–15.

Waterlow, J. (2005) *Pressure Ulcer Prevention Manual*. Taunton: Waterlow.

Waugh, A. and Grant, A. (2006) *Ross and Wilson Anatomy and Physiology in Health and Illness*, 10th edn. Edinburgh: Churchill Livingstone.

Useful web resources

Association for Continence Advice: www.aca.uk.com

British National Formulary: www.bnf.org.uk

Continence Worldwide (website of the continence promotion committee/International Continence Society): www.continenceworldwide.com

Incontact (provides support and information for people experiencing bladder and bowel problems): www.incontact.org

National Advisory Service for Parents of Children with Stoma:

National Institute for Health and Clinical Excellence (NICE): www.nice.org.uk

NHS Direct: www.nhsdirect.nhs.uk

The Continence Foundation: www.continence-foundation.org.uk

www.cancerbackup.org.uk

www.continence-foundation.org.uk/directory

www.continence-foundation.org.uk/intergrated-continence-service.php

www.patient.co.uk/showdoc/267391771

Answers

Scenario 10.2

At 10 years of age the effects of enuresis for Liam can be significant. Most children at this age start to exert some independence, attending school camps prior to the move to secondary school and staying with friends for sleepovers. The need to wear pads and pants will lead to embarrassment and the need for explanations. Furthermore, wetting in the day will make school difficult. Enuresis can lead to bullying and bullying may lead to enuresis. Physical causes such as infection and constipation must also be ruled out.

Activity 10.3

When the patient is unable to offer information initially (as Margaret in the case study), the nurse will assess and plan according to the patient's presenting symptoms. Some information can be sought from relatives.

Activity 10.4

It is important that any urine and faeces in contact with Margaret's skin is cleansed away to prevent irritation and reduce skin breakdown and potential pressure ulcers (see Chapter 11). This will also reduce Margaret's distress. Should diarrhoea be present, this could cause further damage to Margaret's skin due to the presence of chemicals which the body produces to break down food. Prolonged contact and continual wetting and drying of the skin reduce the skin's natural defence barrier and increase its vulnerability to bacteria.

Margaret's skin and perineal area should be gently cleansed with warm water and a neutral pH soap or skin cleanser and then thoroughly rinsed. The nurse should avoid rubbing during cleansing and drying to avoid friction, but should gently pat the skin dry. Emollient therapy and moisturizer can enhance the skin barrier and help to protect and restore it from damage caused by contact with urine and faeces (Ersser *et al.* 2005). During the procedure of skin cleansing to promote comfort and dignity, you would observe, note and record the condition of Margaret's skin on all of her body. A recognized risk assessment tool such as the Waterlow Score (Waterlow 2005) should be used to measure the risk of and assist in the prevention of pressure sore formation. Incontinence and a number of other factors including increasing age and immobility greatly increase Margaret's risk of skin breakdown.

Activity 10.6

You may consider asking patients of a different culture how you can best help them to meet their elimination needs. You could provide a jug by all hand basins which will enable patients to wash under running water. You could develop a resource pack for staff and students which outlines preferences for different cultural and religious groups in relation to personal aspects of care.

Activity 10.9

Your answer may include the following:

- To relieve retention of urine.
- To empty the bladder prior to surgery or during labour.
- To instil bladder washout solutions for irrigation, or cytotoxic drugs as direct therapies.
- To facilitate bladder healing following bladder surgery.
- To assist with urodynamic investigations.
- To relieve the build-up of pressure within the kidneys that can occur during nephritis.

Activity 10.11

Your answer could include the following:

- Ensure Alex drinks a minimum of six to eight glasses of water a day.
- Timed, regular visits to the toilet may help Alex to pass urine. Only visiting the toilet when his bladder has become uncomfortable can lead to infection.
- Encourage general exercise.
- Include fibre in his diet which will help maintain bowel movements.
- Ensure that Alex does not have or develop constipation as this will compound any urinary incontinence difficulties.
- Alex has a lot of information to digest and this information should be given in a way that allows him to ask questions and test his own understanding along with that of any person providing care.
- Positive praise and reward given in a non-condescending manner when Alex demonstrates some ability to contribute to or manage his own care will help Alex feel in control.

Activity 10.12

1 Tom will use simple words which we are all familiar with from childhood. 'Wee', 'poo', 'number 1', 'number 2'. Other terminology may be used at home among the family. It is helpful to ask his mum, dad or carer about this.

2 You need to explain the importance to Tom of being clean and dry to prevent infection, stop the development of pressure ulcers and to promote a feeling of comfort. You should explain to Tom that as soon as he is able you will encourage him to wash and wipe again for himself. It's also important to tell Tom that at all times his privacy and dignity will be promoted. This should be done in language Tom will understand. You could ask who Tom would most feel comfortable with providing this care.

3 Encourage Tom to drink plenty of water and fruit juice and to choose lots of fruit and vegetables from his menu. Encourage him to move about in bed and do some simple exercises and make sure he requests the bedpan as soon as he feels the need to eliminate and respond quickly to his request.

Activity 10.14

1 Analgesics, antibiotics, diuretics, laxatives, iron.

2 The answer is provided in Activity 10.15.

Scenario 10.3

1 You may consider obtaining a specimen of urine and visually observe the colour for cloudiness, debris or blood. It is important to smell the urine as dark-coloured, strong-smelling urine may indicate dehydration and/or infection. A routine urinalysis should be done and the specimen of urine sent for culture and sensitivity to identify any infection present and the antibiotic to be prescribed to treat it.

Both dehydration and infection can lead to confusion. You should note that a confused patient can quickly become dehydrated if not taking in enough fluid. You will need to commence an input and output/ fluid recording sheet and ensure that it is kept up to date at all times.

A blood sample would be taken from Joan by an appropriately trained person, to check her urea and electrolyte balance and also her blood sugar. If Joan's urea and electrolyte balance is disrupted due to dehydration, this may be the cause of her mild confusion, as may a low blood sugar.

General observation of Joan may also indicate dehydration if pallor, lethargy, dry skin, foetid breath and sunken eyes are noted.

Joan should have her temperature recorded to check for pyrexia which again may indicate infection.

2 Joan's agitation may be that having had a fall, she has lost confidence in her mobility. This is often compounded when in a strange environment such as the hospital setting. Becoming dependent on others for assistance to the toilet can be frustrating and embarrassing for patients. It may be that Joan holds on for so long in order to delay 'bothering' the nurses that when she does eventually ask she then experiences overflow incontinence before the nurse responds.

Moving Joan to a bed closer to the toilet facilities and ensuring she has had a falls assessment and input from the physiotherapist may alleviate a lot of stress and give her back some independence with the function of elimination.

You should ensure that Joan is offered toilet facilities regularly. This is particularly advisable before meals, activity and settling for the night. This promotes patient comfort for Joan and reduces her anxiety about requesting assistance. Should Joan request the toilet in between these times you must respond promptly, reducing the risk of an episode of incontinence due to delay and an inability to hold on. Joan's medication should also be reviewed.

11

Pressure ulcers

Melanie Stephens and Helen Iggulden

Chapter Contents

Learning objectives

The aim of this chapter is to discuss the role of the nurse and student nurse in preventing the development of pressure ulcers and in treating pressure ulcers that have developed. Throughout the chapter we will be referring to the accompanying Media Tool DVD. Please watch the video clips as directed as these will reinforce your learning and expand upon the information given in this book. After reading this chapter and interacting with the Media Tool DVD you will be able to:

- Outline the structure of the skin, how a pressure ulcer can develop and the stages of healing that it goes through.
- Carry out a risk assessment under supervision using a recognized screening tool.
- Carry out assessment and grading of a pressure ulcer under supervision using a recognized assessment tool.
- Collaborate with interdisciplinary colleagues in planning and implementing care.
- Involve patients and their families in prevention and treatment planning.
- Identify a range of interventions to prevent and treat pressure ulcers by repositioning patients, selecting and using redistributing support surfaces.
- Carry out, under supervision, an aseptic technique.
- Contribute to the evaluation of care.

Introduction

A pressure ulcer (this is the term that will be mainly used throughout this chapter, but it is sometimes referred to as a pressure sore, bed sore or decubitus ulcer) is damage to a person's skin and underlying tissue caused by pressure together with, or independently from, other factors such as shearing, friction and moisture, physical and psychological well-being, and the care environment (Bick and Stephens 2003). The extent of this damage can range from persistent *erythema* to *necrotic ulceration* involving muscle, tendon and bone (Mallett and Dougherty 2004).

Each year, approximately 412,000 adults will develop a new pressure ulcer in the UK resulting in NHS expenditure of around £1.4 billion (Bennet *et al.* 2004). Pressure ulcers in children are much less common, but they do occur (Willock and Maylor 2004). Infants and children with very acute, chronic or neurological problems or those wearing casts or splints, are particularly vulnerable.

Treating pressure ulcers is expensive. The patient's quality of life and independence are affected and it is also costly to the organization, mostly in relation to nursing time. Not all pressure damage can be avoided, but the incidence can be reduced so the focus of attention should be on the prevention or management of initial tissue damage, the prevention of progression

of an ulcer to a more severe grade and the prevention of infection (Bennett *et al.* 2004; NICE 2005).

Skin integrity and blood flow

It is useful at this point to revise the functions of the skin and these can be seen in Box 11.1.

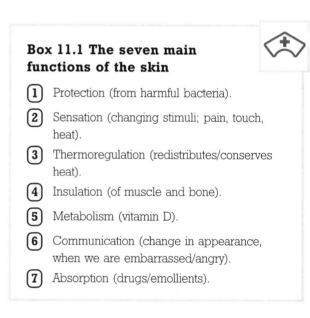

Box 11.1 The seven main functions of the skin

1. Protection (from harmful bacteria).
2. Sensation (changing stimuli; pain, touch, heat).
3. Thermoregulation (redistributes/conserves heat).
4. Insulation (of muscle and bone).
5. Metabolism (vitamin D).
6. Communication (change in appearance, when we are embarrassed/angry).
7. Absorption (drugs/emollients).

A healthy blood supply is essential to the survival of the skin and the blood vessels are the most important structures to consider in relation to a person's susceptibility to developing a pressure ulcer.

Before reading any further it is useful for you to gain some background anatomy and physiology to help you to understand how pressure ulcers can develop, how they are classified and how they heal. Activity 11.1 will help you to do this.

Activity 11.1

Go to the Media Tool DVD, select **Chapter Resources**, then **Pressure Ulcers** and work through Activity 11.1 on the anatomy and physiology of the skin. Then test yourself by completing the accompanying questions before reading any further.

It is also useful to remember that the *capillaries* of the skin are only 8 micrometers in diameter and one cell thick. These allow for the passage of:

- oxygen;
- nutrients;
- carbon dioxide;
- waste products.

If the *arterial blood pressure* drops, there is not enough force to keep these capillaries open, blood flow to the skin is thus obstructed and over time this causes a pressure ulcer to develop. Those who are ill have a much lower *capillary closing pressure* and are therefore more at risk of developing a pressure ulcer.

Activity 11.2

Do you know how to assess a patient's *capillary refill*? Go to the Media Tool DVD, select **Case Studies**, **Adult Health (Margaret)**, then **Nurse checks Margaret's skin** and watch the clip. Did you notice how quickly the skin refilled with blood after the nurse had pressed it? The normal capillary refill time is two seconds.

When blood flow is stopped by external pressure, the skin pales and *blanching* occurs. This is a normal body response. Generally, removal of the pressure

presents as a red flush to the skin and is called erythema, caused by an increased temporary blood flow to the area which was previously *ischaemic*. Normal skin colour is restored quite soon after.

However, if external pressure is prolonged or the circulation is already compromised, local tissue will be damaged and begin to die. In this situation, erythema will also be seen, but the cause is blood leaking from damaged capillaries. Blanching does not occur in this instance when one applies light finger pressure.

Box 11.2 Exposure pressure and tissue damage

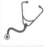

The relationship between exposure to pressure and tissue damage is reliant on two constituents:

- intensity of pressure (the degree of pressure);
- duration of pressure (length of exposure to pressure).

Activity 11.3

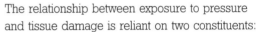

You notice a slightly reddened area, or erythema, on a patient's sacrum. You press it lightly with your finger and the redness does not temporarily disappear. Would this be blanching or non-blanching erythema and would it indicate the need for further assessment? Check your answer with that at the end of the chapter.

Skin pigmentation

Skin pigmentation varies from light ivory, through various shades of brown, to deep black, yellow, olive, light pink and dark ruddy pink or red. Apart from colour change resulting from local damage to the skin such as inflammation, bruising and dead cells, overall differences in skin colour and tone between people's skin are due to four main factors (Bethell 2005):

- carotene pigments in the subcutaneous fat;
- the amount of oxygen circulating in the body;
- the presence of other pigments such as bile;
- the amount of melanin present in the epidermis.

Racial differences in skin tone and colour are due to the amount of *melanin* present in the *epidermis*. In darkly pigmented skin erythema does not appear as redness and it is difficult to detect the rate of capillary refill as only the melanin will be visible (Matas *et al.* 2001). However, when pressure is relieved, heat radiates from the area for 15–30 minutes. To check dark skin for pressure damage, turn your patient over, then, after placing one hand over the 'at risk' areas and another area of skin not at risk, close your eyes and feel for the differences in temperature.

How a pressure ulcer develops

The European Pressure Ulcer Advisory Panel's (1998) definition of a pressure ulcer is: 'an area of localised damage to the skin and underlying tissue caused by pressure, shear, friction and/or a combination of these'. Pressure ulcers can develop from four main 'forces':

1. Tissue interface pressure.
2. Friction forces.
3. Shear forces.
4. Moisture.

Box 11.3 describes what each 'force' is.

Other factors affecting vulnerability

Several other factors, in addition to the pressure, shear, friction and moisture forces mentioned above, contribute to the development of a pressure ulcer. These are separated into *extrinsic* and *intrinsic* factors and are listed in Table 11.1.

The extrinsic factors identify the mechanical forces that deprive the skin and underlying tissue of oxygen by causing traumatic weakening of the dermis and epidermis. Figure 11.1 shows how these forces act in a sitting position while in bed.

The intrinsic factors make a person more vulnerable to pressure damage because of a reduced delivery of oxygen and nutrients to the cells of the dermis and epidermis. A poor blood supply from reduced blood circulation caused by shock, cardiac or vascular disease and reduced mobility all render the skin and supporting structures weaker and more vulnerable to pressure damage.

> **Activity 11.4**
>
>
>
> Go to the Media Tool DVD, select **Case Studies**, **Adult Health (Margaret)**, **Margaret in bed** and then **Child Health (Tom)**, **Introduction to Tom**. List which extrinsic and intrinsic factors you think would contribute to their individual risks of developing a pressure ulcer. Check your list with the answers given at the end of the chapter.

Box 11.3 The four main forces in developing pressure ulcers

1. *Tissue interface pressure* is the pressure on the skin and its underlying structures caused by their compression between bone and the surfaces with which the skin is in contact. The damage here, which occurs deep in the tissues, may not be visible until one to two weeks after the initial injury.

2. *Friction force* occurs when two surfaces rub together. The commonest cause of friction is when a patient is dragged, rather than lifted, off and up the bed. The top layer of skin is scraped off, causing shallow dermal ulcers or blisters.

3. *Shear forces* can disrupt tissue and damage blood vessels. It occurs when tissues are contorted in opposite directions, resulting in angulation or disruption of the capillary blood vessels. Tissue damage from shear forces can be prevented by good positioning.

4. *Moisture* causes more damage to the skin than pressure, shear and friction, due to the stripping of the skin by products of excretion and/or adherence of the skin to the damp surface – for example, bedding, clothing and continence aids.

Table 11.1 Factors contributing to the development of a pressure ulcer

Extrinsic	Intrinsic
Pressure	Cardiovascular status and vascular disease
Shear	Respiratory status
Friction	Reduced mobility
Moisture	Sensory impairment
Medication	Acute illness
Skin irritants	Level of consciousness
	Extremes of age
	Malnutrition and dehydration
	Severe chronic or terminal illness
	Medication

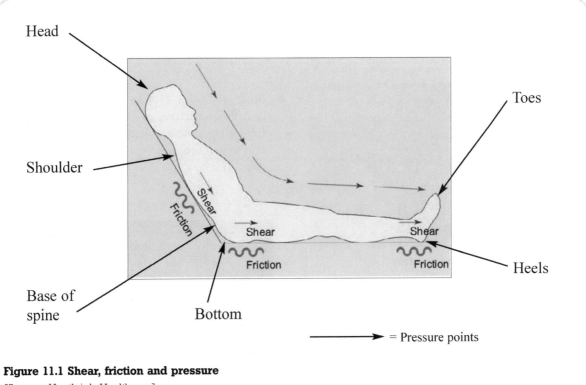

Figure 11.1 Shear, friction and pressure
[Source: Huntleigh Healthcare]

Classification

Wounds

In order to facilitate your understanding of pressure ulcers you need to know that all wounds have a basic classification as follows:

● *superficial wounds* involve the top layer of skin only – the epidermis;
● *partial thickness wounds* involve the top and second layers – the epidermis and the dermis;
● *full thickness wounds* extend into the subcutaneous layer or deeper and may damage muscle, bone and tendons.

Pressure ulcers

Pressure ulcers have a grading system that is more detailed than the general classification of wounds detailed above.

● *Grade 1* (Figure 11.2) is a non-blanchable erythema of intact skin. In this case you will note the discoloration of the skin, and warmth; oedema, *induration* or hardness may also be used as indicators, particularly on individuals with darker skin.

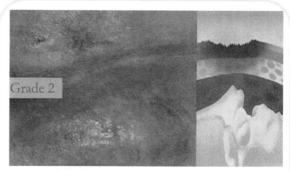

Figure 11.3 Grade 2 pressure ulcer
[Source: Huntleigh Healthcare]

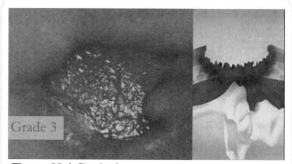

Figure 11.4 Grade 3 pressure ulcer
[Source: Huntleigh Healthcare]

● *Grade 4* (Figure 11.5) involves extensive destruction, tissue necrosis or damage to muscle, bone or supporting structures with or without full thickness skin loss (European Pressure Ulcer Advisory Panel 1998: 1).

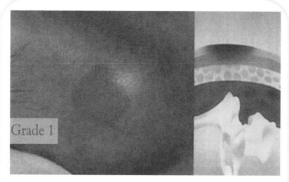

Figure 11.2 Grade 1 pressure ulcer
[Source: Huntleigh Healthcare]

● *Grade 2* (Figure 11.3) involves partial thickness skin loss relating to the epidermis, dermis or both. The ulcer is superficial and presents clinically as an abrasion or blister.
● *Grade 3* (Figure 11.4) is a full thickness skin loss involving damage to or necrosis of subcutaneous tissue that may extend down to, but not through, underlying fascia.

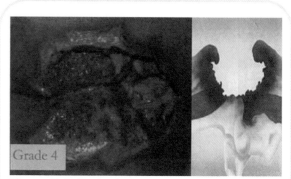

Figure 11.5 Grade 4 pressure ulcer
[Source: Huntleigh Healthcare]

Prevention

Screening and assessment

All patients must have a risk assessment of their susceptibility to develop pressure ulcers. This should involve both formal and informal means and be carried out within six hours of admission to a hospital, or on a first visit in the community. The initial assessment should be followed up by reassessment when the patient's condition or circumstances change, for example, pre-operatively, intra-operatively and post-operatively (NICE 2005).

Several tools are available that highlight the factors that predispose a patient to develop a pressure ulcer. Other tools help to measure and stage an ulcer that has already developed, so that the extent of damage can be assessed and monitored and an intervention and treatment plan developed. It will be useful to review two assessment scales that you might see in practice for assessing patients' risk of developing pressure ulcers.

The most common risk assessment scales are Waterlow (1988, 2005) and Braden (cited in Bergstrom *et al.* 1987). The NICE (2005) guidelines indicate that these tools are useful as an *aide-mémoire*, and that nurses should not rely on them alone. To ensure validity, their use is most effective alongside clinical judgement, a full skin assessment and patient history.

Activity 11.5

The assessment scales are only routinely used in acute general hospitals and some nursing homes. How would you identify risk in care settings where there are no clear guidelines or policies for using these? Go to the end of the chapter and compare your answer to the one given.

The Waterlow Risk Assessment Tool

The Waterlow Risk Assessment Tool was developed following a comprehensive review of research on pressure ulcers as an *aide-mémoire* for nurses working within medicine and surgical departments. The aim was to provide guidelines on preventing pressure ulcers by the selection of the correct pressure-reducing/relieving product as well as the management of pressure ulcers.

There are three degrees of risk identified, which relate to the score calculated:

1 At risk.

2 High risk.

3 Very high risk.

Box 11.4 Waterlow areas of risk

- *Build/weight:* pressure over susceptible areas is increased when a patient is underweight and overweight, as the skin is either less insulated or too insulated and lacks a good blood supply.
- *Continence:* incontinence increases the risk of tissue damage from maceration, imbalance in skin pH and acid from the faeces causing excoriation (burns).
- *Skin type:* skin types can vary from tissue-paper skin (found in the elderly and those on long-term steroidal therapy), very dry skin (that can crack and be infected), to oedematous skin and sweating skin from a high temperature, plastic sheets or a leaking wound.
- *Mobility:* when a patient is mobile and active, they reduce the risk of damage enormously. Restless, fidgety patients increase the risk of shear and friction. Patients who are nursed either in bed and/or a wheelchair are at risk from both intrinsic and extrinsic factors.
- *Sex/age:* due to anatomical differences women are more likely to develop pressure ulcers than men.
- *Appetite:* nutrition is an important factor. Specific nutrients, including some amino acids, vitamins and minerals, are vital in skin repair and healing. It is important to record the nutritional intake of patients at risk of pressure ulcer damage.
- *Special risk:* this segment refers to tissue malnutrition, neurological deficit, surgery/trauma and specific medication (see Box 11.5).

Assessing the level of risk in this way means that you can plan effective, preventative measures and obtain any specialist equipment that you might need. The scoring system of the Waterlow Tool includes six key areas of risk and one special area, as shown in Box 11.4. The special risk section has several terms which you may not be familiar with. They are explained in Box 11.5.

Activity 11.6

What medications do you think might make a person more susceptible to developing pressure damage? Check your answer with that at the end of the chapter.

Activity 11.7

Recalling what you have learned so far what would an early sign of pressure damage be? Check your answer with that at the end of the chapter.

Box 11.5 Areas of special risk

- *Terminal cachexia* is the term used to describe the combination in the later stages of some cancers of: loss of appetite; progressive weight loss; weakness; fatigue; malaise; and loss of skeletal muscle and fat.
- *Peripheral vascular disease* is a hardening or narrowing of the arteries in the legs, which means that the muscles and tissues receive a poor blood supply and hence a poor supply of nutrients and oxygen.
- *Anaemia* is a condition in which the blood has a reduced capacity to carry oxygen to deliver to the cells. This interferes with cell metabolism and tissue viability and can render cells more susceptible to damage from pressure, shear and friction.

Metabolic disorders

- *Diabetes* affects the ability of the body to absorb sugar into the cells, thus interfering with cell nutrition. Patients with long-standing poorly-controlled diabetes can develop peripheral vascular disease and a loss of sensation in the lower legs and feet.

Neurological disorders

- *Multiple sclerosis* is a disease of the nervous system which affects balance, skilled movements and sensation.
- *Cerebrovascular accident* – a blood clot or haemorrhage that damages brain tissue can result in paralysis or weakness down one side of the body, loss of sensation in that part of the body, problems understanding speech, problems producing speech and problems swallowing.
- *Motor/sensory* refers in general to any impairment of the patient's motor or sensory function.
- *Paraplegia* refers specifically to the condition of being paralysed from the waist down.

A neurological disease can modify a person's sensation and awareness of pain and pressure. It can also alter the way a person's weight is distributed over a surface, and the way a person balances and moves.

Surgery/trauma

- Patients who do not have a neurological disease will suffer a temporary loss of sensation and movement when under anaesthesia or having pain relief through a spinal infusion – an epidural.
- Any trauma that affects movement such as a fracture will render a person more vulnerable to developing a pressure ulcer.

Medications

- There are many drugs that have varying effects on the skin.

Medscape® www.medscape.com				
Starkid Skin Scale				
	1	**2**	**3**	**4**
Mobility/ Activity	Confined to bed, minimal spontaneous changes in position	Cannot weight bear but uses chair, occasional spontaneous changes in position	OOB with assistance, frequent spontaneous changes in position. OR if baby, not held by parents more than brief periods	Walks frequently, changes position without assistance OR too young to ambulate but held by parents
Sensory Perception- Ability to feel and respond to pressure related pain	Unresponsive to pain due to injury or continuous sedation OR neuromuscular blockade	Decreased LOC but responds to painful stimuli, communicates by moaning or restlessness OR sensory impairment over > half of body	Responds to commands, can't communicate need to be turned (age appropriate) OR sensory impairment in 1-2 extremities	Age appropriate response to commands, no sensory deficits, able to feel and communicate pain (crying baby)
Moisture Diapers must be age appropriate	Dampness from diaphoresis, drainage, urine or feces noted every time patient moved	Linen changed every 8 hours for dampness OR diaper changes q2 for diarrhea	Linen changed every 12 hours OR diaper changes for diarrhea	Routine diaper changes. Linen change once a day
Friction-Shear From skin against bed surface or cast/ orthotic device. Includes patient and nurse ability to lift	Constant thrashing and friction. Agitated	Unable to lift to reposition (nurse or patient) sliding against sheets unavoidable (ability or size) Slides down frequently	Able to lift but skin slides some Occasional sliding down in bed but maintains position most of time	Easy to lift to change position (baby), OR moves independently, maintains good position
Nutrition	NPO for ≥ 5 days OR rarely eats half of food offered No supplements	TPN or Tube Feedings with inadequate calories even with supplements OR usually eats half of food offered	TPN, Tube feeds of adequate calories OR eats over half of food offered	Eats great
Tissue Perfusion and Oxygenation (use data available)	Hypotensive (MAP < 50, <40 in newborn) does not physiologically tolerate position changes	Normotensive but O_2 sat <92% or < 10 below expected norm CFT > 2 seconds Hgb < 10	Normotensive, O_2 sat <92% or <10 below expected norm, CFT ≤ 2 seconds Hgb < 10	Normotensive, O_2 Sat > 94% or within expected norm, CFT ≤ 2 seconds Hgb normal
				Source: Pediatr Nurs © 2005 Jannetti Publications, Inc.

Figure 11.6 The Braden Scale

The Braden Scale

The Braden Scale is a summated rating scale comprising the six sub-scales identified below and is shown in Figure 11.6.

1. *Sensory perception:* the patient's ability to move position in response to discomfort on their skin from pressure.

2. *Mobility:* the ability to move and change position.

3. *Activity:* the amount and degree of physical activity.

4. *Moisture:* the amount of moisture the skin is exposed to.

5. *Nutrition:* the usual intake of food and the pattern of eating and drinking.

6. *Friction and shear:* the risk from these external forces.

Each sub-scale is scored from 1 to 4, except friction and shear which is scored from 1 to 3, with total possible points ranging from 6 to 23 (Bergstrom and Braden 2002). The lower the score, the greater the risk of pressure ulcer. Generally, a cut-off score is used to classify a patient as 'at risk' or 'not at risk'. The Braden Scale is commonly used in adults and since its adaptation in paediatric units it is important to note that it is the only risk assessment score that has been thoroughly researched for its validity and reliability (Brown 2004).

During any skin assessment it is vital to observe vulnerable sites – for example, any bony prominences such as the sacrum, heels, hips, ankles and elbows to identify early signs of pressure damage.

Repositioning patients

Regular turning reduces the incidence of pressure ulcers (Bonomini 2003). Many practitioners use two-hourly turning regimes, which are recorded on a turning chart (see Figure 11.7.) Although there is no scientific agreement about the time a given amount of pressure can be exerted before injury occurs (Bonomini 2003), the time before turning should not exceed four hours.

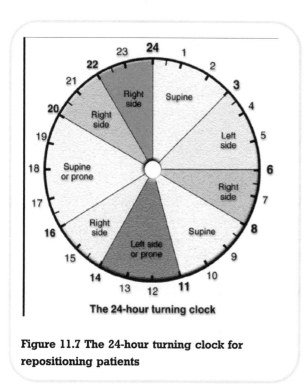

The 24-hour turning clock

Figure 11.7 The 24-hour turning clock for repositioning patients

Turning regimes should be based upon level of risk, skin tolerance tests, the patient's condition, their mental and physical state, the type of support surface and equipment used and general treatment considerations. The approach should be holistic and take into account the patient's other activities such as mealtimes, treatment sessions and personal hygiene. Remember that turning patients is not just for pressure relief, but also a time for you to carry out *therapeutic touch, passive and active exercises* and oral hygiene. All these activities aid *peristalsis*, chest drainage and – most importantly – *social interaction*.

Prevention of injury during moving and handling

A good moving and handling technique ensures that patients are not injured when repositioned or transferred. There are four key factors that can cause a patient harm during repositioning or transfer:

1. *Friction*, particularly between the skin and transfer surface.

2. *Joint damage*, caused by stressing weak joints.

3. *Resistance* from the client, perhaps due to a lack of communication or understanding.

4. *Falls* due to a lack of knowledge of the technique, or the carer exceeding their individual capability during the manoeuvre.

It is important to always refer to local policy for moving and handling.

Moving and handling assessment

It is a legal requirement that every patient has a *risk assessment* regarding their moving and handling requirements. The moving and handling assessment should give comprehensive information about the patient's needs, recommendations about how they should be handled and the best equipment to use, in conjunction with the pressure ulcer risk assessment. Remember too that physiotherapists and occupational therapists can be called upon for advice on correct patient positioning.

Activity 11.8

Go to the Media Tool DVD, select **Case Studies, Child Health (Tom)**. View the case study and answer the following questions.

1. How would you ensure that Tom does not develop an ulcer?

2. Now go to the Margaret case study and watch the video clip **Adult Health (Margaret) Margaret in bed**. What assessments and interventions would you need to make to ensure Margaret does not develop a pressure ulcer?

Compare your answers with those at the end of the chapter.

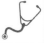

Repositioning a patient in a chair

A chair should be comfortable, support the patient and their posture and allow the patient to stand up and sit down easily.

- The chair height should allow the patient's hips, knees and ankles to be at 90 degrees.
- The depth should support the patient's thighs and allow their bottom to reach the back of the chair leaving a gap of 5 to 8cm between the front of the chair and the back of the knees.
- The chair should be roomy enough to allow the patient to move about a little to relieve pressure, with arm rests to aid sitting and standing.
- It must be firm, but comfortable, and cushions should be used if a patient is at risk of pressure ulcer formation.
- The back should be high enough to support the patient and have lumbar curve to support the back.
- Wheelchairs should be chosen after a full assessment and recommendation for suitability by the occupational therapist.

When sitting a patient in a chair, it is important to ensure:

- the patient's bottom is as far back as possible in the seat;
- where possible, the thigh should be supported along its full length;
- the hips, knees and ankles should be at 90 degrees;
- the lumbar spine should be supported as shown in Figure 11.8;
- the supporting surface is equivalent to the supporting surface when the patient is in bed.

Remember, if you are using leg rests:

- the total height including the pillow should be level with the seat;
- the heel should clear the leg rest.

Types of mattresses and support surfaces

Another key aspect of preventing pressure ulcers from developing is the type of redistributing surfaces on which patients lie or sit. All equipment used for the prevention and treatment of pressure ulcers needs to

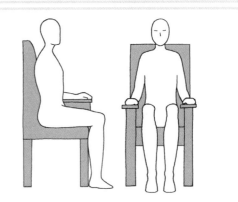

Figure 11.8 How to position a patient in a chair
[Source: Huntleigh Healthcare]

Activity 11.9

Look at Figure 11.9. Why is this position wrong and which force might cause injury? Check your answer with that at the end of the chapter.

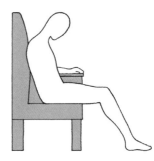

Figure 11.9 How not to position a patient in a chair
[Source: Huntleigh Healthcare]

be suitable to each patient's needs, well maintained in a safe reliable condition and readily available. An ideal support system will:

- distribute pressure evenly;
- provide frequent relief of or low pressure;
- conform to body weight;
- minimize shear and friction;
- provide a well-maintained, comfortable surface that does not restrict movement;
- maintain skin at an optimum temperature;
- be acceptable to the patient;
- not interfere with care;
- be easily operated and allow for height adjustments;

- have a tilt facility, clearance for hoists and be mobile with effective brakes.

Each hospital will have varying access to support surfaces and equipment that can be ordered via in-house or private contract agreements. Each hospital will have a standard foam mattress which will take into consideration its effectiveness, durability, suitability and type of cover. Special products designed to prevent or cure pressure ulcers are generally more effective than standard mattresses (Cullum *et al.* 2004).

You need to clean and maintain mattresses by washing them with hot water and a neutralizing detergent, and drying them thoroughly, inspecting them for signs of wear and tear indicating the need for replacement. These include:

- loss of waterproofing presenting an infection hazard;
- tears and worn areas allowing moisture and dirt to penetrate to the foam, again causing an infection hazard;
- loss of stretch in the cover causing high interface pressures;
- bottoming out, significantly increasing the risk of pressure ulcer formation;
- condition of foam and cover – look for stains, odour, moisture, crumbling and mildew formation.

Box 11.6 Types of mattresses and overlays

- Standard foam
- Fibre filled
- Air filled
- Gel filled
- Fluid filled
- Alternative foam

High-tech devices

- Alternating pressure devices
- Air fluidized devices
- Low air loss devices
- Turning beds/frames
- Low air loss mattresses

There are several different types of mattress or overlay that provide a conforming support surface that distributes the body weight over a large surface area, as detailed in Box 11.6.

Activity 11.10

For your own information purposes, go to the Media Tool DVD, select **Chapter Resources**, then **Pressure Ulcers** and work through Activity 11.10, and read through the descriptions of how these devices are used and see what they look like.

Choosing a redistributing surface

Any patient identified at risk of pressure ulcer damage should be placed on an appropriate mattress in accordance with a holistic assessment and local Trust policy, not just the risk assessment scale alone. Factors to consider when choosing an appropriate piece of equipment will include: identified levels of risk; skin assessment; comfort; general health state; lifestyle and abilities; critical care needs; and acceptability of the proposed pressure-relieving equipment to the patient and/or carer. Low technology support surfaces can reduce the incidence of pressure ulcers better than standard hospital mattresses and some evidence supports the effectiveness of air fluidized and low air loss devices (Bergstrom 2000).

The RCN (2001) advocate the use of alternating systems for those at very high risk and those at risk should not be put on standard hospital foam mattresses. This practice should be reflected when using trolleys, theatre and X-ray tables, as patients are at higher risk due to immobility and hard surfaces.

Should you reposition?

Yes, repositioning should still be carried out for all patients even if nursed on pressure redistributing surfaces. Repositioning not only reduces prolonged pressure on bony prominences, but as previously mentioned also aids peristalsis, chest drainage, allows for social interaction, the building of therapeutic relationships and provides an opportunity to assess personal and oral hygiene needs, and carry out active and passive exercises.

Patients who are at risk and have reduced mobility should not sit in a chair for long periods. Sitting in a chair should be incorporated into the repositioning schedule and linked to mealtimes, interprofessional team activities or visiting. Sheepskins, water-filled gloves and doughnut-type devices should no longer be used (NICE 2005) as they have been shown to be ineffective and sometimes harmful. A good repositioning regime and the correct choice of support surfaces are more effective.

Activity 11.11

Go to the Media Tool DVD, select **Case Studies**, **Adult Health (Margaret)**, **Margaret and her husband choose from the menu**, and watch the clip showing Margaret's food arriving, then Margaret having her lunch sitting in her chair. What are the important points to consider in relation to the prevention of pressure ulcer formation while she is having lunch?

Check your answer with that given at the end of the chapter.

Availability of resources and equipment

When patients are identified as being 'at risk', it is imperative to also assess their need for other resources such as moving and handling equipment, dressings, walking aids, electric beds, frames and seating. This should be carried out in conjunction with other members of the interprofessional team and the patients who are using the equipment should be involved in the decision-making and educated in the correct use of the equipment. With every piece of equipment used, it is imperative that patients and their significant others/carers are assessed on their level of knowledge and then, if appropriate, taught how to use the equipment or told who to contact for help. By informing, involving and educating patients, you are promoting independence; they become experts in their condition and can often educate staff on the care they require.

Within the hospital or community setting there are

several different ways of accessing equipment and you should check your local policy. Box 11.7 details possible sources to access equipment for pressure ulcer prevention.

Box 11.7 Sources for equipment

- *Ward owned* – the ward or department owns equipment and stores it within the clinical area.
- *Loan stores* – access is via a central store. A qualified nurse or healthcare professional would contact them and discuss the patient's particular needs. In turn they would send out within a set time-frame (usually 24 hours) the necessary equipment to aid pressure ulcer management, moving and handling.
- *Contracts with companies* – who then hire and supply equipment on a needs basis.

The equipment available can vary from static and dynamic mattresses to seat cushions, specially adapted chairs, leg rests and electric bed frames, to everything you might need for a patient (IV stands, catheter stands, weighing scales, commodes, etc). Access may be through designated portering staff, administrative staff, or physiotherapy or occupational therapy departments.

Cleaning equipment

Infection control policies are in place within every clinical area and their relevance to equipment cleaning is again dependent on each clinical environment. You must check your local policies in respect of this. However, what is agreed is that each piece of equipment should be decontaminated before the next patient uses it. Decontamination processes vary due to the bacteria that the piece of equipment (mattress, bed, chair, cushion, cot side, moving and handling aids) has come into contact with. Cleaning could be with hot water and detergent or hypochlorite solution, or equipment may be sent for laundering.

If the mattress and/or bed frame is electric, then often the electro-biomechanical engineering department or company will service the pump to British Standard requirements. Again this will depend on Trust policy but often occurs after every single patient use.

If the equipment becomes damaged or stops working, then it must be removed from the patient immediately. Reporting to the appropriate person will depend on each clinical area's policy but the device will be cleaned down, serviced and repaired if appropriate.

Most wards own a static system for every single bed frame, and these should be cleaned after every single patient use or soiling following Trust policy, and turned as per Trust requirements (if a turning mattress).

Every clinical department should have an audit system in place. Every 12 months all static systems should be audited for integrity of the cover, core mattress and signs of staining and bottoming out. These results are recorded and any mattresses identified as problematic will be replaced. Again, you will need to ask a trained member of staff for help, or refer to your local policy for guidance.

Wound assessment

If screening and assessment reveals that a patient has already developed a pressure ulcer you, under guidance, or a qualified member of staff, need to carry out a full and regular wound assessment to help healing and prevent recurrence. The assessment should identify the cause of the wound and, if possible, any underlying pathophysiology, and is essential in planning care and recommending interventions that are effective.

EXAMPLE WOUND ASSESSMENT TOOL (Please circle the appropriate description)	
Type of wound Acute Chronic	
Location	
Date	
Duration	
Sketch the **shape of the wound** and its dimensions (Length x breadth x depth) **Type of tissue on the wound bed** : Granulation Epithelialisation Slough Necrotic Infection	Comments
Type of exudate Clear Blood Purulent Other (state) **Amount:** None Minimal Moderate Heavy **Odour** None Some Offensive **Wound margin** Healthy Macerated Overgranulation Oedema **State colour if different from wound bed**	
Surrounding skin Healthy Flaky Dry Eczema Erythema	

Pain
    None at wound site   Continuous   At dressing change
 	
 Infection
 Signs of infection present Yes/No
 Swab taken Yes/No
 	
 Other comments
  Grade :	

Signature	

Figure 11.10 Sample wound assessment chart

A wound assessment chart is a useful tool which allows a structured approach to assessment and documentation. There are many types of wound assessment charts, but all should include the factors shown in Figure 11.10 (Wound Management Steering Group 2006).

Type of wound

Wounds can be classed as acute or chronic. An acute wound is one caused by trauma, including surgical incisions, that heals without complication in the normally expected time frame. Chronic wounds do not heal in the anticipated time frame.

Location

It is good practice and will be expected that you, under guidance, should always record where on the body a wound is, as the next nurse may not realize which wound it is you are documenting in the care plan.

Shape and dimensions

Tracing the outline of a wound with a clear plastic sheet using an indelible ink marker is one of the simplest methods of measuring a wound. If appropriate, a qualified nurse should use an indelible marker and cling film to protect the plastic sheet from contamination and discard it before attaching the tracing to the patient's notes.

Photography

The use of a photograph with an accurate wound assessment 'speaks a thousand words'. The medical illustration departments in hospitals will, with the patient's permission, produce the best quality photographs.

Volume

When the wound is large, or has a deep cavity, measurement does not always necessarily reflect the healing from the depth of the wound. There is not yet a single system that will measure the volume of a wound accurately but Box 11.8 shows some of the methods (Dealey 2005).

Box 11.8 Measuring the volume of a wound

- Using two sterile probes. One probe is inserted into the deepest part of the wound perpendicular to the wound surface and the other is placed across the wound surface. The maximum depth is then measured.
- Using an alginate to make an impression. Care is needed not to overfill or underfill the wound.
- Using a disposable ruler to measure the maximum length, width and depth.
- Occluding the wound with an occlusive film, then using a syringe and needle fill the cavity with sterile saline; ensure the wound does not have a sinus or fistula and calculate the volume from how much saline is needed to fill the wound.

Type of tissue on the wound bed

The appearance of the wound bed indicates the stage of healing that the wound is at and whether it is infected. Within the documentation it needs to be indicated what type of tissue is at the wound bed and its colour as a percentage. Open wounds healing by *secondary intention* have the varying colours and indicate the subsequent type of tissue – see Table 11.2.

Table 11.2 Different types of tissue

Colour	Significance
Pale pink	Epithelial tissue
Pink/red	Healthy granulation tissue
Dusky pink	Infected or unhealthy granulation tissue
Yellow	Sloughy, dead devitalized tissue, can also be bone or tendon
Green	Sloughy, dead devitalized tissue that is heavily contaminated or infected
Black/dark brown/ blackish green	Necrotic dead, devitalized tissue

Some wounds have more than one category and present as mixed, therefore the amount and percentage of each should be clearly documented.

Type and amount of exudate

It should be clear in the documentation how many times the wound has been re-dressed and the colour of the exudate (clear, green, yellow, blood-stained, red) should be recorded and how much there is (none, low, medium, high).

Odour

If the wound gives off an offensive odour, this should be documented in the assessment (it may be an indicator of a wound infection).

Margin and surrounding tissue

Related problems can be identified by the wound margin and surrounding tissue including:

- trauma to the skin from frequent adhesive dressing removal;
- inappropriate dressing choice;
- allergy to the tape or dressing, which manifests in redness or blistering;
- dryness and flakiness of the skin, when bandages are applied in conjunction with a dressing;
- excoriation or maceration when exudate has not been properly managed or the patient suffers from incontinence or excess sweating;
- not noticing clinical signs of infection – for example, redness, heat, inflammation, swelling, pain, bleeding of granulation tissue not due to dressing removal, malodour and pyrexia.

Scenario 11.1

Read the scenario below and then look at the photograph of Edna's wound (Figure 11.11). How would you describe its appearance?

Edna is 69 and has fallen at home. She was found by a neighbour lying on her left side and had been there for six hours. She was admitted with a left fractured neck of femur and had a dynamic hip screw repair. After the surgery it was noted that a large discoloration had appeared on her left hip above her scar. This broke down and after *debridement* now appears like this on dressing removal which was a *hydrocolloid and hydrofibre.*

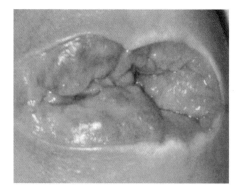

Figure 11.11 Edna's wound

You will probably have noted that the wound margins are slightly macerated, which means that the dressing used is not absorbing a sufficient amount of exudate, is too small or is being left on too long. The wound itself is healthy and granulating, however, looking deeper into the wound there is either sloughy tissue or exposed tendon and bone which would need to be explored by a qualified nurse, tissue viability nurse or doctor.

Pain

It is important to indicate in your care plan any pain the patient may be experiencing from the wound dressing or wound itself, and your actions taken to alleviate the pain and in finding the cause.

Infection

The type of tissue at the wound bed and the exudates will give a visual indication as to whether infection is present. If you suspect infection, you should take a wound swab (under guidance) to send to the lab for analysis.

Grading

Grading a pressure ulcer (as explained previously, see p. 00) gives an objective description of the sore and the amount of tissue damage at the wound bed. It is important to emphasize that the grading system should be used in conjunction with a risk assessment tool and a full wound assessment.

Dressings

Under direction, you should always document the type of primary and secondary dressings used on a pressure ulcer, their size and when they should be renewed.

Box 11.9 Phases of wound healing

1. *Acute inflammatory phase:* the release of histamine and other mediators from damaged cells and migration of white blood cells to the damaged site.
2. *Destructive phase:* the clearance of dead and devitalized tissue by polymorphs and macrophages.
3. *Proliferative phase:* the infiltration of the wound by new blood vessels, supported by connective tissue.
4. *Maturation phase:* re-epithelialization, wound contraction and connective tissue reorganization.

Healing

When skin is broken and breached it needs to heal itself, which it does in four main phases: the acute inflammatory phase; the destructive phase; the proliferative phase; and the maturation phase. Box 11.9 explains each of these phases in more detail.

You will find in practice, however, that these stages overlap and the total length of each phase depends on many factors, such as site, size, the degree of contamination of the wound and the physiological, nutritional and immunological status of the patient.

Types of healing

The four stages may occur in different types of wound healing. There are three main types of wound healing: primary, secondary and tertiary.

- *Primary* (clean cut closed immediately). Skin heals by primary intention when there has been little skin loss and the edges of the tissue are held together by skin tapes or sutures, as seen in a clean surgical wound or minor laceration. Very little granulation tissue is produced and within 10 to 14 days re-epithelialization is normally complete and a thin scar usually remains, which fades from pink to white. Nevertheless it may take many months for the *tensile strength* of the tissues to recover.
- *Delayed primary.* Soiled wounds with linear edges that are closed after three to four days.
- *Secondary* (wounds left to fill with new tissue and re-epithelialize). Healing occurs by secondary intention when there is significant tissue loss in open wounds. Granulation tissue, which is composed of new capillaries, is supported by connective tissue and evolves in the bottom of the wound, while epithelial cells migrate across the centre of the wound surface from the wound edges and islands of epithelial tissue surrounding hair follicles, sweat glands and sebaceous glands. The wound contracts and the connective tissue is reorganized to produce tissue that accrues strength in time.
- *Tertiary* (where there is excessive wound healing and over-granulation, *keloid scarring*). Where the presence of wound infection or a foreign body is suspected, a wound may be left open to commence healing by granulation until the presenting problem

has resolved. The wound edges can then be approximated and healing by primary intention can proceed.

Aseptic techniques

An aseptic technique refers to hand washing, surface cleaning, the use of protective clothing drapes and gloves and the non-touch techniques performed immediately before and during a clinical procedure.

Aseptic techniques are those that do some or all of the following:

- remove or kill micro-organisms from hands and objects;
- employ sterile instruments and other items;
- reduce a patient's risk of exposure to micro-organisms.

Box 11.10 shows the main principles to observe in carrying out any aseptic procedure.

Box 11.10 Main principles of aseptic technique

- Hand hygiene and correct clinical hand-washing technique.
- Use of appropriate sterile protective gowns, aprons, gloves and standard and transmission-based precautions.
- Establishing a sterile field.
- Ensuring that items on the sterile field *are* sterile and transferred to the sterile field appropriately.
- Monitoring the sterile field.
- Monitoring environmental conditions that can influence the integrity of the sterile field.

When performing an aseptic technique you should ensure that all your actions minimize the likelihood of potential *pathogens* being introduced to the site, or being spread to other patients or colleagues. You need therefore to apply fundamental infection control principles. The principles of asepsis need to be carefully implemented during all routine nursing actions, but when performing an aseptic technique strict guidelines should be adhered to.

However, before carrying out a dressing change on a pressure ulcer using an aseptic technique, you need to familiarize yourself with the documentation regarding the wound and the dressings that are prescribed. Box 11.11 shows guidelines for good practice in the treatment of wounds (Newton 2006).

Box 11.11 Guidelines for good practice

- Always employ a holistic approach to wound care (e.g. investigate any underlying problems).
- Wounds should not be routinely cleansed, but if they require cleansing, irrigation should be employed.
- Warm sodium chloride 0.9 per cent should be used for irrigating wounds or, for venous leg ulcers, warm tap water must be the cleanser of choice.
- Wounds should not be routinely re-dressed. An appropriate timescale should be decided upon for each individual patient.
- Wounds should not be left exposed or wrapped in dressing towels. The action of dehydration and the reduction in wound temperature are detrimental to wound healing.
- A multidisciplinary approach must be taken to wound care.
- A clear explanation of the action of certain types of dressings must be given to the patient.
- All dressings must be prescribed.

There is a wide range of dressings and products you can use to aid healing depending on the type of wound and the results of your assessment.

Activity 11.12

Go to Media Tool DVD, select **Chapter Resources**, then **Pressure Ulcers** and work through Activity 11.12. Click on the links in the column beginning **Alginates** to see the wide range of dressings and their uses.

Box 11.12 Dressing change

Step 1

Begin by cleaning your hands using hand gel or soap and water, using the seven-step process. You may wish to refer to Chapter 4.

Step 2

Explain to your patient what you're going to do and gain informed consent, ensuring the person's privacy and dignity.

Step 3

Wash your hands and gather the necessary equipment. Put on non-sterile gloves and an apron. Clean the trolley with general detergent and hot water, making sure to clean the sides and supports, and then dry thoroughly. Then clean with a 70 per cent alcohol solution. Discard your gloves and apron.

Step 4

Check the expiry date of the equipment and sterile packages and place on the bottom of the trolley.

Step 5

Take your trolley to the patient's bedside, put on an apron and wash and dry your hands. Check the integrity of the packaging before opening any sterile packages using non-touch technique

Step 6

Once the sterile field is prepared, clean your hands again with an alcohol gel, put on a pair of non-sterile gloves and turn back the bed covers. Using either the yellow bag from the sterile pack or gloves, remove the dressing according to the manufacturer's instructions. Check the colour, saturation and odour of the removed dressing.

Step 7

After inspection, dispose of the soiled dressing into the yellow bag. Clean your hands again with alcohol gel and perform a wound assessment. After completion of the wound assessment, wash your hands with soap and water, then put on sterile gloves.

Step 8

Draw up the saline into the syringe and clean the wound using a non-touch technique so as not to disturb friable tissue.

Step 9

Dry the surrounding skin to ensure good adhesion of the new dressing. When placing a dressing over the ulcer site ensure that you have at least a 2cm border and a snug fit. Spend time warming and moulding the dressing to the skin. This improves the adhesiveness of the dressing, allowing it to stay in place for longer.

Step 10

Collect all the used equipment from the dressing pack, and together with your gloves and apron place in the clinical waste bag. Tidy up around the patient, make sure they are comfortable, lower the bed and take the trolley to the sluice to throw away all the waste in the clinical waste facility. Clean the trolley down with a general detergent and hot water, dry and return to the clinical room.

Step 11

Document all your care and ask your patient to let you know of any discomfort.

Changing a dressing

Changing a dressing under supervision is a good opportunity to practise interacting with a patient while assessing their wound and general health and developing skills in aseptic procedures. Box 11.12 shows the steps you need to take.

Activity 11.13

To reinforce the information in Box 11.12, go to the Media Tool DVD, select **Skills Sets**, **Wound Care** and watch the clip on **Aseptic non-touch technique**.

Care planning

A nursing assessment of a patient forms the basis on which nursing care is planned and should provide a comprehensive, accurate and current view of the patient's condition. In pressure ulcer management, documentation is an important way in which a nurse can exercise their accountability in prevention and management.

There is a lot to think about as the plan of care must reflect a patient's identified needs and address intrinsic and extrinsic factors, risk status, pressure ulcer assessment, manual handling assessment and patient education with appropriate goals, actions and rationale. Any interprofessional team referrals, support surfaces, repositioning regimes, resources, dressings and aids should be incorporated into the plan and regularly reassessed with the patient, as well as being handed over to qualified staff and the interprofessional team at shift changes, ward rounds, case conferences or as the patient's condition changes. Further discussion on the importance of documentation can be found in Chapter 3.

Implementing the care plan

Once a care plan has been developed, based on the best available evidence and professional and patient choice, the care prescribed is then implemented. Patients and their carers should actively be involved in the care if they so wish, along with other members of the interprofessional team.

Evaluating the care plan

At the end of each intervention and change of shift, as the patient's condition changes or prior to discharge, all care should be documented and reported to the appropriate healthcare professionals, incorporating the patient's and carer's contribution. Only qualified members of staff who are appropriately trained can

evaluate the effectiveness of any intervention. This will include risk and skin assessment, grading, repositioning, support surfaces and equipment used, and other care given in relation to the patient's general condition.

As a student, any evaluations that you have made must be under the supervision of a qualified member of staff. You must insist that before you document anything, they listen to your assessment, plan of care and evaluations, whether they are within normal limits or are highlighting a condition change in your patient. Once you begin to document the care provided, this must always be countersigned by the qualified member of staff.

Interprofessional working

You will probably have already realized that an interprofessional or multidisciplinary approach to the prevention and treatment of pressure ulcers is essential. Nurses need to liaise with other members of the interprofessional team and discuss the appropriate resources, support surfaces and equipment that will meet the patient's needs. Many professionals will be involved in the care of a patient with a pressure ulcer, as identified in the sections below.

Hospital directors and managers

Hospital directors and managers have overall responsibility in ensuring good quality of care through the appropriate allocation of resources, effective systems and the provision of educational support.

Doctors

Doctors have the responsibility of maintaining a patient's optimum physiological condition – for example, hydration, nutrition, circulatory and respiratory function and treatment of infection. Where appropriate, they should refer to other professional disciplines to assist in applying their specialist knowledge to plan appropriate care.

Tissue viability nurses

Tissue viability nurses have a responsibility to provide advice, support, education and promotion of evidence-based practice within the field of pressure ulcer prevention and management.

Product evaluation nurses

Product evaluation nurses have a responsibility to assist in quality trials and evaluations of the latest pressure-reducing/relieving equipment available for the prevention and treatment of pressure ulcers.

General nurses

Nurses have a responsibility to ensure a holistic approach to patient management. They should identify patients at risk of, or who already have, pressure ulcer damage and plan, implement and regularly re-evaluate research and evidence-based care. They, too, should refer to other specialists, after consulting with the medical team of doctors, to aid in effective treatment and prevention strategies.

Student nurses

In your everyday care of patients you have a key role in observing their nutritional intake, fluid intake and output, their level of mobility and activity, whether they are *pyrexial*, have breathing difficulties, their conscious level and mental state and their level of understanding. As you have seen from the risk assessment tools, all of these have an impact on the risk of developing a pressure ulcer. You may also be caring for patients who have already developed a pressure ulcer. Part of that care involves assessing the wound, selecting an appropriate dressing and using an aseptic technique at dressing changes.

Healthcare assistants

The healthcare assistant's role is to act in a responsible manner, implement aspects of the care plan and support the team of registered nurses.

Dieticians

Dieticians are responsible for creating detailed nutritional assessments of patients and for the planning and arranging of an appropriate diet where necessary.

Occupational therapists

Occupational therapists can aid in the assessment of patients' functional abilities and suggest and advise on any problems patients have in carrying out their activities of living, which may increase the risk of pressure ulcer formation or delay wound healing. They can advise on specialist seating and chair requirements, as well as eating and walking implements.

Physiotherapists

Physiotherapists have a dual role: the provision of interventions that promote effective positioning, movement and independence; and teaching other health professionals to handle and position patients so as to reduce the effects of shear and friction to the skin.

Porters

A porter's role is to effectively transfer a patient within a hospital in a timely and safe manner. They are also responsible for the safe and prompt delivery of pressure-reducing/relieving equipment from wards and departments within the hospital.

Bioengineers and estates staff

Bioengineers and estates staff have a responsibility for evaluating and maintaining the performance of equipment used for pressure sore prevention and treatment.

Equipment suppliers

Pressure-relieving/reducing equipment suppliers have a duty to ensure prompt delivery of equipment in response to orders from nursing, supplies and managerial staff. When equipment is on loan, they are responsible for ensuring effective equipment monitoring, maintenance and replacement. They are also responsible for ensuring that users of their equipment are adequately trained to optimize utility.

Activity 11.14

Which other members of the multidisciplinary team could be involved in pressure ulcer prevention and management?

Check your answer with that given at the end of the chapter.

Activity 11.15

Go to the Media Tool DVD, select **Case Studies**, **Child Health (Tom)**. What role will each of the members of the multidisciplinary team play in preventing pressure sore development in Tom?

Check your answer with that given at the end of the chapter.

The patient information in Appendix C of the RCN/NICE (2005) *The Management of Pressure Ulcers in Primary and Secondary Care* has been designed to support nurses and healthcare professionals in providing patients and their families with information that helps them to participate in the prevention and treatment of pressure ulcers. The topics, which are addressed specifically to patients, are:

- What are pressure ulcers and how do they develop?
- How is my risk assessed?
- What care can I expect from healthcare staff?
- What can I and my carers do to help?
- Where can I get more information?

Patient involvement

Patients and carers have a responsibility for furthering their own health gains and avoiding deterioration in their skin integrity. You should involve patients and their significant others with their education and care and in how they can assist in the prevention and treatment of pressure ulcers. Patients and carers can be taught how to assess skin integrity. The Department of Health, your local Trust, NICE, the RCN and various companies all provide booklets, videos, CD-ROMs and leaflets in English and other languages to keep your patients informed. All discussions with patients and their carers or significant others must be documented.

Activity 11.16

Go to the Media Tool DVD, select **Chapter Resources**, then **Pressure Ulcers** and work through Activity 11.16 and click on the link that will take you to the NICE guidelines. Have a look at Appendix C. This is a very good resource to help you educate patients on how they can help.

Summary and key points

Now that you have read the chapter and completed the activities it is opportune to highlight the key areas covered:

- Your knowledge of the structure of the skin and the importance of capillary blood flow to skin integrity will help you risk-assess and plan care.
- Nursing assessment includes the use of structured assessment tools and clinical judgement to identify extrinsic and intrinsic risk factors.
- The interprofessional team and the patient and their family or carers can make a significant contribution to care.
- Care planning needs to include repositioning regimes and the type of redistributing support surface.
- Wound assessment needs to be holistic, detailed and documented.
- Changing a wound dressing involves aseptic techniques.

References

Bennett, G. Dealey, C. and Posnet, J. (2004) The cost of pressure ulcers in the UK, *Age and Ageing*, 33(3): 230–5.

Bergstrom, N. (2000) Review: specially designed products to prevent or heal pressure sores are more effective than standard mattresses, *Evidence Based Nursing*, 3: 54–5.

Bergstrom, N. and Braden, B.J. (2002) Predictive validity of the Braden Scale among Black and White subjects, *Nursing Research*, 51: 398–403.

Bergstrom, N. Braden, B. Laguzza, A. and Holman, V. (1987) The Braden scale for predicting pressure sore risk, *Nursing Research*, 36(4): 205–10.

Bethell, E. (2005) Wound care for patients with darkly pigmented skin, *Nursing Standard*, 20(4): 41–9.

Bick, D. and Stephens, F. (2003) Pressure ulcer risk: audit findings, *Nursing Standard*, 17(44): 63–72.

Bonomini, J. (2003) Effective interventions for pressure sore prevention, *Nursing Standard*, 17(52): 45–50.

Brown, S.J. (2004) The Braden Scale: a review of the evidence, *Orthopaedic Nursing*, 23(1): 30–8.

Cullum, N. McInnes, E. Bell-Syer, S.E. et al. (2004) Support surfaces for pressure ulcer prevention, in the *Cochrane Library*. Oxford: Update Software.

Dealey, C. (2005) *The Care of Wounds*, 2nd edn. Oxford: Blackwell.

European Pressure Ulcer Advisory Panel (1998) *Pressure Ulcer Treatment Guidelines,* www.epuap.org/gltreatment.html, accessed 10 June 2008.

Matas, A. *et al.* (2001) Eliminating the issue of skin colour in assessment of the blanch response, *Advances in Skin and Wound Care*, 14(4): 180–8.

Newton, H. (2006) Prescribing for skin and wound care: the nurse prescribers' perspective, *Nurse Prescribing*, 4(4): 141–5.

NICE (National Institute for Health and Clinical Excellence) (2005) *The Prevention and Treatment of Pressure Ulcers. Quick Reference Guide,* www.nice.org.uk, accessed 10 June 2008.

RCN (Royal College of Nursing) (2001) *Pressure Ulcer Risk Assessment and Prevention Recommendations, 2001, Clinical Practice Guidelines*, www.rcn.org.uk/__data/assets/pdf_file/0003/78501/001252.pdf, accessed 10 June 2008.

RCN/NICE (Royal College of Nursing/National Institute for Health and Clinical Excellence) (2005) *The Management of Pressure Ulcers in Primary and Secondary Care, Clinical Guideline 29,* www.nice.org.uk, accessed 10 June 2008.

Rycroft-Malone, J. and McInnes, E. (2000) *Pressure Ulcer Risk Assessment and Prevention.* London: RCN.

Waterlow, J. (1988) The Waterlow card for the prevention and management of pressure sores: towards a prevention policy, *Care: Science and Practice*, 6(1): 8–12.

Waterlow, J. (2005) *Pressure Ulcer Prevention Manual.* Taunton: Waterlow.

Willock, J. and Maylor, M. (2004) Pressure ulcers in infants and children, *Nursing Standard*, 18(24): 56–8, 60, 62.

Wound Management Steering Group (2006) www.formulary.cht.nhs.uk/Guidelines/MMC/027_Wound_Formulary/00_00_Wound_Formulary_Main.htm, accessed 10 June 2008.

Answers

Activity 11.3

This erythema would be non-blanching erythema. It would indicate that local tissue damage had occurred and the need for further assessment to prevent deterioration.

Activity 11.4

Margaret

Extrinsic factors:

- Dependent on others to reposition her without shear or friction to prevent pressure damage.
- If she gets restless she may be susceptible to friction damage; careful positioning is important to ensure the catheter tube is not causing pressure or friction.
- If she sweats or has a fever, her skin will need to be kept clean and dry.

Intrinsic factors:

- She has lowered awareness and may not feel positional warnings such as numbness or pins and needles.

- She has reduced mobility and a right-sided weakness so will not be able to reposition herself spontaneously.
- She may have risk factors we don't yet know about, such as diabetes, respiratory disease or vascular disease.

Tom

Extrinsic factors:

- He has an immobilizing splint on his left leg which may cause friction or pressure damage from swelling or the risk of compartment syndrome.
- He may be susceptible to shear forces while sitting up in bed.
- He is a 9-year-old boy and could be rather fidgety and restless; this could increase his risk of friction.

Intrinsic factors:

- There do not seem to be any intrinsic risk factors, unless the morphine makes Tom drowsy or forgetful.

Activity 11.5

You need to identify the intrinsic and extrinsic factors, such as assessing the level of mobility and nutritional status, the medication the patient is receiving and any acute illness.

Activity 11.6

Any drugs that may affect the level of consciousness, for instance, sleeping tablets or strong pain killers such as morphine may make a patient more susceptible to developing pressure damage. Some medication such as steroids can affect the condition of the skin. You should check the side-effects of any medications that patients are prescribed.

Activity 11.7

Early signs of pressure damage are redness or erythema, particularly non-blanching erythema, purplish or darkish areas on darkly pigmented skin, discoloration, blisters, dryness, cracking, maceration, induration, localized heat and localized oedema (Rycroft-Malone and McInnes 2000).

Activity 11.8

1 Tom

Pressure ulcer prevention would begin with an assessment of risk using a validated assessment tool, skin integrity followed by Tom's ability to understand and his mobility/activity. Then Tom could be encouraged to change his own position (without causing further damage to his leg) using the monkey pole and aids provided by the physiotherapist. When he is asleep the nurse could use pillows to prop Tom over to the left using a 30° tilt and these could be removed again in the night without disturbing him. Active exercises would be encouraged and the physiotherapist could access different aids to help Tom – i.e. pulling ladders and exercise bands. The electric bed frame Tom is nursed on could also be varied in its position to aid changes in position from sitting upright to semi-recumbent and lying flat. If at any stage Tom's risk status changes, then the qualified nurse or multidisciplinary team member would re-evaluate the suitability of his mattress.

2 Margaret

Pressure ulcer prevention would begin with a risk assessment and skin tolerance test. We know that Margaret has a reduced level of consciousness and this would affect her ability to sense pressure, shear and friction. We would then assess the suitability of the mattress and may decide to use an overlay that is alternating or low air loss in nature. When first placed on the mattress we would make Margaret comfortable. After half an hour we would return and check her skin tolerance. If this was reactive, then we would reposition her and return in an hour; this would continue to a maximum of four hours. However, during this time if her skin did not react, then we would increase the turning. The nurse on the following shift would then change Margaret's position between one- and three-hourly in the day and then four-hourly at night to aid rest and sleep. However, this and other aspects of management would constantly be reassessed in relation to changes in condition.

Activity 11.9

The patient in Figure 11.9 is too tall for the chair and slides forward to over-compensate for their position. This increases the risk of shear forces at the sacrum and pressure on the spinal column.

Activity 11.11

Margaret should be supported in a chair that ensures her knees, feet and thighs are all at 90-degree angles. She should have the use of pillows to aid the position as directed by the physiotherapist. She would also require a pressure-relieving cushion or full chair, which would alternate underneath her.

Activity 11.14

Other members of the team who could be involved in pressure ulcer prevention and management are a speech and language therapist, a podiatrist and the patient's carers.

Activity 11.15

The following members of the multidisciplinary team would assist Tom in the following areas:

- Physiotherapist – aids mobility and activity.
- Occupational therapist – promotes social function and getting back to school, family life and hobbies.
- Pharmacist – reviews medication that may affect the function of the skin and/or activity.
- Dietician – reviews nutritional status and encourages a diet that matches current requirements.
- Porter – ensures smooth transfer to and from departments.
- Community nurse/nurse – carries out nursing duties in relation to activities of daily living but is also the pivotal coordinator of the team, whether at home or in hospital.
- Doctor – ensures the correct medical/surgical management to reduce the risk of intrinsic factors.
- Teacher – maintains level of understanding and offers normal routine and stimulation to Tom's day.
- Play therapist – offers distraction techniques when carrying out dressing/position changes.

Glossary

A

alimentary tract: the tube which extends from the mouth to the anus through which food and liquid are taken in and then broken down into smaller particles for absorption, and waste products excreted.

Alzheimer's disease: a common type of dementia. It is an illness that affects the brain which is characterized by gradual change in memory, behaviour and personality over a long period of time, leading to loss of mental capacity and dependency on others.

amygdala: a small almond-shaped piece of neural tissue which lies deep in the brain. It is involved in our feelings of emotional arousal such as fear. It initiates related and involuntary non-verbal communication such as facial expression and body reflexes.

anorexia: anorexia nervosa is an eating disorder which is characterized by an unrealistic fear of weight gain, self-starvation and conspicuous distortion of body image.

anxiety: a feeling that includes worry and is accompanied by physical feelings such as sickness, racing heart and sweating. For some, this feeling can be disabling and overwhelming.

arterial blood pressure (ABP): the force exerted by the blood on the arterial wall. A good pressure is needed to enable blood to flow to the capillaries supplying all tissue.

assessment tool: see *screening tool*.

attitude: a complex mental state involving beliefs and feelings, values and dispositions to act in certain ways.

auditory hallucinations: a medical description for hearing voices that do not appear to have any external origin.

auroscope: a piece of equipment for looking into the ear canal.

autonomic urination: occurs in infancy when an ability to control emptying of the bladder has not yet developed.

autonomy: the quality of being self-governing. A patient's right to make decisions about their medical care without their healthcare provider trying to influence their decision.

B

balanced diet: consists of carbohydrate, protein, fat, vitamins, minerals, salts and fibre in the correct proportions.

behaviour: the actions or reactions of a person or animal in response to external or internal stimuli.

blanching: in a clinical context this word is usually used in conjunction with *erythematic*. Blanching erythematic means that the tissue turns white under the pressure of a finger.

blood-borne infection: any infection which is transmitted from the bloodstream of one person to the bloodstream of another. Examples include Hepatitis B, Hepatitis C and Human Immunodeficiency Virus (HIV).

British Sign Language (BSL): the code accepted by some deaf people as their first language. It is a visual/spatial language governed by grammatical rules of hand shapes and movements, body postures and facial expressions to communicate meaning.

Broca's area: one of two main areas of the brain, situated in the left temporal lobe, associated with language processing (the other is *Wernicke's*, see below). It is involved in speech and sign comprehension and production. Damage to this area often means that the person is unable to produce grammatical speech.

built care environment: any area where care takes place.

C

Candida albicans: a fungal infection commonly referred to as 'Thrush', usually caused by the Candida albicans fungi.

capillaries: the smallest blood vessels in the body.

They deliver water, oxygen and nutrients to tissues and carry away carbon dioxide and waste chemicals.

capillary closing pressure: the pressure at which capillaries will close and be unable to deliver water, oxygen and nutrients to tissues.

capillary refill: the rate at which blood refills empty capillaries. It can be tested by pressing a finger on the skin and counting how long it takes for the skin to return to its normal colour. This is usually two seconds.

cerebral vascular accident: interference in the blood flow of the brain due to haemorrhage or a thromboembolism.

cognitive-behavioural therapy: a psychological therapy involving clarifying the individual's perception of their problem, and an exploration of how this relates to their feelings and behaviours.

community psychiatric nurses: registered mental health nurses working in a community setting.

confidentiality: ensuring that information is accessible only to those authorized to have access.

consent: permission to carry out an action based upon an appreciation and understanding of the facts and implications of that action.

constipation: the infrequent and uncomfortable passage of a hard stool.

continence: to be continent is to have the ability to maintain control over the emptying of one's own bladder and bowel until an appropriate place is reached.

controlled drugs: drugs which require specific measures to be taken in relation to safe-keeping and record-keeping as stipulated by the Misuse of Drugs Act 1971.

Crohn's disease: often referred to as irritable bowel disease (IBD), characterized by inflammation and ulceration of the bowel (colon). The symptoms include pain, diarrhoea and the passage of blood and mucus rectally.

cross-infection: when a micro-organism is transmitted from one surface to another, or via droplets in the air from one area to another.

D

debridement: the process of removing dead, devitalized or infected tissue from a wound's surface by chemical or surgical means.

deep vein thrombosis: a blood clot which occurs in the deep veins usually in the legs and pelvis. Asso-

ciated with stasis of the blood due to heart failure, altered blood clotting function or immobility.

defecation: the voluntary or involuntary passage of faeces.

dehydration: this occurs when output from the body exceeds input, leading to a loss of water and a urea and electrolyte imbalance.

delusions: a medical term referring to a set of experiences and beliefs that cannot be verified by others (e.g. the belief that everyone is trying to poison you when this is not the case).

dementia: progressive decline in cognitive function due to disease in the brain. The set of symptoms include impairment of memory, language, attention, concentration and problem-solving.

detrusor muscle: the name of the smooth muscle of the bladder wall that contracts to empty the bladder.

diabetes: a condition which is characterized by an increase in blood sugar.

diarrhoea: the frequent passage of a loose, watery stool.

dignity: the quality of being worthy of honour or respect.

discrimination: unfair treatment of a person or group on the basis of prejudice.

Dosett box: a plastic box or wallet which is separated into days of the week. It is loaded with the patient's tablets every week and this can then enable the patient or the carer to take their tablets at the right time and to check that they have been taken.

dual diagnosis: having two diagnoses at the same time. It is often used to refer to people who have a mental illness diagnosis and substance misuse.

E

early warning scoring system: a system used for the early detection of physiological abnormality, therefore reducing the risk of further deterioration.

elimination: the process of excretion of metabolic waste from the blood, kidneys and urinary tract, and the bowel and the gastrointestinal tract.

e-mail system nhs.net: encrypted system providing security for personal identifiable information sent electronically.

emotional experiences: inner personal feelings as a reaction to external events or perceptions.

encopresis: the term given to faecal incontinence in

children. The child will pass a normal consistency stool in a socially unacceptable place.

enteral nutrition: using the gastrointestinal tract for the delivery of nutrients, which includes eating food, consuming oral supplements and all types of tube feeding. The routes of enteral tube feeding are naso-gastric tubes (NGTs) and percutaneous endoscopic gastrostomy (PEG) tubes. Other routes that are increasingly being used include nasojejunal and jejunostomy feeding, which may be the only feasible route if it is not appropriate to feed via the stomach.

epidermis: the outermost layer of the skin. It waterproofs the body, protects it and gives the skin its colour.

erythema: reddening of the skin.

European Convention on Human Rights: known as the Convention for the Protection of Human Rights and Fundamental Freedoms passed by the Council of Europe in 1950.

F

faecal impaction: faeces are so hard and dry that they cannot be passed from the bowel through the anus. Drugs/laxatives may be used to soften the stool or manual removal under anaesthesia may be necessary.

faecal incontinence: an inability to control the passing of faeces from the bowel.

faeces: the waste material eliminated through the bowel.

feelings: the conscious subjective experience of emotion – this may include happiness, sadness, anxiety, guilt, shame or fear.

flatus: a build-up of gas in the bowel which stretches the bowel walls and causes discomfort.

G

gastrostomy tube: a tube which is inserted via the abdominal wall into the stomach.

glans penis: the bulbous end of the penis usually covered by the foreskin.

Grice's conversational maxims: Paul Grice, a philosopher, proposed four maxims that describe our expectations when we listen to others. They include expectations that the speaker will be truthful, informative, relevant and clear.

H

haemophilia: a genetically inherited blood clotting defect where there is a deficiency in factor VIII or IX

which can cause bleeding into deep-lying structures, muscles and joints. It occurs mainly in males.

harassment: repeated and persistent annoyances, threats or demands.

hazardous substances: chemicals present in the workplace which are capable of causing harm.

healthcare environment: the environment within which the care of patients takes place.

housekeepers: personnel responsible for making the ward environment as pleasant as possible, by organizing and directing key services such as catering, cleaning, any laundry and decoration.

hydrocolloid: type of dressing that is able to absorb exudate and form a gel that does not damage healthy tissue.

hydrofibre: type of dressing with similar properties to hydrocolloid dressings but which can be formulated as ribbons for packing wounds.

I

immuno-suppressed: reduced immune system function.

induration: hardening of normally soft tissue. It is associated with inflammation.

indwelling urinary catheterization: the insertion of a self-retaining catheter into the bladder.

infection control: activities aimed at preventing the spread of pathogens within the healthcare setting.

inflammatory bowel disease: the lining of the bowel becomes inflamed and irritable, characterized by diarrhoea, abdominal discomfort and pain, and blood in the stool.

intermittent self-catheterization: a small catheter inserted into the bladder to instil drugs or to drain the bladder of urine intermittently. Individuals can be taught to perform this procedure for themselves.

interpersonal skills: a set of behaviours that allow you to communicate effectively and empathically when interacting with others. They involve knowing when to listen and when to speak, and how to see things from different perspectives.

ischaemic: this describes tissue that has a very poor or absent supply of oxygen.

K

keloid scarring: a type of scar that overgrows the original scar and extends it. The scar is usually red and raised.

L

labelling: a term associated with a rejection of psychiatric classification as unscientific. Instead the person is referred to as being given a 'label', thus emphasizing the stigmatizing nature of psychiatric diagnosis.

language abilities: abilities which include our range of vocabulary and the grammatical structures of understanding and expression we have in our own language, as well as the ability to speak other languages.

laxatives: drugs used to evacuate or relieve constipation of the bowel.

learning disability: a disorder that can affect a broad range of academic and functional skills, such as spoken and written language, reasoning or organizing information. A learning disability is not necessarily an indication of low intelligence.

M

malnutrition: a lack of adequate nutrition resulting in ill health.

medicine brand or trade name: the name given to a drug by the manufacturer.

medicine generic name: a drug name not protected by a trademark.

melanin: pigment that gives skin its colour.

metabolism: the burning of nutrients to produce energy, measured as the basal metabolic rate (BMR).

micturition: see *urination*.

minerals: essential inorganic elements. Trace minerals are those elements that are needed in smaller amounts.

multidisciplinary team: a group of professionals working together towards the same objective of helping the patient to their optimum condition. They plan and carry out treatment and rehabilitation and may include doctors, nurses, physiotherapists and occupational therapists.

multiple sclerosis: a condition of the auto-immune system when the immune system attacks the central nervous system and causes demyelination.

N

nasogastric tube: a tube which is inserted via the nasal passage into the stomach.

necrotic ulceration: the stage of ulceration that follows redness, swelling and inflammation. The skin tissue dies and reveals fat and damaged tissue beneath.

nutrition: food (balanced diet) and liquid which are taken in.

O

obesity: an excess of body fat that frequently results in a significant impairment of health.

observation: a term used to indicate that someone is being watched or their whereabouts, behaviour and interactions with others are being monitored.

observations: term commonly used to describe the measurement of vital signs (e.g. body temperature, pulse, blood pressure, respirations).

occupational therapist: a health professional and member of the multidisciplinary team who works with the patient to help them achieve a satisfactory lifestyle through activity and interventions aimed at developing, sustaining and achieving functional abilities leading to the highest possible level of independence.

osteoporosis: a bone disease which leads to an increased risk of fractures.

oxygen saturation levels: the amount of oxygen transported by haemoglobin in arterial blood.

oxygen saturation monitor: device used to measure oxygen saturation levels, often referred to as a pulse oximeter.

P

pantomime: the same as mime, but of a more exaggerated nature. The use of gestures and movements without words to entertain or convey meaning.

paranoid schizophrenia: see *schizophrenia*. This is one type of schizophrenia characterized by suspiciousness and paranoid feelings and experiences.

parasympathetic sensory nerves: these form part of the autonomic nervous system.

parenteral nutrition: providing nutrition via an intravenous line.

Parkinson's disease: as in Parkinsonism, this is a disease of the brain, characterized by tremor, rigidity and slow movement.

passive and active exercises: passive exercises are those that are facilitated by a therapist who, for example, lifts a client's limb and takes it through a range of motion. In active exercises the client initiates the movement and uses energy against gravity.

paternalistic: a system, policy or style of management

providing for someone's needs without granting them their rights, responsibilities or choices.

pathogens: organisms that cause disease, such as bacteria or viruses.

perceptions: individual interpretations of situations, people or events. Perception of the same event may be different for different people.

peristalsis: rhythmic contraction and relaxation of the gut that moves food and waste through the digestive system.

personal environment: the immediate area surrounding the patient. For example, this can be the hospital bed space, consulting room, patient's home or any treatment or clinic area.

personal protective equipment (PPE): any equipment which protects a worker from exposure to germs, chemical and other hazardous substances. Examples of PPE include gloves, masks, goggles or appropriate headwear and footwear.

physiotherapist: a healthcare professional and member of the multi-team who treats people of all ages who have soft tissue injuries and a range of disabilities, using a range of manual and technology-based techniques in order to enhance the body's natural healing mechanisms.

physiotherapist's risk assessment: physiotherapists need to consider 'risk' in terms of the patient, the therapist, the treatment/technique and the environment.

prejudice: a preconceived opinion or feeling.

primary care: healthcare provision in the community as opposed to in the hospital.

privacy: the ability to seclude oneself or selves or to selectively disclose information about oneself.

proxemics: the study of how human beings perceive their personal and public space. This influences many of our daily encounters.

psychological equilibrium: a sense of emotional harmony and balance.

psychological safety: the feeling of being able to express and occupy one's self without fear of negative consequences to self-image or status.

psychosis: a medical concept referring to the experience of hallucinations and/or delusions.

pyrexial: a body temperature above the patient's normal (usually 36.5°C). A raised temperature usually indicates infection.

pudendal nerve: plays a part in controlling the external anal sphincter to allow defecation to occur.

R

re-epithelialize: the outer layer of the skin grows back.

risk assessment: identification of potential hazards.

S

schizophrenia: a medical psychiatric classification referring to a set of experiences including psychosis and often associated with difficulty with social and interpersonal skills.

screening tool: a tool which is used to measure certain parameters.

secondary intention: a type of wound healing which allows the edges of the wound to close naturally rather than by suturing them together.

self-esteem: relates to our feelings of worth and to our feelings of competency and effectiveness, and importantly, to the interconnectedness between those two feelings, which will impact on how we act and behave.

service users: people who access or use medical services.

sharp injuries: percutaneous injury with a sharp object which may potentially be contaminated with blood or body fluid. These sharps include needles, scalpels, lancets or broken glass.

social carers: people who care for individuals but are not paid for the work they do. They can include family, friends and neighbours.

social interaction: communication between people for pleasure and leisure.

social worker: a professional and member of the multidisciplinary team who is primarily concerned with dealing with social problems, exploring their causes, solutions and the impact they have on society. They work with individuals, groups, families and communities as well as organizations.

sociolinguistics: the study of how social factors such as class, ethnicity, age, sex and language are related. It also considers the significance of language in all social contexts and cultural groups, and features such as slang and dialect.

sphygmomanometer: device used to measure blood pressure.

stereotype: an oversimplified, exaggerated and fixed

notion, image or preconception about a certain type of person, group or society.

stigma: the negative effects of a label placed on an individual or group, often as a result of ignorance, prejudice and discrimination.

stimulus: something that causes or encourages a given response.

stool: semi-solid faecal mass evacuated from the bowel.

stress: a normal human response to anxiety-provoking situations. Also used as an umbrella term to describe a complex set of feelings often experienced as a result of intolerable pressure.

stressors: situations or events that cause an individual stress.

substance misuse: excessive use of drugs or alcohol usually to the extent of addiction.

supra-pubic indwelling catheterization: the surgical insertion of a self-retaining catheter into the bladder through the abdominal and bladder wall.

T

tensile strength: the strength of a material in relation to the force required before it breaks or is damaged.

therapeutic relationship: the relationship between a healthcare professional and a patient or client. The relationship is based on trust, respect, empathy and professional intimacy, and contributes to the client's health and well-being.

therapeutic touch: involves a variety of approaches to using touch as a means of comfort and healing.

thrombosis: a blood clot formed in the blood vessel.

triggers: particular events or experiences significant to an individual that cause a reaction in that individual.

tympanic thermometer: a thermometer to measure temperature that takes its recording from the area around the eardrum (tympanic cavity).

U

ulcerative colitis: often referred to as irritable bowel disease (IBD), characterized by inflammation and ulceration of the bowel (colon). The symptoms include pain, diarrhoea, and the passage of blood and mucus rectally.

urinary incontinence: an inability to control the passing of urine.

urination: the voluntary or involuntary passage of urine.

urine: the fluid excreted by the kidneys, containing waste products of nitrogen, urea, uric acid and creatinine.

V

Valsalva manoeuvre: a forced expiration against the closed glottis, to increase the intra-abdominal pressure and force faeces downwards to aid the defecation process.

victimization: being unfairly singled out for bad treatment.

vital signs: indications of the body's physiological state.

vitamins: essential organic compounds (nutrients) that the body needs for normal functioning.

W

warfarin: a drug used to slow the blood clotting speed and prevent thrombosis.

Wernicke's area: an area of the brain (in the left temporal lobe) which is important in language development and the comprehension of speech. Damage to this area can cause natural-sounding rhythm and grammar in speech, but the utterance may not have any meaning.

wound classification: wounds can be classified in different ways, such as whether chronic or acute, what has caused the wound, what depth and width it is or whether it is infected. There are many different wound classification systems. The main aim is to assist in assessing the wound, wound healing and the effectiveness of treatment.

Index